Colonialism and Transnational Psychiatry

ADVANCE REVIEWS

'As a solidly researched corrective to the psychoanalytic bias of many histories of psychiatry in colonial India, this book represents an invaluable contribution toward the institutional grounding of transcultural psychiatric historiography.'

—*Eric J. Engstrom, Humboldt University of Berlin*

'Ernst has shown that decolonisation and globalisation of psychiatry in India went almost hand in hand, creating practices which were both nationalistic and internationally standardised.'

—*Akihito Suzuki, Keio University*

'An in-depth account wherein individual and institutional histories coalesce, a work of honest scholarship which will be useful by medical historians, sociologists and lay readers alike.'

—*Deepak Kumar, Jawaharlal Nehru University*

'A very important and original contribution to the growing literature on psychiatry and colonialism, notable for its tight focus on a single mental hospital for Indians rather than the imperial ruling class.'

—*Andrew Scull, University of California, San Diego*

'In *Colonialism and Transnational Psychiatry* Waltraud Ernst makes an exceptionally valuable contribution to our understanding of colonial medicine. Beyond providing a critical perspective on the practice of psychiatry in early twentieth-century India, and the many tensions and contradiction reflected in the Indianisation of a colonial mental hospital, this book breaks new ground by providing a deep, nuanced and rich analysis of transnational psychiatry. In other words, Ernst insightfully contextualizes the problem of mental health in India in terms that relate to, but are not limited by, the power structures of empire or the postcolonial priorities of area-specific studies. She paints a fascinating picture of a mental hospital in India where doctors and patients struggle with the problems and paradoxes of modernity during an era of dramatic political change and medical innovation on a global scale.'

—*Joseph Alter, Pittsburgh University*

Colonialism and Transnational Psychiatry

The Development of an Indian Mental Hospital in British India, c. 1925–1940

WALTRAUD ERNST

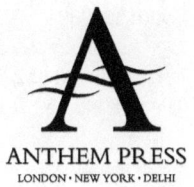

ANTHEM PRESS
LONDON · NEW YORK · DELHI

Anthem Press
An imprint of Wimbledon Publishing Company
www.anthempress.com

This edition first published in UK and USA 2014
by ANTHEM PRESS
75–76 Blackfriars Road, London SE1 8HA, UK
or PO Box 9779, London SW19 7ZG, UK
and
244 Madison Ave #116, New York, NY 10016, USA

First published in hardback by Anthem Press in 2013

Copyright © Waltraud Ernst 2014

The author asserts the moral right to be identified as the author of this work.

Cover images courtesy of the Digital South Asia Library, http://dsal.uchicago.edu.

All rights reserved. Without limiting the rights under copyright reserved above,
no part of this publication may be reproduced, stored or introduced into
a retrieval system, or transmitted, in any form or by any means
(electronic, mechanical, photocopying, recording or otherwise),
without the prior written permission of both the copyright
owner and the above publisher of this book.

British Library Cataloguing-in-Publication Data
A catalogue record for this book is available from the British Library.

Library of Congress Cataloging-in-Publication Data
The Library of Congress has catalogued the hardcover edition as follows:
 Ernst, Waltraud, 1955– author.
 Colonialism and transnational psychiatry : the development of an
 Indian mental hospital in British India, c. 1925–1940 / Waltraud
  Ernst.
    pages cm
 Includes bibliographical references and index.
 ISBN-13: 978-0-85728-019-0 (hardcover : alk. paper)
  ISBN-10: 0-85728-019-8 (hardcover : alk. paper)
  1. Psychiatry–India–History–20th century. 2. Psychiatric
hospitals–India–History–20th century. 3. Psychoanalysis and
   colonialism–India. 4. Psychoanalysis and
racism–India–History–20th century. 5. Medical policy–Great
   Britain. I. Title.
  RC451.I6E76 2013
  362.2'10954–dc23
    2013032094

ISBN-13: 978 1 78308 352 7 (Pbk)
ISBN-10: 1 78308 352 2 (Pbk)

This title is also available as an ebook.

CONTENTS

Acknowledgements   ix
Abbreviations   xi
Tables and Figures   xiii

Introduction   xvii

Chapter 1   **Indianisation and its Discontents**   1

    Towards Indianisation   3
    Structural Inequities   5
    Medical Politics and European Racial Prejudice   6
    The Medical Market and Indian Competition   8
    Professional Discrimination   8
    Professional Closure and the Pathologisation
        of a Successful Community   11
    The Decline of the 'Good Parsi'   15
    Collaborators, Competitors and Ambivalence   17
    Indianisation and Histories of Medicine   20
    Subalterns   21

Chapter 2   **The Patients: The Demographics of Gender and Age, Locality, Occupation, Caste and Religion**   27

    Gender Confined   29
        'Chronic patients' and long-term confinement   30
        'Private' and 'public' patients   33
    'Criminal Lunatics'   35
        Political prisoners   38
        Petty crimes and the criminalisation of the mentally ill   39
    Intellectual Disability and Patients' Ages   41
    Occupational Background and Caste   45
    Religion   55

Chapter 3 Institutional Trends and Standardisation: Deaths, Diseases and Cures 67

- Mortality 68
- Death and Illness by Gender 69
- Causes of Death 74
- Towards Standardisation 76
- Mortality and Morbidity 78
- Disease Prevalence 81
  - *Influenza and malaria* 81
  - *Airborne diseases* 84
  - *Waterborne and parasitic diseases* 87
  - *General paralysis of the insane (GPI) and syphilis* 91
- Accidents and Injuries 91
- Suicide, Escapes and Patients' Freedom of Movement 94
- Cures 99

Chapter 4 Classifications, Types of Disorder and Aetiology 105

- Standardisation and Variation of Classifications 106
- Ruptures and Continuities 108
  - *'On the omnibus': Dementia praecox and schizophrenia* 111
  - *Identifying mania* 112
  - *Framing melancholia and circular/manic depressive insanity* 114
  - *Delusional insanity – paranoia* 120
  - *Dementia, delirium and confusion* 122
  - *From idiocy and imbecility to mental deficiency* 126
  - *A culture-specific syndrome: Cannabis insanity* 128
  - *General paralysis of the insane (GPI): A Western culture-bound condition* 137
- Male and Female Maladies? 141
  - *Confusional insanity and female reproduction-related disorders* 142
  - *Cannabis and alcohol insanity* 143
  - *Epilepsy* 145
  - *Male melancholia – female mania and schizophrenia* 149
  - *Institutions compared: Longitudinal trends in gendered diagnoses* 155
- Aetiology – 'the outstanding problem of psychiatry' 159

Chapter 5 Treatments 173

- Indigenous Herbs 174
- 'Modern' Drugs 178
- Wonder Cures 180
- The Shock Therapies 182
  - *Sulfosin therapy* 182
  - *Insulin coma and Cardiazol shock therapy* 183

Malaria shock therapy	185
Justifying the Need to Shock and Sedate	186
Psychoanalysis	188
Western and Indian Tubs: Hydrotherapy	189
Dutt's *Bratachari*	191
Feasts and Religious Therapy	192
Work and Occupational Therapy – 'useful both to the patients as well as to the State'	193
Diet – 'one of the most important methods of mental treatment'	197
Sports and Entertainment – 'helps enormously towards socialisation and rehabilitation of patients'	199

Conclusion 205

Notes 209
Bibliography 247
Index 259

ACKNOWLEDGEMENTS

My sincere thanks to Dr Subhash Gupta of Peninsula Medical School, Teignmouth and Dr Veenu Pant of Jaipur for having kindly put me in touch with staff at Ranchi Institute of Neuro-Psychiatry and Allied Sciences (RINPAS, the former Ranchi Indian Mental Hospital at the centre of my analysis) and the Central Institute of Psychiatry at Ranchi (CIP, formerly Ranchi European Mental Hospital). Their help in opening doors at supposedly 'closed institutions' has been invaluable. Professor S. Haque Nizamie of CIP and Professor Amool R. Singh of RINPAS enabled me to pursue my research on location. Mr J. Kumar and Mrs T. K. Prasad assisted with archival queries at CIP and RINPAS respectively. Many thanks to all of them for their support.

I am also grateful for the opportunities I was offered to give talks during 2009 on some aspects covered in this book. I greatly benefited from the comments and criticisms of colleagues from different academic disciplines. Particular thanks are due to staff at RINPAS; the Department of History at Delhi University; the Nehru Memorial Museum and Library, New Delhi; the Indian Council for Historical Research, New Delhi; the Department of Social Sciences at the University of Calicut; and the Centre for Studies in Social Sciences, Calcutta.

I believe my study to be interdisciplinary and firmly imbedded within the paradigm of the social history of medicine. Reference to existing work in the fields of history of South Asia, transnational studies, medical anthropology, medical demography and European medical history has been vital. Guidance by and collaboration with colleagues of varied academic backgrounds was therefore highly appreciated. I would like to thank Professor Biswamoy Pati (History, Delhi University), Assistant Professor Projit Bihari Mukharji (History and Sociology of Science, University of Pennsylvania), Dr Saurabh Mishra (History, University of Sheffield) and Dr Samiksha Sehrawat (History, Newcastle University) for their challenging comments and patient guidance on aspects of social, cultural and economic Indian history.

Professors Debasish Basu and Ajit Avasthi (Department of Psychiatry, Postgraduate Institute of Medical Education and Research, Chandigarh) lent invaluable assistance in clarifying present-day issues concerning the meanings of cannabis-induced psychosis and mania and kindly let me have copies of their own research and of the classic study by L. P. Varma. Professor Hashimoto Akira (History, Aichi Prefectural University Japan) kindly assisted with locating O. Berkeley-Hill's autobiography. Dr Alok Sarin (New Delhi), who became fascinated by Dhunjibhoy's life and work after my talks in Delhi in 2009, has been of immense help by tracing the great man's daughter and letting me have some of the ensuing correspondence. I have learnt much about Dhunjibhoy and the

Parsi community in Mumbai and Karachi from Dr R. M. Kalbag FRCS, Newcastle, and Dr Kershaw Khambatta FRCS, Karachi, and greatly appreciate their willingness to pass on to me their knowledge and some of their personal memories.

Professor Bernard Harris (History and Social Policy, University of Southampton) and Professor Steven King (Economic and Social History, University of Leicester) have rendered valuable assistance on aspects of quantitative analysis and the history of classifications and statistics. A number of colleagues specialising on the history of psychiatry in Britain and Germany kindly responded to my queries, pointing me in the right direction regarding their own and others' work on early twentieth-century institutions, psychiatric nomenclature and pharmaceuticals. Many thanks are due to Dr Pamela Michael (Social Sciences, University of Wales, Bangor), Dr Leonard Smith (Health and Population Studies, University of Birmingham), Dr Steven Cherry (History, University of East Anglia), Professor Hilary Marland (History, University of Warwick), Dr Thomas Mueller (History of Medicine, Ravensburg – University of Ulm), Dr Andrea Dörries (Centre for Health Ethics, Hanover), Professor Cay-Ruediger Pruell (University of Mainz), Dr Heike Liebau (Centre for Modern Oriental Studies, Berlin) and Dr Viviane Quirke and Professor John Hall (History, Oxford Brookes University). Any failures of analysis in this work are of course my own. Professors Volker Roelcke (History of Medicine, University of Giessen) and Eric Engstrom (History, Humboldt University Berlin) kindly let me have their latest writings on Kraepelinean classifications. I am particularly grateful to Professor Engstrom for alerting me to correspondence between Dhunjibhoy and Kraepelin and putting me in touch with Professor M. M. Weber and Dr Wolfgang Burgmair of the Max Planck Institute for Psychiatry at Munich who generously let me have copies of the existing letters.

The guidance provided by Professor German Berrios (Epistemology of Psychiatry, University of Cambridge) on conceptual issues relating to classification and diagnosis has been greatly appreciated, inducing a steep learning curve. I am deeply grateful also for the material sent and the prompt and patient responses to my endless requests for further information.

As ever, particular thanks to Dr Michael Williams who reads all my work and never fails to remind me of my PhD supervisor of some thirty years ago, Professor Kenneth Ballhatchet, who said that I never fail to use one word when several would do.

ABBREVIATIONS

Report 1925 — J. E. Dhunjibhoy, *Report on the Working of the Mental Hospitals for Indians in Bihar and Orissa for the Year 1925* (Patna: Government Printing, 1926)

Report 1926 — J. E. Dhunjibhoy, *Report on the Working of the Mental Hospitals for Indians in Bihar and Orissa for the Years 1924–27* (Patna: Government Printing, 1928)

Report 1927 — J. E. Dhunjibhoy, *Report on the Working of the Ranchi Indian Mental Hospital, Kanke, in Bihar and Orissa for the Year 1927* (Patna: Government Printing, 1928)

Report 1928 — J. E. Dhunjibhoy, *Annual Report on the Working of the Ranchi Indian Mental Hospital, Kanke, in Bihar and Orissa for the Year 1928* (Patna: Government Printing, 1929)

Report 1927–29 — P. C. Das, *Triennial Report on the Working of the Ranchi Indian Mental Hospital, Kanke, in Bihar and Orissa for the Years 1927–29* (Patna: Government Printing, 1931)

Report 1930 — J. E. Dhunjibhoy, *Annual Report on the Working of the Ranchi Indian Mental Hospital, Kanke, in Bihar and Orissa for the Year 1930* (Patna: Government Printing, 1932)

Report 1931 — J. E. Dhunjibhoy, *Annual Report on the Working of the Ranchi Indian Mental Hospital, Kanke, in Bihar and Orissa for the Year 1931* (Patna: Government Printing, 1932)

Report 1930–32 — J. E. Dhunjibhoy, *Triennial Report on the Working of the Ranchi Indian Mental Hospital, Kanke, in Bihar and Orissa for the Years 1930–1932* (Patna: Government Printing, 1933)

Report 1933 — J. E. Dhunjibhoy, *Annual Report on the Working of the Ranchi Indian Mental Hospital, Kanke, in Bihar and Orissa for the Year 1933* (Patna: Government Printing, 1934)

Report 1934 — J. E. Dhunjibhoy, *Annual Report on the Working of the Ranchi Indian Mental Hospital, Kanke, in Bihar and Orissa, for the Year 1934* (Patna: Government Printing, 1935)

Report 1933–35	J. N. J. Pacheco, *Triennial Report on the Working of the Ranchi Indian Mental Hospital, Kanke, in Bihar, for the Years 1933, 1934 and 1935* (Patna: Government Printing, 1936)
Report 1936	J. E. Dhunjibhoy, *Annual Report on the Working of the Ranchi Indian Mental Hospital, Kanke, in Bihar, for the Year 1936* (Patna: Government Printing, 1938)
Report 1937	J. E. Dhunjibhoy, *Annual Report on the Working of the Ranchi Indian Mental Hospital, Kanke, in Bihar, for the Year 1937* (Patna: Government Printing, 1939)
Report 1938	J. E. Dhunjibhoy, *The Fourteenth Annual Report of the Ranchi Indian Mental Hospital, Kanke, in Bihar, for the Year 1938* (Patna: Government Printing, 1940)
Report 1939	J. E. Dhunjibhoy, *The Annual Report on the Working of the Ranchi Indian Mental Hospital, Kanke, in Bihar, for the Year 1939* (Patna: Government Printing, 1940)
Report 1940	P. C. Das, *The Annual Report of the Ranchi Indian Mental Hospital, Kanke, in Bihar, for the Year 1940* (Patna: Government Printing, 1942)
Madras Report 1928	J. W. D. Megaw, *Annual Report on the Working of the Mental Hospitals in the Madras Presidency for the Year 1928* (Madras: Government Press, 1929)
Madras Report 1929	J. W. D. Megaw, *Annual Report on the Working of the Mental Hospitals in the Madras Presidency for the Year 1929* (Madras: Government Press, 1930)
Madras Report 1930	C. A. Sprawson, *Annual Report on the Working of the Mental Hospitals in the Madras Presidency for the Year 1930* (Madras: Government Press, 1931)
Madras Report 1921–23	T. H. Symons, *Triennial Report on the Working of the Mental Hospitals in the Madras Presidency for the Years 1921, 1922 and 1923* (Madras: Government Press, 1924)

TABLES AND FIGURES

Tables

Table 2.1.	Number of 'criminal lunatics' detained in jails in the provinces of Bengal, and Bihar and Orissa, 1930–1932	35
Table 2.2.	'The following table shows the analysis of offences committed by the criminal population in this hospital'	38
Table 2.3.	Number of patients admitted to and confined at Ranchi, 1939, and overall population numbers in Bengal, Bihar and Orissa, 1941 (male, female, total)	63
Table 2.4.	Gender ratio for selected religious groups, for Bengal, Bihar and Orissa, Census 1941.	219
Table 2.5.	Percentages for main religious groups calculated for Ranchi, 1928–1939.	219
Table 4.1.	Particular types of disorders attributed on admission as a percentage of the total of conditions identified (male and female) at Ranchi and Denbigh mental hospitals, 1930	106
Table 4.2.	Form of mental disorder (main categories used from 1934)	114
Table 4.3.	'Types of insanity commonly met with in India', listed in order of frequency	118
Table 5.1.	Results of *Rauvolfia Serpentina* trial, 1935	176
Table 5.2.	Results of experiments on 140 cases, with sulphur injections, 1930–1932	240
Table 5.3.	Result of Cardiazol experiments in 42 cases of schizophrenia	241

Figures

Figure 2.1.	Percentage of 'criminal patients' in mental hospitals (1924–1925 for Dacca, Patna and Berhampore; 1926 and 1940 for Ranchi)	36
Figure 2.2.	Age groups of patients admitted to Ranchi, by gender, as percentage of total male and female admissions, 1927–1939	44

xiv COLONIALISM AND TRANSNATIONAL PSYCHIATRY

Figure 2.3.	Age distribution of population in Bengal, Bihar and Orissa, by gender, census 1931	45
Figure 2.4.	Main male occupational categories assigned as percentage of average total admissions, 1929–1932	51
Figure 2.5.	Religious affiliation of patients at Ranchi (average percentage 1927–1939), and in population of Bengal, Bihar and Orissa as a whole (census 1941)	58
Figure 2.6.	Average gender ratio by religion (patients admitted, 1927–1939)	60
Figure 2.7.	Ratio of females to males, India overall, Bengal, Bihar and Orissa (census 1941)	61
Figure 3.1.	Average percentage of death to daily average of patients in different mental hospitals in British India, 1930–1932	68
Figure 3.2.	Average percentage of sick patients admitted to the infirmary, for males (mainly upper graph) and females (mainly lower graph), for all diseases, 1927–1939	72
Figure 3.3.	Mortality: Aggregate disease categories and diseases assigned to those who died, in per cent, 1926–1933	75
Figure 3.4.	Morbidity: Aggregate disease categories and diseases assigned to those admitted to the infirmary, in per cent, 1926–1933	79
Figure 3.5.	Percentage of patients admitted to the infirmary for influenza, by gender, 1927–1935	81
Figure 3.6.	Percentage of sick treated in the infirmary out of total number of both male and female patients at Ranchi, based on average daily number, 1927–1939	82
Figure 3.7.	Percentage of infirmary patients admitted on account of malaria, 1927–1935	83
Figure 3.8.	Percentage cured of daily average strength (lower line) and percentage cured of total admission during the year (upper line), 1927–1939	101
Figure 3.9.	Percentage of infirmary patients admitted on account of malaria, by gender, 1927–1935	223
Figure 3.10.	Percentage of infirmary patients admitted on account of all other diseases of the respiratory system, by gender, 1927–1935	223
Figure 4.1.	Percentage of patients assigned circular insanity/manic depressive insanity (mainly lower line) and mania (mainly upper line), 1925–1939	119

Figure 4.2.	Percentage of men and women (of total number treated) assigned the diagnosis 'melancholia, other forms', 1933	152
Figure 4.3.	Percentage of men and women (of total number treated) assigned the diagnosis melancholia, 1939	156
Figure 4.4.	Percentage of men and women (of total number treated) assigned the diagnosis manic depressive insanity/psychosis, 1933	157
Figure 4.5.	Percentage of men and women (of total number treated) assigned the diagnosis manic depressive psychosis, 1939	157
Figure 4.6.	Percentage of men and women (of total number treated) assigned the diagnoses melancholia (other), and circular insanity/melancholia and manic depressive psychosis, combined, 1933	158
Figure 4.7.	Percentage of men and women (of total number treated) assigned the diagnoses melancholia, and manic depressive psychosis, combined, 1939	158
Figure 4.8.	Percentage of men (lower graph) and women (upper graph), resident at end of year, assigned the diagnosis dementia praecox/schizophrenia, including dementia praecox, 1925–1939	235
Figure 4.9.	Percentage of men (upper graph) and women (lower graph), resident at end of year, assigned the diagnosis delusional insanity (acute or chronic)/paranoia and paranoid states, 1925–1939	236
Figure 4.10.	Percentage of men (lower graph) and women (upper graph), resident at end of year, assigned the diagnosis circular insanity/manic depressive psychosis, 1925–1939	236

Unless otherwise indicated, figures have been calculated from the relevant Ranchi reports.

INTRODUCTION

This book focuses on the Ranchi Indian Mental Hospital, the largest public psychiatric facility in colonial India during the 1920s and 1930s. Although it does not cover the views of the patients and their families, its scope is wide-ranging in other respects and it breaks new ground in the fields of history of colonial medicine in South Asia and of the history of psychiatry more broadly. The latter has been a mixed blessing on account of the relative dearth of material that would have allowed a comparison of trends at Ranchi to those in other institutions in India and Britain. Historians of Indian colonial medicine as well as of psychiatry have hitherto tended to focus on earlier periods. Only very recently have they begun to investigate institutions during the early twentieth century. To date, the few existing studies on particular mental hospitals in Britain do not consistently and comprehensively deal with the full range of institutional data here examined. In particular, information on the types of mental disorders assigned, variations in classifications and conceptual changes are rarely discussed. Nor do they frame local developments in relation to global and transnational ones. It will be left to subsequent scholarship to assess how the local affairs and transnational connections discussed in the current study on Ranchi compare with a wider range of institutions in, and medical exchanges between, South Asia, Western countries and other parts of the world.

Five themes drive the analysis of the Ranchi material. The first relates to the question of how psychiatry fared within a colonial setting that was newly reconstituted in the 1920s and 1930s following demands for local self-government and decolonisation. The main issue discussed concerns the gradual replacement of European doctors with Indians – a process also known as 'Indianisation'. Ranchi's superintendent, J. E. Dhunjibhoy, was one of the first Indians admitted to the prestigious Indian Medical Service (IMS) and appointed to a senior position with responsibility for a newly built medical institution. How did the reconstituted imperial order that established formal parity between Indians and Europeans affect Dhunjibhoy's career trajectory? Was there any continuity with the way the nineteenth-century colonial state had affirmed its governance and influenced institutional developments? These questions will be assessed in relation to the varied professional connections Dhunjibhoy established across the globe and his reference to European and North American medical discourse. The aim is to establish how the trajectories of colonialism, Indianisation and transnational connections intersected and impacted Ranchi, its staff and patients.

The second theme concerns the socio-demographic characteristics of the patients admitted to Ranchi. Did they come from the lower orders of Indian society? Were there any gendered trends? Were particular communities represented disproportionately?

The statistical evidence will be probed to assess whether the institution was instrumental in the control and disempowerment of the socially undesirable and politically inconvenient during a period of nationalist strife and anti-British feelings. It is also important to examine the role of Ranchi as a facility for the medical care of particular groups within the wider context of social welfare and health provision. The limited accessibility of the institution to voluntary patients, its restrictive admission policies and the high percentage of 'criminal patients' among the inmates will emerge as important features. Above all, the numerical insignificance of available mental hospital beds compared to overall population numbers in the three provinces of Bengal, Bihar and Orissa (Odisha) that Ranchi catered for requires assessment. This is pertinent in light of contemporary demands for the expansion of state-sponsored healthcare facilities. Whether we are inclined to see a lack of institutional provision as a curse or a blessing depends on how we resolve the issue of psychiatry as a means of social control or care.

The third theme focuses on the outcomes of institutional confinement and treatment, as revealed in death, illness and cure statistics. The different sets of causes that had a bearing on patients' likelihood of dying or falling ill from physical causes will be charted, with particular emphasis on the most frequent among them: malaria, influenza and airborne, parasitic and waterborne diseases as well as accidents and injuries.[1] The rare incidence of suicides and escapes and the favourable cure rates deserve particular attention as they are seen as vital indicators of a well-managed medical institution. The difficulties faced by historians when they attempt to relate an individual institution's vital statistics to those available for others and to general population figures will be mapped. Despite the apparent streamlining of forms and standardisation of disease classification, the doubtful reliability and validity of data compiled during the 1920s and 1930s imposes considerable restrictions on their interpretation and comparability.

The standardisation of disease categories is also important to the fourth theme. Changing diagnostic classifications and official nomenclatures are scrutinised. The extent to which new terms implied new concepts, and retention of old ones signalled conceptual continuity, is investigated. Dhunjibhoy drew on a number of different strands of diagnostic thinking prevalent in Britain, continental Europe and North America, as well as local ideas on culture-specific syndromes such as cannabis insanity. The different meanings attributed to specific terms at Ranchi and other institutions in India requires critical attention, as seemingly similar incidence rates of particular mental conditions may hide highly diverse conceptualisations. The main categories, including schizophrenia, mania, melancholia and dementia, will be assessed in terms of their history within Western psychiatric thinking, their prevalence at Ranchi and their shifting meanings during a period of rapid change. Gender-specific trends for particular disorders, such as male melancholia, will be traced within the wider context of other conditions and in relation to gender discrimination and selective admission procedures. Ideas on the causes of particular disorders and race- and gender-specific aetiological rationales will be set within the wider context of mental and racial hygiene, which framed the thinking of Dhunjibhoy and his colleagues.

The final theme pays particular attention to treatments and the extent to which they were conceptualised as 'modern'. Similar treatments to those applied in Britain were also practised at Ranchi. Among these were newly developed sedatives (barbiturates) and shock therapies. There was also a range of other treatments that had a considerable impact on patients' experiences, such as organotherapy, hydrotherapy and dance therapy. These will be assessed alongside activities that structured institutional life at Ranchi and were considered by Dhunjibhoy to be important aspects of therapeutic provisions: feasts and diet, religious engagement, sports and entertainment as well as work therapy.

The main sources used were produced within the context of institutional record keeping and administrative scrutiny, namely the annual and triennial superintendents' reports submitted to the inspector-general of civil hospitals and to the local government. The numerical data appended to these have been evaluated and statistical trends and averages identified. Unless otherwise indicated, all statistical data are based on the author's calculations, drawing on the tables provided in the superintendents' and inspector-generals' reports. Further primary sources consist of census reports, medical journals and textbooks, and official as well as private correspondence.

Chapter 1

INDIANISATION AND ITS DISCONTENTS

The Indian gentleman, with all self-respect to himself, should not enter into a compartment reserved for Europeans, any more than he should enter a carriage set apart for ladies. Although you may have acquired the habits and manners of the European, have the courage to show that you are not ashamed of being an Indian, and in all such cases, identify yourself with the race to which you belong.
—H. Hardless, *The Indian Gentleman's Guide to Etiquette*, 1919

During the early part of the nineteenth century, most senior positions in the colonial medical services were occupied by Europeans. Only from 1855 were Indians allowed to occupy higher-level roles. However, public proclamations and official regulations did not always reflect British officials' sentiments and unofficial practices. In his book *Race, Sex and Class*, Ballhatchet discusses the case of a highly qualified, mixed-race (Eurasian) doctor who had been made assistant surgeon in the mid-nineteenth century.[1] He soon fell foul of European prejudice, becoming the victim of a scandal. Although the allegations against him were eventually shown to have been groundless, if not malicious, the director-general of hospitals recommended that in order to avoid similar occurrences in the future, Indians and Eurasians ought not to be appointed to senior positions, regardless of their qualifications. Instead of being given a commission they should be made warrant officers, as:

> this course would not [withdraw] them from their own class, or [place] them in a false position, one in which though equals in virtue of holding Her Majesty's Commission, they are, nevertheless, not looked upon by the other Officers of the service as on an equality in a social sense.[2]

The career of S. G. Chuckerbutty, an Indian from Bengal, highlights similar issues.[3] He sat and excelled at the first competitive exams organised in London in 1855, and had converted to Christianity. He has been celebrated as the first, and one of only a few in the late nineteenth century, who had managed to 'remove from his race, the stigma of a proscription which denied them a career of honourable ambition in their own land'.[4] However, his dire experiences prior to his eventual senior appointment as professor of *materia medica* at Calcutta Medical College, and even afterwards, attest to the many structural obstacles he had to contend with, and the considerable social prejudice and outright hostility he experienced from Europeans.

The practical and social obstacles that stood in the way of Indians and Eurasians aspiring to positions in the colonial service led to them being present almost exclusively in the subordinate uncovenanted service (at the level of 'subassistant surgeon') during the nineteenth century. This dovetailed with the contemporary need for employment opportunities for British professionals. The Raj constituted an attractive career outlet for the British middle classes, offering not only secure employment (as long as colonialism prevailed) but also a far more luxurious lifestyle than that available to them in their motherland. This phenomenon is well documented. British civil servants and the upper strata of the military were aptly described as belonging to a distinct social category: a kind of 'middle-class aristocracy'.[5] Much of the imagery of Raj lore reflects this. India is depicted as an exotic playground for Britons, presenting its own environmental tribulations (the 'heat and dust'), attractions (hunting, sports, club life) and displaying a distinctive social etiquette (calling cards and seating orders) that governed relationships between the various strata among the 'Anglo-Indians' (that is, the British in India), and the official rules of social engagement between them and Indians.

As long as Europeans were allocated senior positions, with Indians relegated to subservient, even menial, activities, the imperial social pecking order remained largely circumscribed in terms of European seniority and supremacy on the one hand and Indian subalternity on the other – even though both sides were highly heterogeneous, with their own social hierarchies based on social class, ethnic origin, caste and religious affiliation. The decades around the turn of the nineteenth to the twentieth century could be considered the ideological heyday of this formal constellation. The announcement of Delhi as the new imperial capital in 1911, 'undertaken in large part to enable the government to escape the uncomfortable political atmosphere of Calcutta, marked by continued and often violent demonstrations of nationalist sentiment', could be, as Metcalf put it, considered as 'the beginning of the end'.[6] Following increased anti-British political agitation from the late nineteenth century and the formation of the Indian National Congress in 1885, Indians (and some Europeans) gradually began to challenge the prevalent imperial, political and social order. From 1892 Indian medical degrees were finally recognised, removing the requirement to sit exams in Britain. The formal rules of engagement between Europeans and Indians of the middle and upper echelons of colonial society began to change. This was particularly pronounced from the second decade of the twentieth century, when the number of Western-trained Indian medical practitioners increased noticeably, leading to what the authorities termed the Indianisation of the Indian medical services.

Indianisation, alongside the decentralisation of some of the colonial services in 1919 (via the devolution of medical administration to individual provinces) and the establishment of local self-government in the various provinces in 1935 changed the administration of the colonial state considerably. These developments bring into relief a number of important issues and questions. Foremost among these is whether members of the gradually emerging group of Indians in senior positions should be most appropriately pigeonholed as mere collaborators with the colonial project, who fulfilled Macaulay's earlier nineteenth-century vision of the British colonial state and its educational institutions of raising an Indian middle class that could interpret 'between us and the millions whom we govern – a class of persons Indian in colour and blood, but English in tastes, in opinions, in morals, and in intellect'.[7] The experiences of colonial subjects and mediators between the indigenous uneducated 'masses' and the rulers were, in the context of French North Africa, described by Fanon in 1952 in his *Black Skin, White Masks*. Being a psychoanalyst by training, Fanon focused on the 'psychopathology of colonisation', namely the feelings of dependency and inadequacy that he considered to be the consequence of 'black subjects' embracing the culture of the colonial power. Fanon's work developed from earlier debates on negritude, which had also grappled with the social and psychological consequences of French colonialism during the 1920s and 1930s. This is, significantly, also the main period with which this book is concerned.

The role of, and the psychological impact on, Macaulay's indigenous mediators – or members of what Marxist and dependency-theory scholars in the 1970s and 1980s have termed the 'comprador bourgeoisie'[8] – has received considerable critical attention throughout the twentieth century among historians of colonialism and those involved in colonial liberation and postcolonial movements. More recently there has been a conceptual shift towards questions of 'identity' and in particular 'multiple identities', allowing for a more comprehensive and nuanced assessment of the condition of the colonised.[9] However, in the history of colonial psychiatry, the issue of how to conceptualise the gradual incorporation of Western-trained indigenous practitioners into the senior ranks of the colonial medical service has rarely arisen.[10] This is partly due to the fact that only very recently have historians of psychiatry begun to shift their focus from the nineteenth to the twentieth century, with 'no narrative in sight which can explain the psychiatry of the 20th century, comparable to the authoritative coherence achieved for the 19th century'.[11] The history of psychiatry in British India has been written mainly by reference to nineteenth-century colonial culture. On the other hand, existing work by medical historians on the important role of 'intermediaries', 'middles' or 'subalterns' within colonial settings has concerned itself mainly with those appointed to positions at the intermediate, subordinate or auxiliary level,[12] or with the development of medical research and science.[13]

Towards Indianisation

Dhunjibhoy had been trained at Bombay Medical College, graduating with a fully recognised MBBS (Bachelor of Medicine and Surgery). He was also a fellow of the College of Physicians and Surgeons (FCPS), a distinction considered highly prestigious among medical practitioners. Dhunjibhoy was made a member of the Indian Medical Service, the supreme medical service on account of its strong link with the British Medical Association (BMA). As was common practice at the time, the appointment was both military and civilian; Dhunjibhoy was therefore given a military commission on joining the IMS.[14] No suitable vacancy being available at the time in Bombay, his services were 'placed temporarily at the disposal of the Government of Bengal', some sixteen hundred kilometres across the subcontinent, where a position needed to be filled at the mental hospital in Berhampore, almost two hundred kilometres northwest of Calcutta (Kolkata).[15] When the building work at the new institution in Ranchi was completed, Dhunjibhoy was appointed as its first superintendent.

An appointment such as that at Ranchi was highly coveted among doctors. Not only did it entail taking over a large, brand-new purpose-built institution, but well-paid vacancies at senior-management level were few and far between, especially at a time of financial retrenchment such as the decades following the First World War. What is more, Dhunjibhoy was among the first few 'native' medical officers to head a major medical institution. At the three old mental hospitals from which Ranchi got its first intake of patients, high-ranking Europeans had been in charge: Lt. Col. H. R. Dutton at Patna, Lt. F. E. Knight (following Dhunjibhoy's reposting) at Berhampore, and Lt. Col. M. Mackelvie at Dacca (Dhaka). Dhunjibhoy's appointment promised to put an end to European pre-eminence in senior IMS positions. His practical achievements were acknowledged locally and in Britain. H. Ainsworth, the most senior medical officer in the province and the inspector-general of civil hospitals, Bihar and Orissa, announced in relation to the successful transfer to Ranchi of 1,226 patients in 1925: 'I think Captain Dhunjibhoy and his staff deserve much credit for the success which has attended the opening of the hospital.'[16] This view was echoed in the *Journal of Mental Science (JMS)*:

> The organization necessary to safely effect the transport of such large numbers can be better imagined when it is stated that the distance, for instance, from Dacca is some 300 miles, and involves a journey of 51 hours by steamer and rail and road. ... Great credit is due to Capt. Dhunjibhoy and those who assisted him, in that the transport of this large number of patients was carried out without hitch or mishap.[17]

The colonial government facilitated Dhunjibhoy's further training and specialisation. He was sent to Europe and North America on a number of occasions prior and subsequent to his appointment at Ranchi. He was put in charge of the training of students from Patna Medical College and the Department of Psychology at the Universities of Calcutta and Dacca. When the mental hospital was recognised in 1936 for postgraduate study by the Universities of London and Edinburgh, he was responsible for students working for 'diplomas in Psychological Medicine'.[18] In regard to his formal career development, Dhunjibhoy had the official support of the colonial government at the highest level. This was in line with the Indianisation of government services pursued during this period – enforced, not least, to appease increased anticolonial strife.

There is however evidence that Dhunjibhoy's lot was not an easy one and that his achievements were not acknowledged by all of his European colleagues. Although the colonial government actively facilitated Dhunjibhoy's career at the highest level proportionate to his training and experience, he became the target of criticism and discrimination – not so much despite his elevation to a senior position but because of it. The new government policy of Indianisation within the colonial service did not instantly do away with discriminatory practices and ingrained adverse attitudes among European practitioners. New terms of reference were supposed to govern working relationships between European and Indian practitioners but, as will be shown, notwithstanding the official requirement for equity between European and Indian senior officers, issues of race, class and professional competition for scarce jobs were rife. Structural inequalities that had affected staff in earlier decades persisted, ensuring the continuation of an employment hierarchy favouring European staff.

Structural Inequities

The IMS pay scales for Europeans and Indians were seemingly on a par, being based, as before, on formal qualification and length of service. Dhunjibhoy, for example, was paid Rs.1,350 per month in 1925, when he started at Ranchi as a captain. On reaching, in due course, the rank of major in 1928, he earned Rs.1,500 per month, and then Rs.1,650 from 1931. This was apparently in line with what his European counterpart, Owen Berkeley-Hill, superintendent at the neighbouring mental hospital for Europeans and higher-class Eurasians, who was paid as a major (that is, Rs.1,200 per month in 1920 and Rs.1,350 in 1921). However, Dhunjibhoy was in charge of the largest mental hospital in India (confining, on average, 1,400 patients). His European counterpart was responsible for a much smaller number of Europeans and higher-class Eurasians (a maximum of 102 men and 96 women).[19] Berkeley-Hill also had the benefit of working in an institution that provided care on a superior scale, commensurate with the higher social standing of its patients (the institution's admission restrictions clearly specified that only Europeans and higher-class Eurasians were eligible for treatment). A range of discretionary payments and special allowances were common. Dhunjibhoy himself seems to have been acutely aware of the pay differential. One of his daughters noted, 'I know my father complained from time to time about racism. He received about Rs.1000 less than his British counterparts.'[20]

Another problematic structural issue concerns the extent to which Indians of the lower ranks, such as Dhunjibhoy's attendants and subordinate staff, did not appear to profit from the Indianisation of the medical service. They remained, as before, subservient, being graded according to the proximity of their position to European structures of management and command. Hence, attendants who looked after Indian patients at the Ranchi Indian Mental Hospital received a lower remuneration than those caring for Europeans and Eurasians at the Ranchi European Mental Hospital. In 1921, European male attendants (later to become psychiatric nurses) were paid Rs.150 or Rs.160 per month in the former, and at the latter, Indian male attendants received Rs.24, Rs.21 or Rs.18. At Madras (Chennai), Indian attendants received between Rs.15 and Rs.27 (with eight salary points for males, and four for females), while 'Attendants, Superior Grade', employed in the adjoining but separate premises reserved for European patients, earned considerably more, namely between Rs.84 and Rs.100 (with five salary points).

Pay scales also varied between different provinces, some qualifications were considered less deserving than others, and members of the IMS were generally paid more. The fairness of this system was contentious. For example, in the province of Madras, another non-European, of Sri Lankan Tamil heritage, Dr H. S. Hensman, started as superintendent at the Madras Mental Hospital in 1924 on only Rs.900. He had obtained his licentiate in medicine and surgery in Madras (LMS). This was a lesser certificate awarded after a shorter course than Dhunjibhoy's MBBS from Bombay. However, Hensman also held the LRCD and the MRCS (Diploma or Licentiate of the Royal College of Physicians and of the Royal College of Surgeons in Britain, a conjoint initial qualification in medicine). The government had also posted him to England for one year for specialist training in the treatment of mental diseases (in 1922–23).[21] His starting salary was low in contrast to his immediate predecessor at Madras, W. R. J. Scroggie, a European who had trained in London some ten years earlier, who was paid over double Hensman's rate for doing the same job (Rs.2,000 in 1923). Scroggie was then a lieutenant colonel and a member of the IMS. Hensman, in contrast, despite his additional diploma from a British institution, was not made a member of the IMS.

The Indianisation of the colonial service was certainly an important official step towards equality – but it was an 'equality' that maintained de facto discrimination against the higher sections of Indian society by means of special allowances and recognised the services of lower-grade Indians on the basis of their closeness to European staff.

Medical Politics and European Racial Prejudice

Both Dhunjibhoy and Hensman were good advertisements for the Indianisation of the colonial services. However, their positions in the imperial pecking order were very different. Dhunjibhoy had been admitted to what the BMA considered to be the 'superior civil medical services',[22] the IMS, while Hensman had not. At the time, the Westernised medical marketplace in British India was wide ranging – encompassing, alongside the IMS, civil medical practitioners, such as Hensman, medical missionaries, and members of the Royal Army Medical Corps (RAMC). Following the Montague-Chelmsford Reforms, 'provincialisation' was introduced from 1919. This meant that some government functions were deferred or devolved to the local governments of Bengal, Madras, Bombay and the remaining six provinces of British India.[23] Other functions, considered politically and economically more essential for the continued British administration of India (such as finance, revenue and home affairs), were retained as reserved or imperial areas by the central government of India, based in Delhi. European medical practitioners, especially members of the IMS (backed by the BMA and hence the *British Medical Journal* (*BMJ*)), resented the resulting decentralisation of medical power. The new system meant that the Government of India, and thus the IMS, had only an advisory role in regard to medical matters.

The apparent plurality of medical politics was still subject to a highly hierarchical order, with Indians practising indigenous medicine being relegated to the bottom rungs. In addition, Indians were subject to severe hostility from European colleagues who feared Indian 'encroachment' both within the IMS (like Dhunjibhoy) and by independent medical professionals (like Hensman). For Europeans, Indianisation entailed increasing competition for jobs, both within the IMS and in the other medical services. It also implied a reduction of income from private practice that had previously been linked with particular positions.

There was also the sensitive issue of whether Indianisation would lead to Indians being permitted to treat Europeans and to examine them during training. As Jeffery and Chakrabarti have shown, Europeans held strong views on this and expressed them in no uncertain terms, at the highest level during the 1910s and 1920s.[24] For example, the governor of Bombay, George Lloyd, wrote to the secretary of state, Lord William Peel, in 1923: 'I need scarcely add that I should never dream of allowing European patients in our hospitals out here to be used as clinical material for the study of Indian medical students.'[25] This kind of view echoed earlier ones, expressed prior to the passing of the Ilbert Bill of 1883, for example, when Indian judges and magistrates were to be allowed jurisdiction to try British offenders in criminal cases at district level. In regard to medical matters, the BMA expressed its grave objections to Indian demands put forward by the Bombay Union,[26] in 1913, for equal pay and privileges for independent medical practitioners and an end to the IMS monopoly, arguing:

> Those who know the Indian most intimately, and who admire most intelligently his many excellent qualities as a profession[al] man, cannot blind themselves to the fact that his standards are still far from being those of his British brother.[27]

Sentiments such as these coloured the context within which Dhunjibhoy and Hensman received their training and had to function on a professional and personal level in leading medical positions. Even if equity of sorts was officially prescribed, European prejudice and hostility on account of fearing loss of control, income and status persisted. As Sinha put it, in relation to mixed-race gentlemen's clubs, which gradually emerged during the early twentieth century alongside the traditional 'whites only' clubs, the former were the 'product of a new political expediency demanded by a reconstituted imperial order'.[28] This new order encompassed not only the Indianisation of the colonial services, but also the policy of provincialisation, namely the devolution of the powers of the central colonial government in particular areas (such as medicine and education) to individual provinces. Provincialisation, introduced in 1919, was loathed by many Europeans, as any decentralisation of colonial power potentially threatened monopolies such as that of the IMS.

This newly reconstituted imperial order often failed to reach the level of the 'everyday life' of social sentiment and personal relationships between the gentlemen and ladies of the upper echelons of the Indian and European communities. For example, the Bankipore Club, then called 'The European Club', in Patna, some three-hundred or so kilometres from Ranchi, had previously been an exclusive meeting place for rich European planters and officials in Bihar. It was obliged to open up membership to Indians such as A. K. Sinha, the first Indian inspector-general of police.[29] This was not a proactive decision to abolish the racially discriminatory admission policy but arose because local officials of the higher grades automatically became, on the basis of their position, not only members but also part of the executive committee of the club located in the area they had been posted to. Dhunjibhoy, too, attended the local Ranchi Club, located some twelve miles from the mental hospital in the heart of the city, on what is still called 'Club Road'.

It is doubtful that the official policy of parity between Europeans and Indians had overcome the deeply rooted 'whites only' sentiments of European fellow members. As M. K. Sinha, points out, other prominent clubs such as the famous 'Bengal Club' in Calcutta retained their apartheid policy until Independence in 1947, a persistently challenging and painful circumstance for elite Indian society. As Memmi pointed out in his work *The Colonizer and Colonized*, those working for and identifying with the colonial rulers would be aware that they were not well respected regardless of how well they tried to excel in their work and to fit in with polite colonial society.[30]

The Medical Market and Indian Competition

Professional competition and fears of outsider infringement on career opportunities and private medical practice were present not only among European practitioners. They prevailed also between Indians aspiring to find a foothold in the medical marketplace, in particular at a time when Western medicine was the mode of healing preferred by central and provincial governments, marginalising indigenous practices. As South Asia is a large subcontinent, divided into separate provinces under British control (and about six hundred Indian States under indigenous rulers), each region encompassed its own socio-cultural traditions and diverse communities. Dhunjibhoy's hospital catered for patients from three very different regions, namely Bengal, Bihar and Orissa. As Bara has shown in regard to teaching and education, there existed a certain tension between the Bihari and Bengali elite in the area surrounding Ranchi (then part of Bihar) as they were competing for jobs in the colonial service, with the former feeling squeezed out by the latter.[31] In Bengal and particularly in Calcutta, local elites had become Westernised earlier than in other provinces, with Bengalis taking up highly coveted positions also in neighbouring Bihar. The appointment of an outsider from Bombay to one of the few existing positions involving superintendence of a medical institution could not but induce displeasure among Indian Western-trained doctors from all three provinces. Potential candidates from Bihar and Orissa missed out yet again, while on this occasion a contender from the major rival northern province pursuing elite Westernisation sidelined Bengalis. Structurally, Dhunjibhoy's arrival at Ranchi was therefore not particularly welcomed by the Indian colleagues who had to work with and under him.

Dhunjibhoy would of course have been well aware of this situation and the potential problems he might face from Indian deputies and colleagues on his transfer to Ranchi. However, he was successful in managing the institution's affairs, including its staff. It may well be that being an outsider from a distant region, across the other side of India, helped him to stay aloof from rivalries among elite local groups. As his daughter pointed out, Dhunjibhoy and his wife led an active social life, meeting regularly with Europeans as well as members of the local Bihari elite, thereby facilitating good relationships. At the same time, Dhunjibhoy had very good contacts in Calcutta. He frequently received visitors from there and was in touch with some eminent Bengali reformers and professionals. According to his daughter Roshan, Dhunjibhoy attempted to rise above interethnic and communal strife. To what extent this also ameliorated hostility and ill feelings on the part of potential professional competitors is difficult to gauge.

Professional Discrimination

The experience of social discrimination for senior Indian medical officers, such as Dhunjibhoy, was real and tangible. His daughter noted, 'My father understood racism and discrimination very well.'[32] There is indeed evidence of discrimination against

Indians in senior positions. For example, in regard to professional matters, medical authorities sought European rather than Indian superintendents' expertise, even in cases when the latter's experience may have been more relevant. In 1929, for example, when Dr Hensman had been in charge of the Madras Mental Hospital for about five years, improvements in this province's three mental hospitals were planned and consultation with an expert arranged. Hensman and his colleagues from the other two institutions in the Madras province were sent to Ranchi.[33] Given that the majority of patients in Madras province were Indian (namely 492 out of 510, or 96 per cent), and that no Europeans at all were confined in two of the three institutions (Calicut and Waltair), we might well expect that the appropriate expert to consult would have been the one person at Ranchi whose treatment of Indians was as successful as no other superintendent's had been at any institution in India (including the Ranchi European Mental Hospital).[34] However, Dhunjibhoy was not even mentioned. In the official records, 'going to Ranchi' meant a visit to Berkeley-Hill's institution for Europeans, where, so it was reported, 'Lt. Col. Berkeley-Hill is carrying out modern methods of treatment'.[35]

In colloquial language, too, the phrase 'going' or 'being sent to Ranchi' has implicitly come to relate to the former European Mental Hospital (now Central Institute of Psychiatry). Berkeley-Hill's institution has retained a high profile in north India – unlike the Ranchi Indian Mental Hospital (now Ranchi Institute of Neuro-Psychiatry and Allied Sciences), which declined steadily after Independence, being subject to underfunding and scandals about bad conditions. Even scholars and practitioners working on Indian psychiatry have neglected the history of Dhunjibhoy's institution, some of them unaware of the fact that there were (and still are) two psychiatric facilities at Ranchi. The enduring marginalisation of the Indian Mental Hospital and Dhunjibhoy is a legacy of colonial and postcolonial developments as well as current historiographic preferences. First, Dhunjibhoy was recalled in 1940 to Bombay for wartime service in Karachi where he stayed on, becoming part of the newly formed Pakistan following Partition in 1947. Apart from a few appearances at meetings and conferences, Dhunjibhoy more or less disappeared from the purview of Indian psychiatry – not least because of the development of almost completely separate traditions of medical organisation and historical writing in India and Pakistan.

Second, the existence of the European institution next door distracted attention from its Indian counterpart and the achievements of its Indian superintendent. Berkeley-Hill was more successful in publicising his institution and treatment methods within a colonial context that continued to favour – albeit unofficially – European agency and its institutions. What is more, Berkeley-Hill practised psychoanalysis on his patients. Psychoanalysis was highly fashionable during the interwar period, attracting much attention on the part of elite European and Indian society in Calcutta. Historians too have been much more fascinated by the development of psychoanalysis in India than by mainstream psychiatry.[36] The latter was at the time focused on medical treatments (such as insulin, Cardiazol and malaria shock, and sedation by paraldehyde) as well as water and work or occupational therapy; all of which is far less appealing to social and cultural historians than engagement with the role of sexuality, the unconscious mind and mechanisms of repression in regard to individual, cultural and political processes.

Third, the administration of the European institution was, 'fortunately', as Berkeley-Hill remarked, 'taken out of the hands of the Government of Bihar and Orissa' in the early 1920s. Mental institutions had been under provincial control since 1919, but responsibility for any IMS staff associated with them lay with central government. Following Berkeley-Hill's complaint and subsequent newspaper reports in the *Statesman* that the European Mental Hospital was 'worse than a kaffir's kraal', the provincial authorities demanded from central government his immediate removal.[37] However, the European lobby in the IMS and among the local and all-India European communities was strong and inclined to disapprove of provincial influence over the fate of a European medical officer and an institution dedicated to the care of Europeans. Besides, Berkeley-Hill had good connections with influential people, such as Colonel J. P. Murray, a member of the IMS and the civil surgeon of Ranchi, and 'Miss Caroline Hubback', sister of the governor of Orissa, Sir John Austen Hubback (1936–38).[38] What is more, a number of vocal interest groups such as the European Association, the European Trades Association and the Anglo-Indian and Domiciled European Association got involved, and the European Mental Hospital was eventually removed from provincial control, ensuring funding and control by central government.

This setup meant that Berkeley-Hill's European Mental Hospital received funding from central government even after Independence, on a much higher scale than Dhunjibhoy's Indian institution, which remained under the purview of the provincial authorities. Consequently, the latter suffered from underfunding and deterioration of services like many other institutions in this region. In the case of the Indian Mental Hospital, the provincialisation of health services from 1919 and provincial self-government from 1935, which had been designed to empower Indian local governments, resulted in the decline of service provision after Independence in this particular region.[39]

Djunjibhoy and his institution experienced a certain degree of marginalisation. Even Berkeley-Hill, described as a 'good friend' of the Dhunjibhoys, did not appear to have paid them much attention in his autobiography. It is doubtful that he was able to empathise with his Indian colleague. Marrying an Indian woman, whom he regarded as 'one of the dearest creatures I have ever known', clearly did not exempt him from disdain for Indians more generally. While bestowing on his wife Karimbil Kunhimanny the distinction of having been 'the only Indian I have ever met who can be relied on consistently to do things promptly and properly' and pointing out that she had 'an infinite capacity for taking pains', he deftly combined a patriarchal compliment with a sweeping racist criticism of Indians.[40] It is doubtful that Dhunjibhoy would have missed Berkeley-Hill's derision for Indians' abilities and his ambition to keep himself aligned with the powers that be, even if from the protected position of an eccentric or 'a pariah' (in the words of Dhunjibhoy's daughter) who had, in his own words, 'incurred the displeasure of many members of [his] family, as well as that of many of [his] friends' by marrying an Indian woman from Cannanore in south India.[41] He had also come 'within an ace of being expelled' following minor incidents such as when he was 'ordered to grow a moustache' and generally rebelled against 'elderly men' and the 'mob of gentlemen-employees who know very little and who do even less'.[42]

Within the context of the Indianisiation of the colonial service, it is significant that Berkeley-Hill was able to mock his seniors' narrow-mindedness, and – as a European – he largely got away with it. He did gain a reputation as a colourful, if cantankerous, eccentric – a role up to which he seems to have been happy to live, albeit with occasional bitterness and sarcasm. Overall, it does not appear to have done him much harm in terms of his professional career. In contrast, Indians exposed to systemic prejudice and parochial narrow-mindedness had to bear it – lest they got the sack or, in light of the wider political context of anti-British agitation, fall under Europeans' suspicion about their loyalty. The official records are full of court cases against Indians employed by the British who were dismissed and/or imprisoned when they displayed anti-British sentiments and were engaged in nationalist pro-Independence activities. Even Indian employees' children had to toe the line. Dhunjibhoy's daughter remembered:

> The British, at the time, were also threatening higher Indian officers and functionaries, if their children joined the Freedom movement. They were warned that they would lose their pensions. My sister [celebrated Pakistani poet and professor of literature, Maki Kureishi] was actively supporting the Congress [Indian National Congress Party, active in the Independence movement] and I, at twelve, had paid my four annas to the CPI [Communist Party of India]. It was a time of tension and many arguments at home.[43]

Dhunjibhoy and Berkeley-Hill were reportedly powerful characters with, what would nowadays be called, 'strong egos'. This might not have facilitated any close relationship. Furthermore, a strong personality and views were desirable attributes of a superior British 'character', encouraged if displayed by Europeans of the higher orders supposedly attuned to the correct hierarchical circumstances within which they could find expression. Lapses by middle- and upper-class Europeans who overstepped the line, venting their feelings and views, were, as Berkeley-Hill's case shows, politely ignored and attributed to gentlemanly eccentricity – they were but mildly rebuked. It was however an altogether different situation if Indians (or lower-class Europeans) displayed similar traits.

Professional Closure and the Pathologisation of a Successful Community

In 1928, an article published in the *BMJ* on seemingly narrow clinical matters led to a flurry of exchanges between its author, Lt. Col. W. S. J. Shaw and two readers. Shaw had been superintendent of the mental hospital near Poona (Pune), in Bombay presidency, and had written on the prevalence of dementia praecox among the Parsi (Zoroastrian) community of India. The Parsi were a small community of not more than one hundred thousand people at the time, and most of them lived in Bombay. From the 'Western point of view', they were, as Shaw put it, 'far more in touch with our civilization than any other Indian people', and had a strong ethos of philanthropy – being, incidentally, engaged also in the provision of mental healthcare facilities in Bombay.[44] During his time at the mental hospital, Shaw had seen a number of public and private Parsi patients and on the basis of his general observations (but no reliable qualitative or quantitative data) postulated that Parsi patients had a higher incidence of dementia praecox than Hindu and Muslim patients.

The issue that particularly irked two readers of his article was that he not only claimed that there was consensus among researchers that schizophrenia was indeed a hereditary disease, but also that marriage between cousins among the Parsi – or 'inbreeding' – was 'a very definite cause', adding that 'moral imbecility', 'feeble-mindedness' or 'mental deficiency' as well as epilepsy were also implicated.[45] Shaw held that, 'Nowadays at all events, the common Parsee [Parsi] stock is seriously tainted with *Dementia Praecox*' and, because of the Parsi 'proverbial' trait of 'jealous family secretiveness', he suggested, quite offensively, that research ought to be 'carried out by a Parsee of an unusually altruistic type'.[46] Shaw concluded saying that he considered the subject of 'immense importance sociologically and eugenically'.

The first letter of outrage and criticism was printed just a week later. Its author, Arthur Brock, argued that Shaw had in fact, 'inadvertently', demonstrated a 'more important cause' for the high incidence of dementia praecox, namely '"Western" education and civilization generally'.[47] Brock was a medical doctor with an MD from Edinburgh and also an advocate of the emergent field of sociology. He was the author of *Health and Conduct* (1923) in which he argued that there were 'parallels between human diseases and diseases of the body politic' and that current discontents were mainly a mental condition – a 'psycho-sociological upset comparable to "shellshock"'.[48] Brock had close connections with the renowned Scottish biologist, sociologist and town planner Patrick Geddes, who wrote the introduction to Brock's book. Geddes had also been professor of civics and sociology at Bombay University from 1920 to 1923, when Shaw still worked in nearby Poona.[49] He claimed a relationship between spatial form and social processes (or 'regionalism' and 'civics') and, in his role as town planner, believed that Indian cities ought not to simply imitate European ones but should find their own expression of civic pride. Brock mirrored Geddes's contention when he suggested that not inbreeding but Western education was to blame for the 'breaking up of these young people's minds'. Furthermore, he noted, 'If we are to advise the Parsees against anything, it is rather against their too wholesale acceptance of Western civilization.'

Shaw was quick to respond. In a letter written the day after Brock's views were published, he rejected the Brock–Geddes position and affirmed that 'the peculiar incidence of schizophrenia among Parsees was not traceable to any faulty education or environment'.[50] He took issue also with the sociological habit of putting quote marks around particular phrases, even if these were not direct quotes but referred to the gist and implicit assumptions of an opponent's argument. Brock's reference to Shaw's alleged view that, in contrast to Parsis, Hindus and Muslims were at a 'lower' stage of civilisation, was strongly refuted. Other comments by Brock, based on speculation and inference, but capturing the flaws and prejudice that underpinned Shaw's argument and characterised the wider debates on eugenics and the heredity of particular races' assumed predispositions, were also dismissed.

The most significant comment, intended as a *coup de grâce* by Shaw, was his reference to Brock as 'a correspondent, who does not appear to have any personal knowledge of Indian conditions'.[51] The argument that those lacking first-hand experience of 'Indian conditions' ought to abstain from discussion of India-related matters had a long tradition and was put forward especially when certain interest groups in Britain questioned the continuation of British colonial rule or the ways the empire was run by their compatriots on the ground in India. Only 'old India hands' had the relevant experience. As Shaw had worked at the mental hospital near Bombay from 1912 to 1926, he had known of many challenges by outsiders to imperial and medical policies – not least by Geddes during his time at Bombay.[52] He was also familiar with Indian demands and political agitation for political and medical reforms, for example in relation to the provincialisation of medical services in 1919. Debates had been particularly heated in Bombay during the 1910s and 1920s, as the Bombay Medical Union, the interest group of independent medical professionals, with support from the Indian National Congress, had challenged the IMS monopoly. Shaw would have known very well how contentious the ideas were that he had published in the mouthpiece of the BMA, even if these were clothed in the language of clinical debate on the heredity of mental illness and popular eugenics thinking. Given the wider political, medical and social context at the time, Shaw's views could not but be read as allegations of inferiority levelled against the Parsis, a community that had acquired the necessary skills, expertise and social influence to compete at the highest level for medical and political positions with Europeans. Brock had put his finger on Shaw's underlying agenda and was discredited for it by reference to his lack of Indian experience.

However, the story did not finish there. Dhunjibhoy contributed to the debate as soon as he received the relevant copies of the journal some weeks later. His intervention might be expected to have been considered as most appropriate by the editors of the *BMJ*. Unlike Brock, being an Indian, Dhunjibhoy did have 'personal knowledge of Indian conditions'. He was also an expert in psychiatry and, as he belonged to the 'superior' IMS, he was officially well qualified. What is more, he was also a Parsi, and hence belonged to the very community Shaw had speculated about and from whom he had elicited a volunteer to shine more light on the matter of the alleged heredity of schizophrenia. However, despite Dhunjibhoy's merits and qualifications, the journal printed only a highly abbreviated extract in the 'Letters, Notes, and Answers' section from the well-evidenced criticism that he had advanced in response to Shaw's full article, which was based on mostly anecdotal and impressionistic accounts.

One of the central arguments in Dhunjibhoy's brief published extract was that the incidence of dementia praecox was high also in England, Germany, France, Italy and America – 'yet none of these nations is known to practise inbreeding like the Parsees'.[53] Dhunjibhoy was able to back this up with statistics – but the *BMJ* did not publish these. Shaw had selected one potential causative factor, attributing it to one select group only. Dhunjibhoy, too, could only speculate about the possible cause for schizophrenia. His assumption was that it was related to 'the stresses of present-day civilization and education', but he warned against undue generalisations, pointing out that this may not be 'the sole cause', but may 'at least have something to do with it'. Dhunjibhoy also quite correctly argued that the relationship between inbreeding and schizophrenia 'has never been definitely established'. His objections were well grounded in the scientific evidence available at the time. He also did not fail to point out that researchers assumed a 'greater hereditary predisposition in manic-depressive psychoses than in *Dementia Praecox*', so that inbreeding was more likely to produce a higher incidence of the former condition – not seen in the diagnoses of Parsi patients.[54] And, finally, referring to statistics from the various mental hospitals, Dhunjibhoy pointedly noted that schizophrenia was not as rare within other communities in India as Shaw 'imagined'.

Shaw did not respond to the issues raised by Dhunjibhoy. Instead he published an amended version of his original *BMJ* piece in yet another renowned British journal, the *JMS*, one year later. Although Shaw provided a good literature review in the amended article, his evidence on the Parsi was still based on conjecture and highly selective observations. Again he repeated the same questions, admitting that his observations were 'pure speculations' and that there were as yet no answers: 'I have come across no reference to inbreeding in any of the ordinary text-books.'[55] Despite this acknowledgement, he concluded: 'In any case the Parsi stock is now so seriously tainted with *Dementia Praecox* that the propriety of their abandonment of the mating of cousins should be seriously considered.'

Again Dhunjibhoy responded as soon as volume 76 of the *JMS* had arrived at Ranchi. His response, which was, as previously, well grounded in existing research and backed up by statistical data, was again published only in the 'Notes and News' section, but this time in a full version that included data sets from Indian institutions. In his last sentence, Dhunjibhoy hinted at what had been an important issue in relation to the whole, seemingly purely scientific, exchange between experts:

> However, if Col. Shaw will satisfy me as to why the incidence of [schizophrenia] is high amongst other communities and nations who follow western education and culture but are free from 'in-breeding', I am quite prepared to adopt his suggestion, and take up research work in order to determine the cause or causes of the alleged high incidence of [schizophrenia] amongst the Parsees.[56]

Like Brock, Dhunjibhoy again put his finger on one particular flaw of Shaw's logic. A specific diagnosis shared by highly educated Indians and Westerners had been attributed to an inherited defect (based on custom) in the former but not the latter. An Indian community like the Parsi that had competed successfully with Europeans, operating at the same level with them, was considered by Shaw to be tainted by virtue of persistent cultural preference, inevitably leading to hereditary decline. Shaw's pathologisation of a particular ethnic community on the grounds of its cultural habits resonated more closely with the tenets of racial hygiene than those of mental hygiene subscribed to by Dhunjibhoy. Like Brock, Dhunjibhoy too had identified the agenda implicit in Shaw's arguments: although some Indians may have been equals in terms of their formal positions and achievements within the imperial order, they were still, as has been noted above in relation to the nineteenth-century colonial context, 'nevertheless not looked upon by the other Officers of the service as on an equality in a social sense'.[57] Shaw merely provided a seemingly scientific rationale for his social sentiments at a time when mental and racial hygiene were part of mainstream scientific thinking. The publication of Shaw's views on the mental profile of the Parsi community, in two of the most high-profile British expert journals, pathologised the very group that had closely interacted and collaborated with the British since the late eighteenth century and had become their single most successful competitor in trade and industry.

The Decline of the 'Good Parsi'

The debate on the alleged high incidence of mental illness among the Parsis, and its supposed relationship with endogamy sparked off by Shaw's article, were part of a wider discourse on the decline of this particular community from the 1920s onwards. Elite Parsis and their European colleagues alike were well aware of this, making it potentially more precarious for Parsis in senior positions in the colonial services, like Dhunjibhoy, to assert their authority *vis-à-vis* European colleagues. Unfortunately for Dhunjibhoy, his rise in the supreme medical service occurred after the zenith of Parsi success, dating from the late nineteenth century to the first two decades of the twentieth century. As Guha has argued, members of this small community had been the 'earliest to enter modern industries, and they were able to maintain their lead in this field well until the end of World War I'.[58] Reasons cited for the community's success have been its religiously grounded work ethic (whereby Zoroastrianism is seen from a Eurocentric perspective as mirroring Weber's 'protestant work ethic'); close community spirit and endogamy; lack of caste barriers; production-orientated peasant–artisan background and, 'above all, their acceptability to British patrons as stable collaborators'.[59] In the first decade of the twentieth century, Parsis were consistently portrayed as more Western in appearance than members of other communities and about one-quarter spoke English (compared to less than 1 per cent of Jains and 0.5 per cent of Hindus).[60]

Given the common perception that the Parsis' destiny was 'bound up with the British in India', and their ambition to 'see themselves as like the British and as unlike other Indians', it is not surprising that the attributes ascribed to a 'good Parsi' were similar to those of an English gentleman.[61] These included virtues such as rationality, honesty and loyalty, as well as physical prowess. In 1896, R. P. Karkaria proclaimed that 'In physical matters, too, Parsis are rapidly developing robuster qualities of body, which will in the long run make them the equals of many Western nations, and on which Western supremacy rests'.[62] H. D. Darukhanawala reiterated this point in 1935 in *Parsis and Sport* where he considered the Parsi as 'the most physically vigorous men in India'.[63] However, by then the discourse of Parsi decline had become a mainstream trope among European and Indian communities in British India. S. F. Markham, for example, noted in his report to the trustees of the Sir Ratan Tata Trust: 'There seems to be a feeling […] in certain quarters that the community has reached or passed its zenith.'[64] Mirroring Shaw's impressions, he argued that the birth rate and literacy had declined, while insanity and unemployment were on the increase. To back up his claims that there had been a 'steady fall of the prestige of the community', he cited the renowned Parsi scientist and director of the Colaba Observatory, Dr N. A. F. Moos.[65]

The rise and fall of the Parsi community has received much attention from historians, and attempts have been made to answer N. B. R. Kotwal's question in 1937, 'I say, in Education the Parsis were the first and foremost in India. How then came the decay, when and where from, it is necessary to know.'[66] There have been two strands of answers relevant to our context. One focuses on the role of the Parsis as 'compradors' or collaborators with the cause of colonialism and the community's decline along with the death throes of British power from the period following increased anti-British agitation.

This fits in with Fanon's contention that 'for the black man there is only one destiny. And it is white.'[67] The implication is that feelings of abandonment, painful ambivalence and self-criticism as well as unacknowledged anger ensue at the loss of the colonial father figure. The earlier mimetic mirroring of the British representation of self and identification with the coloniser become problematic once the coloniser's authority itself declines.

The other explanations for the Parsi decline focus on aspects that had been particularly prominent in scientific and popular discourse since the late nineteenth century, namely racial factors and 'deterioration of moral fibre',[68] or, as Guha put it, issues such as 'ethnic qualities' and 'value systems'.[69] This line of argument contends that the Parsi rhetoric of asserting similitude to the European entailed an assertion of distance from other non-Parsi Indian communities, which was expressed in terms of racial and cultural difference. Dhunjibhoy's daughter noted that, 'many Parsis of his generation did not feel particularly "Indian" [. . .] Most [...] when asked: "Where do you come from?" would answer "I am a Parsi – from India"'.[70] The trope of Parsi racial purity and cultural distinction from other Indian communities changed into a narrative of racial decline and genetic corruption from the 1920s onwards: endogamy or 'inbreeding' was now seen to have led to degeneration of the racial stock, inducing a reduced entrepreneurial spirit, alongside reliance on easily accessible communal charity, reduced fertility and madness. As J. F. Bulsara affirmed, this resulted in 'the alarming problem of growing economic misery and the physical, intellectual and spiritual impoverishment of an increasing section of the community',[71] It is within this kind of debate, which ascribed social and political changes to biological factors, that Shaw's publication on the alleged higher incidence of mental illness among Parsis must be set.

Guha has indicated another important factor in the rise and subsequent decline of Parsi fortunes: the changing economic trajectory of industrial and financial capital following the world economic crisis of 1929. He suggests that the success of the Parsis as a community was linked to their entering into modern trades and industries including joint-stock trading, banking and manufacturing corporations during the late nineteenth century, following earlier engagement in shipbuilding and in the opium and cotton trade with China. The Parsis maintained their economic lead until the end of World War I. To explain this success, Guha points at 'the exigencies of circumstances' or rather at a 'conjuncture of favourable circumstances': like other trading communities from Gujarat (in the west of India), the Parsis not only belonged to one of 'the economically most advanced region[s] of India', but, in contrast to Bengal (in the east of India), to an area that saw much later British imperial expansion and hence 'allowed for large-scale survivals of pre-British administrative structures'.[72] Consequently, 'colonial capitalism was forced to leave more room to its partners in empire in western India than in eastern India'.[73] However, such local interweaving with world economic developments implied also being subject to its repeated cyclical crises. Changes in the development of international trade and British monopoly capitalism during and following the period of the Wall Street crash of 1929 posed considerable problems to Parsi entrepreneurs, which led to a shift in the community's self-perception, much soul searching and the frantic and anxious identification of a variety of social, cultural and biological factors that could be considered as plausible causes for the shift in fortune.

Both the comprador and the racial-decay theses that have been mooted to explain the decline of the Parsi from the 1920s onwards are highly problematic, and, judging from his responses to Shaw's articles, Dhunjibhoy for one would have been uncomfortable with either of them (although he contended that inbreeding was 'undesirable').[74] Of course, the assumption of degenerated racial stock or 'bad genes' as a result of 'inbreeding' was common during the heyday of mental hygiene and constituted, in its extreme form, a mainstay of racial-hygiene protagonists during the 1930s. Intriguingly, endogamy was encouraged when allegedly superior racial purity was considered the aim (Nazi Germany in regard to the 'Aryan race'), but was considered to have engendered corrupted stock in regard to particular communities that were discriminated against and persecuted, such as the Jews. In a similar vein, it is, as Luhrmann points out, 'a weird and telling argument, in India, where endogamy is taken for granted, that in Parsi endogamy the blood of the community should be said to fold in upon itself and implode'.[75] The reason for Parsis' self-perception from the early twentieth century onwards as a community subject to 'decadence and degeneration',[76] 'decline in numbers' and 'decline in quality also',[77] which was repeated and reinforced by the British in India (for example, by Shaw), requires further research.

Collaborators, Competitors and Ambivalence

The Parsi community's mirroring of the rise and subsequent fall of the British led commentators at the time, as well as postcolonial writers, to consider the Parsi as 'compradors' or collaborators with the cause of the empire whose downfall was inevitable once British rule was challenged and eventually terminated. Many elite Parsis were indeed beneficiaries of British rule. However, those who made a career in the colonial services in the wake of Indianisation during the 1920s and 1930s were both 'collaborators' with the ongoing albeit fading cause of the empire, on a structural level, and, in practice, allies of those Indians who pressed for the replacement of British with Indian agency in preparation for Independence. On account of this double role they were subject to divided loyalties and to mistrust as well as celebration from both sides, British and Indian.

Authors such as Memmi and Fanon, whose experience of colonialism was of French North Africa, focused mainly on the psychological cost of identification and collaboration with the aggressor: self-loathing and self-criticism as well as loss of identity. As Memmi put it: 'So goes the drama of the man who is a product and victim of colonialism. He almost never succeeds in corresponding with himself.'[78] There are traces of this in Dhunjibhoy's experience as narrated by his daughter. The pessimistic comprador or collaborator trope also partly explains the earlier self-confidence and later self-criticism of the Parsis as a community and Dhunjibhoy's experiences of continued professional marginalisation by British colleagues even while Indianisation was progressing rapidly. The various hurdles that were put in his way when he attempted to initiate new procedures or recommend a change in health policies attest to the continued discrimination towards highly qualified Indians despite their senior roles in the colonial service. However, an emphasis on Indianisation as a mere ploy of colonialism and as an inherently doomed attempt at a 'march through the institutions' by those involved in it, is problematically narrow, as is the assumption that a 'loss of self' is always inevitable and terminal. In regard to the latter, Dhunjibhoy may have been, as his daughter put it, 'a disappointed man', but he also regained a former identity and inner world into which he apparently 'slipped comfortably'.[79]

The role of those who profited from colonial rule and Indianisation could of course not but be full of conflict, contradiction and 'ambivalence'. Considering the structural consequences of Indian actors' ambivalent position, Nandy emphasised the potential for subversion. He sees the colonised subjects not just as 'simple-hearted victims of colonialism' but also as 'participants in a moral and cognitive venture against oppression'.[80] Most importantly: 'They make choices.' As Bhabha explained: 'ambivalence' is inherent in colonial discourse and in the attempt by the colonised to copy the coloniser. 'Mimicry' is therefore 'at once resemblance and menace.'[81] Roshan Dhunjibhoy, too, noted that the experience of divided loyalties, or ambivalence, affected individuals deeply, creating heartache for them, but still offering the opportunity to eventually settle – even comfortably in her father's case – into a life world of their choice. Maki Kureishi, Dhunjibhoy's second daughter, encapsulated her and her sister Roshan's experience of postcolonial ambivalence in a poem.[82]

....

Always the long, repeated journeys looking for
something you've left behind.

When we meet, all the doors swing open
for this is where you live; but the rooms

are empty, echo to our timid
grown-up voices; and this old child
who lifts a broken-toy face, is she
you or me? Only our scars mark where we built

our personal and nursery planet.
Still, we've kept the knack. I, middle-aged, fidget

with make-believe; you, homesick and not
eager to come home, are foreign everywhere. Live European,

stay haunted by the image of
that makeshift geography we share.

....

The role and experience of specific individuals and particular communities in colonial settings is multilayered and complex. Guha emphasises the economic and political dimensions in relation to the Parsis as a community. He suggests that they were not only beneficiaries of British rule but 'also victims of its policies' since the British did not 'tolerate rivals in the same market'.[83] He provides evidence for this contention in regard to Parsi trade and industry, concluding that 'the Parsi business-men were "comprador" only in a limited sense', as they also pursued their independent business, alongside working for the British.[84] Unlike indigenous elites in other colonial settings, the Parsis were both collaborators and competitors, so that both 'collaboration and conflict were reflected in the [Indian comprador's] vacillating political stand and economic position'. This was also true of Dhunjibhoy who constituted a competitor in the medical marketplace to European as well as Bengali and Bihari colleagues. Colonial discrimination and ill feelings between different communities trying to carve out a living within the parameters set by the British on the one hand and the nationalist movement on the other made no exception of the Parsis.

Dhunjibhoy's career can be seen as a showcase of successful Indianisation of the medical services. From a moderate Indian nationalist point of view, Dhunjibhoy belonged to a group of Indians trained to take over from the British on their imminent departure from South Asia; from the perspective of radical nationalists, he was collaborating with the enemy. For the British he was an excellent exemplar – particularly at international events – of the British promise to entrust an increasing number of Indians with high-profile positions in the move towards decolonisation. Dhunjibhoy was clearly grateful to the colonial government. Coming from a lower Parsi background, he reportedly felt 'that he owed everything he had achieved to the Army and the British'.[85] This does not imply that he had any anti-nationalist inclinations or was in political allegiance with the British. His daughter described him as 'not political' and, despite having met Gandhi and received visitors who were protagonists of the Independence movement, such as the president of the Indian National Congress, Dr Rajendra Prasad,[86] he 'was not particularly nationalistic'.[87] Like other Parsis, Dhunjibhoy sat on the fence of pre-Independence politics and upheaval. The eminent industrialist Jamsetji Tata, for example, maintained close links with the Congress and the Swadeshi movement while proclaiming that the Parsis had 'benefited more than any other class by English rule' and that 'their gratitude to that rule is, as it ought to be, in due proportion to the advantage derived from it'.[88] Reflecting this nonpartisan position, he had named one of the Tata textile mills after the Empress and another *Swadeshi*.

Like many others who benefited from the Indianisation of the medical services – Parsi or not – Dhunjibhoy followed a tactical line of noncommitment that may be read negatively as evidence of collaborators' bourgeois self-interest or, perhaps more pragmatically, as attempts at self-preservation and endeavour to assure one's family's prosperity during a time of political turmoil. Unlike their children's generation, which 'was the first generation of Parsis that identified completely with India', many of those who lived as adults through the 1920s and 1930s did not have a strong affiliation with the politics of Indian nationalism and separatism (neither Hindu nor Muslim), as they felt Parsi first and Indian second.[89] As Roshan Dhunjibhoy put it, they thought of themselves as Parsi and 'did not feel particularly "Indian"'. Consequently, Dhunjibhoy would stay on in Karachi, which became part of Pakistan after Independence and Indian Partition in 1947 – although, 'like many Parsis', he 'disliked Muslims' – because there was 'a good Parsi community and [he had] friends and [knew] no one, any more, in Bombay'.[90]

Despite the 'torn self' and 'white masks' that have been ascribed to the 'black skin' in colonial contexts, it seems that for Dhunjibhoy 'Parsiness' continued to remain the essential reference point. As his daughter pointed out:

> I think [my father] died a disappointed man, who did not understand the world around him, any more. I remember when he retired and took off his uniform for the last time – it was like an actor taking off his make up. Everything changed: his accent, his clothes, his hobbies. He slipped comfortably into becoming an old, orthodox Parsi.[91]

Dhunjibhoy's ambition to stay clear of political involvement and avoid jeopardising his family's wellbeing may have been particularly pressing for him also because he had married 'upwards', coming from a lower family background than his wife. Also, he had second-hand experience through his in-laws of the ways in which political contingencies could detrimentally impact family life and threaten one's professional survival. His wife had grown up in Berlin, where her father, A. M. Vacha, had been engaged from 1893 to 1934 as a researcher and teacher of Persian, Gujarati and Hindi at the oriental seminar at the university.[92] He had been threatened with dismissal in 1916 when he refused 'to teach German soldiers', because as a British Indian citizen who had crossed enemy lines, he feared future repercussions back in Bombay. Given that the Dhunjibhoys travelled to Europe on a regular basis, the Vachas' problems in Germany during the First World War would have constituted a cogent reminder to them of the fickle fortunes of life during politically unstable periods.

Dhunjibhoy's marriage to Shirin Vacha points us to another important aspect. Just as he identified as Parsi first and Indian second, Dhunjibhoy was not an anglicised Indian but a cosmopolitan Parsi, familiar with the life and customs of people in Britain as well as in other European and North American countries. His wife was also a Parsi but had been 'born and brought up in Germany', in the vibrant atmosphere of pre–World War I Berlin.[93] Her four brothers and sisters 'were brought up completely European and the only son in the family never saw India', except once, for a few weeks, when he was sent as a child to Bombay – significantly, to confirm his 'Parsiness' and 'have his Navjote ceremony'.[94] As Shirin Vacha's upbringing was European, she 'did not really regard herself as Indian.' This would undoubtedly have shaped Dhunjibhoy's own cultural identification. When Dhunjibhoy had to leave Ranchi (a social backwater, where, according to Berkeley-Hill, the hospital was located at a 'dismal spot' surrounded by 'wilderness'),[95] to be posted to the vibrant metropolis of Karachi during the Second World War, his wife was 'glad to get back to "civilisation"'.[96] In this context, civilisation was neither British nor Indian, but the kind of imaginary cosmopolitan place inhabited by an elite versed in the social ways and customs exhibited by the privileged of all ethnic and religious stripes in many of the large cities around the world.

Indianisation and Histories of Medicine

Dhunjibhoy's professional career and personal life choices reflect the new opportunities opened up by the colonial government during this period in response to nationalist demands for Indian self-government. Dhunjibhoy's experiences during his posting in a region characterised by economically based communal tension as well as strong anti-British sentiments, points to the importance of local factors in which senior officers were embroiled. The persistence of European racial prejudice, resistance on the part of senior European medical staff and British professional associations in abdicating their privileged position in the medical marketplace, and competition among Indian Western-trained practitioners in different locations all go to show that Indianisation was an officially decreed policy aimed at the abolition of British predominance and professional monopoly, which did away necessarily neither with ingrained colonial attitudes among colonial servants nor continued attempts at the 'institutionalization of medical dependency'.[97] It also exacerbated competition among Indian doctors for key positions in the customarily supreme IMS, continuing the marginalisation of other medical service providers and their staff. Despite formal equity, there was continued discrimination. How the latter manifested itself and stamped the experience of senior Indian staff depended on their varied medical qualifications, their specific service affiliation and local parameters. All of these factors require attention, not least in order to avoid a medical history that focuses on official policies and homogenising proclamations rather than the continuities (as well as changes) and the multifaceted experiences and contradictory trends concomitant with the 'constitution of a new imperial order' in varied localities during the period of Indianisation.

The wider administrative framework within which Dhunjibhoy pursued his career was characterised by the provincialisation of the medical services from 1919 and the move towards provincial self-government from 1935 onwards. European doctors resented these measures as they entailed loss of centralised power and the eventual Indianisation of command structures. They also exacerbated existing differences between the various regions in South Asia. The common nonchalance with which medical developments in particular states, such as Bengal and Bombay for example, have been taken by historians of medicine as representative of other areas in India, is even less appropriate for the twentieth than for the nineteenth century.

Subalterns

The extent to which colonial divisions continued to prevail is exemplified by the fact that European or Eurasian senior staff were employed at the European Mental Hospital, while an institution dedicated to the treatment of Indians only, like Dhunjibhoy's mental hospital, could be headed by either Indians or Europeans. In 1935, for example, J. N. J. Pacheco was sent to officiate during Dhunjibhoy's absence. The first- or perhaps even the second-assistant superintendent could have acted as locum. After all, the assistants were familiar with the management of the institution and the peculiarities and needs of patients. Officiating for the superintendent would also have raised their career profile (as well as their pay during their locum period). In fact, the first-assistant surgeon had filled in for Dhunjibhoy on an earlier occasion, in 1933. Instead of being put in charge again, he was sent on a training course for two years. It is not clear whether the arrangements made in 1935 were due to a potential need to provide a posting for Pacheco, as it became increasingly difficult to find vacancies even for senior positions once Indianisation had gained momentum.

Apart from Pacheco, only Indian staff assumed senior medical positions at the Indian Mental Hospital. Throughout the period there was one first- and one second-assistant superintendent. There were also a matron, nurses, subassistant surgeons and compounders.[98] The salary and status differential between assistant surgeons, who were appointable as assistant superintendents, and subassistant surgeons, who were trained at medical colleges in India rather than in Europe, was considerable.[99] In 1925, the monthly wages for the former ranged between Rs.300 and Rs.400, and for the latter between Rs.120 and Rs.150. As Hochmuth has shown in regard to subassistants' career trajectories during the nineteenth century, their title signified subordination to, and lower status than, assistant surgeons trained in Europe or nonvernacular medical schools in India. These discrepancies were a consequence of enduring colonial discrimination. The situation was more complex in regard to the pay differential between trained nurses and subassistant surgeons. Nurses earned between Rs.6 and Rs.16 more than the senior and junior subassistant surgeons. The matron was commended by Dhunjibhoy in 1925, for 'the perfect working of the female section', which was seen by him to be due to her 'masterly handling'.[100] She was paid over double a subassistant surgeon's rate.

At the bottom of the pay scale for the auxiliary medical and care staff were the four compounders (on Rs.35–45 per month) and the 302 male and female attendants (Rs.18–24 per month). In comparison, the cooks earned Rs.20, the typist Rs.40 and the 'sweepers' or waste-disposal staff Rs.14 per month. Attendants had an important role in the day-to-day care of patients, yet their pay scales were diversified, with the majority of them working at significantly reduced rates during the later period.[101] In fact, they not only belonged to the group of employees where payroll savings were made but they also seem to have been a continued concern for Dhunjibhoy during the early years of the hospital. In his first report of 1925 he complained:

> The attendants staff was mostly required from the Indian Christians of the Ranchi district. With few exceptions [the] majority of them were found to be illiterate and unsuited for the work of this hospital. Every effort was made to impress upon them the responsibility and the nature of their duties but our efforts met with little success.[102]

The newly recruited staff had clearly not undergone any training and their duties would of course have been strange to them. However, attendants transferred from the old institutions and hence familiar with work in a mental hospital, were apparently no longer acceptable. Dhunjibhoy considered them 'not satisfactory' and wished to 'replace many of them by male nurses'. The following year an 'informal conference' met and recommended that the appointment of 24 male and 4 female nurses ought to be 'sanctioned as early as possible'.[103] He pointed out that there was 'at present no skilled nursing arrangement in the male section' and that 'the nursing is inadequate in the female section'.[104] Nursing had to be 'entrusted to the attendant staff' with a 'disappointing' result as they were 'unsuited for responsible and delicate nursing work'.[105] Despite an admission that a 'slight improvement was noted in their work as compared with 1925', Dhunjibhoy continued his disparaging comments, stating that 'much cannot be expected from this class as the majority of them are lazy, ignorant, illiterate and with little native intelligence'. Apparently 48 attendants were discharged 'as incompetent to carry out hospital work' and fines amounting to the exorbitant sum of Rs.210 were inflicted 'for slackness of work'.[106] Like many superintendents before him, Dhunjibhoy had little good to say about attendants.

The lack of qualified nursing staff continued to irk the superintendent. It interfered with his ambition to provide efficient and 'modern' care in the hospital. There is a clear tension in his report of 1927, for example, between his assertion that the 'treatment received by the patients in this hospital is up to the level of the latest modern methods employed in all the modern mental hospitals' on the one hand and the concern that there was 'still a complete lack of nursing in the Male Section and inadequate in the Female Section' on the other.[107] When only two more nurses were sanctioned in 1928, bringing the total up to four, with no more being likely in the foreseeable future, it was decided that training the attendants was the only way forward. The second-assistant superintendent and the matron began to run 'classes in mental nursing, first-aid and hygiene'.[108] By the early 1930s the 'standard of work of the attendant staff' was reported to have steadily improved every year. However, Dhunjibhoy attributed this not to ongoing training, but to 'steady efforts at weeding out the incompetents'.[109]

At the same time it had become clear how difficult it was to attract 'suitable nurses of any nationality' to Ranchi for the two available positions, despite 'advertising in almost all the leading newspapers of India' during 1930 and 1931.[110] The standards for nursing care had risen but there was a shortage of appropriately qualified nurses. Given these problems, training for 'new recruits of the attendant staff' became a standard feature at Ranchi, leading to allegedly 'ignorant', 'lazy' and 'illiterate' Indian Christians drawn from the local community to benefit from hands-on vocational education. There also emerged a new focus on the continued on-the-job training of medical staff and the four nurses. From 1931 onwards, they were 'allowed to attend by turn a full course of training with clinical demonstrations in psychological medicine'.[111] This was part of the course that was run twice a year for the students of the Patna Medical College during their practical placement at Ranchi. The courses were meant to 'permit the staff to acquire a knowledge of the elementary principles in psychological medicine', which was expected to help them 'considerably in their work'.[112]

From the late 1930s the skills and attitude of subordinate staff no longer appear to have been a matter for concern. When the prominent Edward Mapother of the Maudsley Mental Hospital visited Ranchi on New Year's Day in 1938, he commended the institution and its staff. Given that Mapother was known for his uncompromising ideas on research-led psychiatric management and medical care, his evaluation constitutes evidence for Ranchi's high standard.

> I visited the Indian Mental Hospital at Ranchi on January 1st 1938, and was most favourably impressed by all I saw. It is evident that under the direction of Lt.-Col. J. E. Dhunjibhoy the greatest care and skill is exercised in the diagnosis and treatment of new cases upon arrival there, so that all such patients may be given the best possible chance of recovery.

With regard to more long standing cases, the arrangements for occupational treatment and recreation such as will render their lives as happy as possible are strikingly good. The physical condition of the great majority of the patients seemed excellent: they appeared as content with their lot as could possibly be expected and appreciative of the kindness and sympathy which inspired the Staff of the hospital and particularly the medical staff. The whole state of the hospital seemed, so far as I could judge, to reflect the greatest credit upon the Administration of Colonel Dhunjibhoy.[113]

The following year, Dhunjibhoy reiterated Mapother's positive assessment of the staff, noting that 'the work and general conduct of the staff as a whole were of the usual high standard'.[114] The record of success, which had been achieved by means of fines, training and 'weeding out of the incompetents', persisted also in 1940. Dhunjibhoy's former first-assistant superintendent, Dr P. C. Das, replaced him, and although many changes in medical personnel occurred, 'the general conduct of the staff was satisfactory and discipline was well maintained, as in previous years'.[115] Das noted that 'only in a few cases' was 'severe disciplinary action' called for.[116] Both carrot and stick continued to be important in quality assurance at Ranchi.

In addition to early concerns about the standard of nursing care at Ranchi, other staffing deficiencies were reported in the early years. While the number of attendants increased by 106 within one year of the hospital's opening, the shortage of medical staff was not rectified.[117] This meant that five surgeons had to deal with a total of 1,564 patients during 1926, for example. As Dhunjibhoy pointed out, 'each Sub-Assistant Surgeon in the male section has nearly 400 patients under his charge and each Assistant Surgeon has 700 patients'.[118] Permission to recruit one more subassistant surgeon was therefore asked for, but the request was not sanctioned until 1929. This put considerable stress on the senior medical officers and their subordinates, and, presumably, had a negative impact on patients. However, staff-to-patient ratios are difficult to ascertain, not least because staffing levels varied according to the demands of the different wards, with the suicide and infirmary wards being the most labour intensive. Furthermore, there were two different types of staff who looked after patients: 'jemadars' and 'keepers' or 'attendants'. The former were paid more and were responsible for a considerably higher number of patients than the latter.[119] It is however, difficult to ascertain what exactly the duties of these two groups were. The patient-to-staff ratio, calculated on the average number of patients per day, stabilised from 1929 onwards at around 58 and 38 for jemadars on the male and female wards respectively, and at three patients per attendant.

Hierarchy and enforcement of discipline by means of punishment and positive encouragement are arguably part of the fabric of any medical institution. Except in cases when subordinate members of staff were considered 'incompetent' and had to pay fines or were severely disciplined for misconduct or dereliction of duty, employees seem to have benefited from reasonably good working conditions at the hospital. Subordinate staff employed at Ranchi benefited from accommodation made available for them in married and single quarters. They also had access to treatment at the outpatient clinic, and vaccination and antimalarial measures.[120] The latter had become necessary when vegetable and paddy cultivation was increased during the early 1930s, temporarily leading to a significant increase in sickness.[121] A range of sports and leisure activities, as well as a co-operative-style loan scheme, devised in 1935 to deal 'a severe blow to the local money-lenders' and help 'some of the Attendant Staff and majority of the menial staff' who had been 'heavily involved in debts and were entirely in the clutches of some heartless Marwari and Pathan money lenders', would have constituted additional attractions.[122] There were also opportunities, albeit limited in the case of subordinates, for further medical and vocational education, as when staff were sent to Calcutta for training in the Bratachari Movement or in the operation of technical equipment.[123] Medical and nursing staff were 'by turn' allowed to attend the training course that was run at Ranchi for medical students from Patna University. Attendance by in-house staff of these university-level events was reported to impart on them 'a knowledge of the elementary principles in psychological medicine which helps them considerably in their work'.[124]

The fact that students from outside the hospital came and went throughout the year may have encouraged a vibrant work atmosphere at Ranchi. From 1927, an 'intensive training in mental diseases as required by the curriculum of the Patna University for the degree of M.B.B.S.' was run in April for two batches of final-year medical students of the Prince of Wales Medical College, for a fortnight each.[125] In 1931, a group of '13 passed students of the Darbhanga and Cuttack Medical Schools were also sent for intensive training in Mental Diseases'.[126] From 1934, postgraduate students of experimental psychology from the Universities of Calcutta and Dacca visited the hospital and were given short lectures on the subject of abnormal psychology, with 'demonstration on interesting cases'.[127] In contrast to medical students at Patna, those at the University of Calcutta had their training at the Bhowanipur Mental Observation Ward, to which Ranchi sent in 1935, for example, a 'batch of about 12 patients with the classical signs and symptoms of various Psychoses for demonstration purposes'.[128] In 1936, Ranchi gained recognition for its practical training, as part of the postgraduate diplomas in psychological medicine awarded by the Universities of London and Edinburgh.[129]

It seems that by the early 1930s, things had settled down for staff at Ranchi, with training for subordinate recruits and opportunities for continued learning and career development in the case of medical and nursing staff. Treatment, teaching and learning (as well as research, as will become evident later) were well integrated. Moreover, the standards of diagnostics, therapeutics, patient care and institutional management lived up to the reputedly high demands of the ever-critical Edward Mapother.[130] In regard to hospital management at the Ranchi Indian Mental Hospital, Indianisation was certainly a full success.

Chapter 2

THE PATIENTS: THE DEMOGRAPHICS OF GENDER AND AGE, LOCALITY, OCCUPATION, CASTE AND RELIGION

Knowledge linked to power, not only assumes the authority of 'the truth' but has power to make itself true.
—Michel Foucault, 1975

One of the most pertinent questions in relation to any mental hospital is: who were the people who ended up in it? Who were they prior to becoming 'patients' with a particular diagnosis attached to them? Were they 'village idiots' and 'half wits', as is often assumed; 'the morally disreputable, the poor, and the impotent, […] vagrants, minor criminals, and the physically handicapped', as the sociologist Andrew Scull suggested in 1979 for the period prior to the mid-nineteenth century in England?[1] Or were they dangerous psychopaths, religious fanatics and 'mad axmen', as many fear when they hastily walk past a mental institution? Were the inmates merely somewhat strange 'eccentrics' who had developed the Indian version of the British colonials' 'doolally tap' syndrome where they went '*pagal*' ('mad')? Were they just a mixed bag of inconvenient family members and depressed women, political rebels, uncooperative Indian princes or intractable tribals who were locked away?

Evidence for each of these characterisations can be found in hospital records and medical, official and patient accounts all over the world. Sociohistorical analyses that set themselves apart from previously preferred 'Whig' narratives that celebrated the progress of biomedicine in Western science-based psychiatry have tended to focus on mental institutions as means of social, political and gender control, where formerly autonomous people were forced into the role of the 'passive patient'. In relation to Europe and North America, the suggestion that those who ended up in mental hospitals consisted of the 'rabble' and of political and social outcasts has been a pervasive trope among historians, especially in the wake of the antipsychiatry movement of the 1960s. Although the assumption of social and political control as the predominant purpose of psychiatric confinement has been challenged in more recent historical accounts, its tenor has resonated particularly strongly among historians working on colonial South Asia.[2]

For example, in his study of the 'native only' lunatic asylums of British India during the late nineteenth century, James Mills looked at the 'disciplinary functions of the asylums'. In accordance with the precepts of postcolonial theory and Foucauldian thinking, he argued that asylum medicine 'functioned to drill and produce bodies that could prove useful in a colonial system'.[3] He focused on how inmates 'may have lost their freedom as they were incarcerated in a colonial institution but [...] were determined to resist the imposition of an alien order on their bodies'.[4] In their work on the incarceration of members of the various Indian royal courts of formally independent princely states, Shruti Kapila and Fiona Groenhout also highlight the element of political control. Groenhout showed how the 'medicalisation of princely misconduct provided one of the few means by which control could be asserted' over Indian royalty, and that 'the notion of princely insanity was of political value to the British' as it 'depoliticised' the behaviour and actions of Indian contenders to power.[5] Kapila argued, in relation to Indian rulers who did not conform to British political schemes and social expectations, that the 'sciences of the mind – especially colonial psychiatry – were deployed to resolve contestation'.[6]

There is also evidence that, alongside the repressive Criminal Tribes Acts of 1871, 1876, 1911 and 1924, admission to a psychiatric institution was used to dispose of troublesome tribal leaders in locations earmarked for 'pacification' and 'development' by the British.[7] Religious sages, too, sometimes ended up in mental hospitals, as in the case of Hazrat Tajuddin Baba, a Muslim Sufi *qutub* (master) who was much revered even during his confinement at Nagpur Mental Hospital from 1892 to 1908, when people visited to receive his blessings.[8] Furthermore, Showalter's gendered version of the 'social control' thesis, which suggests that women in northwestern Europe and North America were between two and seven times more likely than men to be diagnosed as mentally unstable, has been applied by many historians to characterise the inmates in a variety of institutional settings, including in India.[9]

Whether these kinds of characterisation apply across each and every institution is doubtful. They may reverberate with a wider public, as they complement common suspicions about medical experts who spuriously label people as mentally ill. Certification implies the enactment of medical and legal authority over the patient. As Ivan Illich put it provocatively in his *Medical Nemesis* in 1976: 'Professional power is the result of a political delegation of autonomous authority to the health occupations.'[10] While psychiatrists may prefer to believe that their power is exclusively based on medical expertise and professional authority, there is clearly a potential for, and evidence of, abuse. The medical personnel who worked in the Gulag and in Nazi extermination camps justified the atrocities they committed by reference to medical and purely scientific rationales. This provides a stark reminder that while mental hospitals are claimed to be caring medical sanctuaries or 'asylums' for people 'like you and me' who suffer from mental breakdown, they may also be used for other, sinister purposes and may be inhabited by the ostracised, inconvenient, vulnerable, oppressed, rebellious and quirky.

The tension between, on the one hand, appreciation of mental institutions as places dedicated to those who need care and cure and, on the other, fear and suspicion that particular groups and communities are being cruelly and unjustly disposed of, has been evident ever since the rise of the asylum as the officially preferred option for the confinement of the 'mad' – whoever they may be. Concerns were reflected as early as the eighteenth and early nineteenth centuries in Britain in extended debates on 'unlawful confinement'.[11] Legal provision was made to safeguard against it in Britain and British India, but speculation and unease continued to prevail among the wider public about the identity of those confined in closed institutions – no doubt fuelled by the widely reported cases of abuse that continued to emerge.

In the face of these various concerns, the question of the identity of those who ended up in the Ranchi Hospital is clearly relevant. However, it is also difficult to answer as the available evidence comes mainly from sources produced by medical and administrative staff connected with the very institution under scrutiny. To avoid stereotyping and sweeping generalisation, individual testimonies from those not connected with the hospital, as well as institutional statistics and official reports, need to be examined. The scope of individual cases is clearly limited by concerns about the potential for bias. The researchers' interests and conceptual categories are also bound to have a bearing on the analysis. Furthermore, institutional statistics on patients' backgrounds and identity are of course sensitive to changes in admission criteria and institutional procedures. There are also issues about the consistency with which different members of staff employed particular categories over time. Ideally, assessment of a wide range of evidence would ameliorate such shortcomings. If an analysis of the hospital population is, as here, based mainly on institutional records, particular care is vital in the interpretation of the data, and sustained critical reflection on the limitations of any claim is imperative.

The problem of how to make sense of the immense volume of information produced by hospital staff on inmates, and how to extract details on who they were, will be a central feature of this chapter. A good part of the data is based on reasonably 'hard' demographic details (such as age, sex, and number of public and private patients), while some of the statistical material is more problematic in terms of the validity of the categories that were employed (such as 'caste', 'occupation' and 'religion'). The viability of interpretative extrapolations from both kinds of material will frequently need to be assessed carefully – in particular when we are aiming to identify patients' social class background. It is also necessary to discuss the data in relation to themes and topics that have emerged in recent historiography. Hence issues of gender, social and political control will receive particular attention.

Gender Confined

When the Ranchi Mental Hospital was opened in 1925, the first batch of patients arrived from Patna 'in time for their lunch' on 4 September.[12] By 18 January the next year, a total of 1,342 patients had been transferred from the three dilapidated institutions in Dacca, Berhampore and Patna. By the end of 1926, Ranchi provided for 1,389 patients. It was the largest psychiatric institution in South Asia and was to provide for the mentally ill of three populous regions under British control (Bengal, Bihar and Orissa[13]). As in other similar institutions, the overall number of patients confined was constrained by the number of beds available. At Ranchi capacity was already overstretched when all inmates had been relocated from the three institutions it replaced. Only 1,014 beds were available for men, while the maximum number treated on any one night in 1926 was 1,391. This led to considerable overcrowding, which was to remain an ongoing problem resulting in severe restrictions being imposed on admissions.[14]

It is striking that far fewer women than men were confined at Ranchi. The bed ratio was 1,014 for males to 272 for females; women were clearly expected to constitute only about one-fifth of the total. Similar ratios prevailed at other mental institutions in India. What is more, unlike in the case of men, the number of women admitted was not restricted by scarcity of beds, as vacancies were available for most of the period in the female quarters, which were located within their own grounds across the road from the men's. It was not until 1938 that the need for extra accommodation arose on the female side, too. Although there is much evidence of enduring gender inequality among many communities in South Asia, repression of women in India appears not to have been enforced on any great scale by means of psychiatric institutionalisation.[15]

The average percentage of women in the hospital from 1929 to 1939 was 18 per cent, less than the target of 20 per cent. It seems that colonial policies did not result in disproportionate incarceration of women. During the whole period admission was restricted to those who had attracted police and magistrates' attention for dangerous and disruptive acts. Apparently Indian women's behaviour in public places was not judged to constitute a danger to the public quite as much as Indian men's. Frequently, colonial officials and critics attributed this to Indian women's lesser visibility, cultural factors such as the practice among some communities of excluding their women from the public eye, and social restrictions on single as well as married women's free movement in public places. The significantly lower rate of institutionalisation for women does not therefore indicate a low incidence of mental illness among Indian women per se. It is much more likely to be due to prevalent public-order priorities and socio-cultural practices. Colonial administrators aimed to keep down the cost of psychiatric institutions and so avoided filling them up with socially harmless mental patients – male or female. Nevertheless, the feminist suggestion that women's behaviour at home and within their communities was more likely than men's to be labelled as aberrant, may still be valid. This aspect and the question of how women were dealt with in a culturally and socially congruent way within their families requires further assessment beyond the scope of the current chapter.

'Chronic patients' and long-term confinement

For England and Wales, the overcrowding of mental hospitals with 'chronic' cases, from the 1870s onwards, has been identified as the real beginning of the 'great confinement of the mad'.[16] Those who consider mental illness as a social construct and 'chronicity' as no more than a stigmatising label and a sinister attempt by the medical profession to keep people unjustly locked away tend to see long-term confinement as a major feature of the 'warehousing' of hopeless and incurable cases in 'mammoth asylums' or 'museums for the collection of insanity', where the 'maintenance of order' rather than attempts at curing was the main driver and 'many patients were simply left to rot'.[17] The assessment of patients' length of hospitalisation is therefore an important issue for a variety of reasons. Were women, for example, institutionalised for longer periods?

Unfortunately, no composite or sex-specific data on patients' duration of stay at Ranchi are available in the hospital reports. The only available quantitative data relate to those inmates who died or were discharged (as cured, improved or not improved). Most of the women (96 per cent) who were discharged in 1930 for example, had not spent more than three years in the hospital. In contrast, only 65 per cent of the men discharged during that year had been confined for less than three years. In other words, 35 per cent of men discharged, compared to only four per cent of women discharged, had spent more than three years at Ranchi. This could be interpreted as indicative of highly favourable conditions for women. Admittedly, data pertaining to the group of people discharged do not, of course, allow us to assume that those who stayed behind shared their characteristics. It is therefore not possible to conclude that overall women were not subject to prolonged confinement. The higher rate of discharge following longer-term confinement for men could have been due to women having been less likely to be released once they had been confined for more than three years. Alternatively, it might have been the case that they were less likely to be confined for as long as men. We simply cannot tell on the basis of these data.

Similar problems prevail in relation to the statistics on the duration of confinement of those who eventually died in the hospital. In addition, the low numbers in mortality rates allow us only to speculate with much caution about trends among the deceased. With these caveats in mind, some intriguing features can still be discerned among the 332 patients who died from 1930 to 1940. First, the ratio of male to female deaths is almost exactly congruent with the overall male to female population ratio, roughly 80 per cent to 20 per cent. This implies that there was no sex-specific trend in men's and women's likelihood to die during their stay at Ranchi.

Second, about 10 per cent of newly admitted patients died within one year. About one-third of those who died had been at Ranchi for more than twenty years. If we disaggregate the Ranchi rates, it emerges that 10 per cent of men and 14 per cent of women died within the first year, while an equal proportion of men and women who died had been confined for over twenty years. The only sex-specific feature of note in these mortality statistics was a higher proportion of women being confined for between one and five years (26 per cent of females in contrast to only 14 per cent of males). Men were more likely to have been institutionalised for between ten and twenty years (27 per cent of males versus 19 per cent of females).

What can we conclude from the limited statistical data on the length of institutionalisation at Ranchi in relation to any gender-specific trends? It seems that of those discharged, the majority of women were released earlier than men. Further, women were no more likely than men to die in the hospital, nor had women who died at Ranchi been hospitalised for longer than their fellow male inmates. Thus women do not appear to have been discriminated against.

To put the statistical data into context, we need to introduce further evidence. Lacking statements by patients, their families or the wider community, we are left to rely on medical officers' analyses. Despite professional differences and personal animosities between different doctors, they all shared the same sentiment on 'chronic patients' (those confined for long periods). These were not considered the most desirable of patients, even when they drew doctors' sympathy. Doctors considered a high rate of 'long timers' or chronic patients among hospital inmates generally as having a detrimental impact on work and living conditions for both staff and inmates, leading to be related to low cure rates, bleak outlooks, low staff morale and deteriorating service provision. This led to a negative public image of the institution and disinclination on the part of families to have relatives admitted to it. As today, psychiatrists during the early twentieth century were keen to employ their medical expertise to attempt to cure patients. However, effective treatments for mental illness – then as now – were hard to come by. As J. N. J. Pacheco put it:

> The chronicity of some mental disorders is inevitable in spite of the many forward strides of modern mental science, and it is not surprising therefore that a fair majority of patients in most mental institutions are in a state of advanced dementia.[18]

In 1935, for example, a 'large majority' of patients at Ranchi were 'in an advanced state of chronic mental disorder' and hence had been 'resident over a number of years' without having 'progressed in spite of all attention bestowed from every aspect of therapy, physical, psychological and sociological'.[19]

Medical officers invariably noted with apprehension that patients were kept in their homes by friends or relatives 'as long as possible till management of him (or her) at home becomes intolerable or impossible'.[20] If there was no hope for recovery, the main regime that medical staff could pursue was 'custodial and occupational'.[21] This kind of institutional treatment was not the approach favoured by doctors as it reduced them to mere custodians of 'hopeless cases' and overseers of inmates' occupational and recreational management. During an age when research, expertise and specialist skills became evermore highly valued, engagement in management rather than medicine was not attractive. It was clearly not in the interest of medical superintendents to unduly retain patients for long periods of time. Just like medical professionals today, practitioners were outcome orientated and interested in cure efficiency whenever feasible. It is therefore not surprising that attempts were routinely made to get rid of as many chronic inmates as possible. For example, in 1932, Dhunjibhoy, reported:

> Special efforts were made to discharge 43 chronic and harmless patients to the care of their relatives who could be traced out by the Magistrates of their districts. As a result, 18 patients were discharged and in 14 cases no friends or relatives could be found in spite of vigorous enquiries instituted by the Magistrates concerned. In 11 cases inability for financial reasons to take charge of the patients was accepted by the enquiring Magistrates and they were, therefore, not discharged.[22]

Despite such efforts, the number of chronic patients confined for long periods remained high right up to the beginning of the Second World War. Pacheco reported this in 1935, and Dhunjibhoy noted in 1939 that the 'so-called "new admissions" in spite of our giving them all the known modern scientific treatment of mental disorders' were 'chronic cases beyond any hopes of recovery'.[23] This had been so ever since the hospital was established in 1925. Dr P. C. Das had reported that on the opening of Ranchi, the 'majority' of patients were 'chronic cases and merely transfers who had been for years already in residence in other Mental Hospitals'.[24] Consequently, a 'large number of infirm, incurable and homeless cases' had accumulated.[25] Das referred to several patients who 'have been continuing as inmates for more than 30 years' and mentioned one who had died at Ranchi at the age of 80. He had been in mental hospitals, Das pointed out, for 46 years.[26]

Long-term patients were also a thorn in the side of government officials because of the cost of maintaining them in an institution. Administrative restrictions were therefore imposed to reduce the tendency for chronic patients to accumulate over the years. However, this was only partially effective as only the 'harmless' and 'not dangerous' could be excluded from admission from 1928 onwards. As the secretary to the government of Bihar and Orissa put it:

> A serious attempt has been made, not without success, to discharge to the care of friends and relatives the class of incurable but harmless patients who formed such a large proportion of the inmates when the institution was opened.[27]

He noted that 'Magistrates have also been given definite instructions to avoid sending this type of patient for admission'.[28] Institutional care remained restricted to those who constituted a threat to the wider community. It is unlikely that patients – including the women among them – would have been locked away unduly.

'Private' and 'public' patients

Private patients made up a relatively small percentage of the overall hospital population, fluctuating between 11 per cent and 22 per cent from 1929 to 1939. Their number would certainly have been higher had the provincial governments been willing to finance a separate building for them as Dhunjibhoy had requested at Ranchi's inauguration in 1925. Every year thereafter he noted with regret that 'several applications' for admission had to be refused to those willing to pay for the upkeep of their relatives.[29] Demand clearly outstripped supply.

In the case of public patients, eligibility for admission was regulated by government and hence reflected to a large extent the state's priorities towards the Indian mentally ill. Admission patterns in private patients, in contrast, partially indicate communities' preferences and concerns. In regard to the latter, the question then emerges whether women were over-represented among the private hospital population and may have been victims of their relatives' inclination to keep them out of sight for long periods. Among private patients, too, women were in a minority, making up only one-quarter of them. It is intriguing that in comparison to public patients the female ratio was slightly higher (25 per cent for private in contrast to 18 per cent for female patients overall). We do not know if the admission restrictions imposed on public patients were applied also in regard to those presented for certification by their relatives. Given that there were never enough vacancies for private patients, it may have been the case that the superintendent primarily confined those who were difficult to restrain and care for within family settings.

On the other hand, Dhunjibhoy frequently mentioned that families presented their relatives for institutional treatment far too late, only once all other options had proven unsuccessful. By then the mental condition, he pointed out, had often become chronic, reducing the chance of cure. It is possible that the superintendent may have elected to admit those for treatment whose mental affliction was still in the early stages and who were therefore more likely to benefit from psychiatric treatment. As we do not know the criteria on which Dhunjibhoy based his admission decisions, it is difficult to explain why women constituted a slightly higher percentage of private patients than of those referred by magistrates. However, the overall numbers involved were much less for the former, so that even percentage ratios need to be interpreted with appropriate caution. On average, 222 women were confined at Ranchi as public patients, whilst on the private wards the average was only 16.[30] Despite the low numbers, some intriguing trends deserve to be scrutinised. For example, the average rate of discharge was 7 per cent for males and 10 per cent for females, while it amounted to 29 per cent and 44 per cent for private male and female patients respectively. Clearly, both men and women in private wards were far more likely to be discharged (as cured, improved or not improved) by a factor of roughly four. Yet, about two out of three discharged public or private inmates were women. If we consider early discharge from a mental hospital as desirable, then the pattern at Ranchi was clearly in favour of women, regardless of whether they were private or public patients. However, other issues would need to be considered, too, such as the severity of patients' conditions on admission and the quality of care and conditions that discharged patients could expect inside and outside the institution.

From the present-day perspective, which currently tends to favour treatment within the community, discharge rates of 7 to 10 per cent, and perhaps even of 29 to 44 per cent, sound very low. There are no details available on the condition upon discharge of private patients (that is, if 'cured', 'improved' or 'not improved'). It also remains an open question whether patients' relatives insisted on their beloved ones' early release even if their condition had not improved, whether more therapeutic attention was paid to private patients (especially the women among them), inducing higher cure and improvement rates or if private patients (particularly women) suffered from less severe and/or chronic conditions on admission than those on public wards.

Whatever the reasons for the variation in discharge rates with gender and private/public status, there was one great equaliser: death. As highlighted earlier, mortality rates were almost identical for patients overall, private inmates, men and women. They amounted to an average of two per cent. This is a strikingly low percentage for any institution in India at the time and in particular for one like Ranchi – a large public facility for inmates who had been ill for prolonged periods, had often been admitted with poor general health and displayed symptoms of violence. The consistently low mortality rate at Ranchi will require further analysis. To return to the original questions: Who were the people who ended up at Ranchi? Were they from the higher or lower sections of Indian society? Did they belong to particular religions or social, cultural and occupational communities? Where had they lived before, how old were they and had they suffered from any particular afflictions?

'Criminal Lunatics'

A large number of people sent to Ranchi as public patients had committed some kind of crime, most commonly murder or grievous bodily harm. Unlike any other feature, the reception of this group determined the treatment that could be pursued by hospital staff. There was no specialist facility available in Bengal, Bihar and Orissa comparable to England's Broadmoor Hospital (previously Broadmoor Criminal Lunatic Asylum, established in 1863). Therefore, any person charged with a crime and considered mentally ill had to be put forward by magistrates and jail officials for admission to the region's general mental hospital. The Indian Lunatic Asylums Act of 1858, the Indian Lunacy Act of 1912 and subsequent amendments – in conjunction with the Code of Criminal Procedure of 1898, amended in 1923, and the Prisoners Act of 1900 – provided for the detention of violent and dangerous mentally ill persons.[31] These provisions were based largely on similar legislation in England and Wales.

As in England and Wales, in British India, too, a 'lunatic asylum' or mental hospital was seen to be the most appropriate place of confinement for mentally deranged people who had committed a crime. Jails were considered inappropriate, not least because prison discipline was not easily enforced on those who behaved in erratic and irrational ways, leading to situations where the imposition of order among other prisoners was compromised. This was unacceptable for an institution designed to discipline and punish. Reports from the nineteenth century onwards also refer to the better care that could be provided for this group, as 'criminal lunatics' were seen to require a distinct vigilance (no violence or punishment) from staff. By the early twentieth century, the need for medical treatment increasingly predominated. However, confinement at Ranchi was not resorted to for all criminal lunatics; on account of persistent accommodation problems, some continued to be detained in jails. The inspector-general of civil hospitals, Col. L. Cook, provided information on their overall numbers in the provinces' prisons for the period 1930 to 1932 (see Table 2.1).[32]

Table 2.1. Number of 'criminal lunatics' detained in jails in the provinces of Bengal, and Bihar and Orissa, 1930–1932

	1930	1931	1932
Bengal	53	53	65
Bihar and Orissa	10	20	29

Cook considered the measures in place adequate, noting that 'the administration has accomplished a difficult task with a minimum of expenditure and a commendable modicum of efficiency'. He was aware of the 'pitfalls in trying to collate these figures', as they did not include 'habitual "B" class prisoners' who suffered from 'a mental kink, viz., anti-social tendencies'. But even were they included, he surmised, 'the aggregate compared to the total population is not such an one as to call for any drastic change in the administrative methods or to bring down upon us', he added in a facetious aside, 'the condemnation of that critical body of Cosmopolitan Evangelists known as the League of

Nations'. Cook clearly was no friend of international agencies passing critical judgement on colonial health and penal policies in India.

It was however correct of Cook to point out that the number of those certified as 'criminal insanes' [sic] confined at Ranchi and the provincial jails was indeed very small in relation to overall population figures. The latter were at the time about fifty million in British Bengal and nearly forty million in British Bihar and Orissa. The total number of criminals certified with mental illness amounted on average to only 73 in jails and 467 at Ranchi. In England and Wales, in contrast, 757 patients were confined at Broadmoor Hospital in 1937, while 75 people classified as 'criminal lunatics' were sent to county or borough mental hospitals during that year, at a time when the population was less than half of the catchment area of Ranchi (about forty million in 1931).[33]

However minor the Ranchi numbers may have been in relation to the overall population, 'criminal lunatics' were still over-represented among patients confined at Ranchi, preventing the admission of other mentally ill people who might have benefited from the treatment or the care and provisions available to inmates at the psychiatric hospital. Their percentage fluctuated between a high 44 per cent in 1926 to a somewhat lower, but still significant, 37 per cent in 1940. In the old institutions the ratio had been even higher, with Dacca leading with about 55 per cent of its inmates, whilst Patna's and Berhampore's ratio was around 45 per cent (see Figure 2.1).

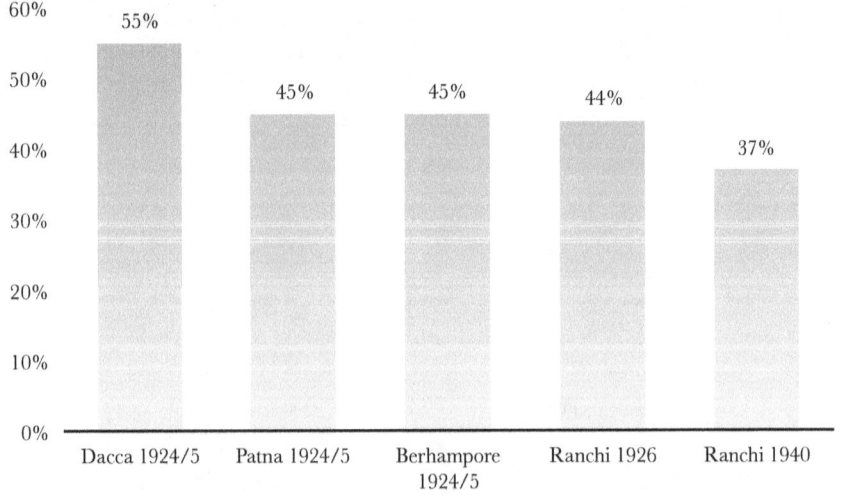

Figure 2.1. Percentage of 'criminal patients' in mental hospitals (1924–1925 for Dacca, Patna and Berhampore; 1926 and 1940 for Ranchi)

Although the 'criminal insanes' constituted the single largest group among hospital patients, their number declined somewhat over the period. This may be a local trend, partly related to the administrative autonomy granted to provincial governments during the 1930s that gave local officials some discretion in regard to admission policies and procedures. This in turn had a diversifying effect on municipality and district officials' enforcement of law and order. Provincial governments, on Dhunjiboy's instigation, had issued advice to local police and magistrates against the criminalisation of mentally ill people who had committed 'minor acts of nuisance' such as pilfering. A number of mentally disturbed people, who might previously have been admitted to Ranchi as 'criminals', were therefore received as ordinary patients.

Last but not least, for the period from 1927 to 1929, the superintendent pointed out that the 'gradual decrease in the number' of criminal patients was 'partly due to the fact that several old patients charged with petty offences were subsequently transferred to the non-criminal class with the sanction of the Government concerned'.[34] The apparent decline of the number of 'criminal lunatics' in the institution's statistics therefore reflects to a considerable extent wider changes in colonial policies, administrative procedures and institutional specifics. The fact that the makeup of the patient population was largely determined by administrative factors is evident also in relation to many other aspects of hospital management.[35]

Gender was also important. As in Western institutions, the majority of 'criminal lunatics' were men. As Busfield has pointed out, 'hospitals for the criminally insane tend to have more male than female inmates'.[36] At Ranchi, on average about 43 per cent of men confined in the hospital were classified as criminals.[37] Among women patients, the figure was much lower (17 per cent). The ratio of men to women (about 10 to 1) at Ranchi does not match statistics from other parts of the world. For example, in England and Wales, the ratio of men to women at Broadmoor was about three to one.[38] At Ionia State Hospital in the US, in contrast, the numbers were 576 men and 74 women in 1930 (namely 89 per cent and 11 per cent respectively, or roughly nine men to one woman). This figure is clearly more in line with Ranchi's; Ionia was however described as 'somewhat unusual'.[39] Patients were 'made up of representatives of 33 peoples (counting native born whites of many generations back, and negros) and natives of 31 states'. This was supposed to be 'due to the fact that this part of Michigan, being the center of the automobile industry, draws to itself roamers and wanderers from all over the United States'. In fact, unlike Ranchi, 'minor crimes' at Ionia and four other mental hospitals for the 'criminal insanes' in the US accounted for the second largest category (29 per cent), after 'crimes committed against person' (41 per cent) and well ahead of 'crimes of acquisition' (20 per cent).[40]

The kinds of 'criminals' admitted to some US institutions were therefore very different from those sent to Ranchi – though Dhunjibhoy continually bemoaned magistrates' practice of transferring people who had committed 'petty crimes' as 'criminals' rather than just 'patients', for institutional treatment. In contrast, Michigan's response to loafers and to behaviours such as 'disorderly fighting' engendered confinement in an institution for the 'criminal insanes'. It is clearly the case that changes and differences in the policy towards 'criminal lunacy', and in particular towards petty crimes and vagrancy, play a key role in determining the social character and thereby also the gender balance of patient populations.[41]

What kind of crimes had been committed by those who ended up at Ranchi? The majority of criminal patients (more than 50 per cent in 1930–32, for example), were murderers, 'some of whom', according to Dhunjibhoy, had 'more than one murder to their credit'.[42] He provided a table (see Table 2.2) that revealed the incidence and range of crimes committed from 1930 to 1932.

Table 2.2. 'The following table shows the analysis of offences committed by the criminal population in this hospital'[43]

Class	Murder	Culpable homicide	[Grievous] hurt	Rape	Mischief by fire	Attempt to commit suicide	Exposure and abandonment of child	Petty offences	Total
I	105	33	53	2	6	3	1	26	*229*
II	131	22	16	–	4	1	1	11	*186*
III	46	7	1	–	–	–	1	2	*57*
Total	*282*	*62*	*70*	*2*	*10*	*4*	*3*	*39*	*472*

The different 'classes' identified in Dhunjibhoy's table were based on those used in relation to prisoners more generally. Prisoners were not classified in relation to the severity or nature of the crime they had committed, or the extent to which their escape would be dangerous to the public or the security of the state. Instead it was their socio-economic status, education and previous 'habit of life' that was considered crucial. Thus, prisoners in class I and II were those who 'by special status, education and habit of life have been accustomed to a superior mode of living'.[44] The distinction between classes I and II related to whether or not a person had committed a previous offence: the former were designated as 'nonhabitual' and the latter as 'habitual prisoners'. In jails, these two classes would have been entitled to superior and more lenient treatment, and even to services provided by those unfortunates in class III, which was made up of the uneducated and those whose status in society and 'habit of life' were low.

These definitions were based on the Prison Act of 1894 and subsequent revisions.[45] Clearly, even before colonial and postcolonial law, equality did not exist within Indian society. At the time, the criteria employed were considered a happy marriage between modern principles of penology and the ancient Hindu Code of Manu. The Dharmashastras also ordained punishment in relation to learning and economic position of the offender (as well as motive and nature of offence, time and place, strength, age, conduct and reoffending).[46]

The different class categories were assigned to prisoners by legal officials and magistrates prior to confinement in the mental hospital. Dhunjibhoy engaged in vain in debates against the prevalent practices in relation to the 'criminal insanes', preferring medical criteria to take precedence. He also commented on the predominance of murderers among the patients, noting that this engendered 'a very grave responsibility' for the administration of the hospital and its 'limited staff' charged with housing and guarding these 'acute homicidal insanes'.[47]

Political prisoners

At least two major issues require further assessment in this context: first the question of whether Indian political agitators ended up as 'criminal lunatics' at Ranchi. The definition of what constitutes a danger to the public, the police or the security of the state is always socially and politically fraught, particularly within a colonial context and especially during a period of considerable anticolonial strife such as the 1920s and 1930s. As Walsh has argued in regard to Ireland (another British colonial setting), 'legislation governing lunacy was shaped within a highly politicised environment, in which issues of security, and the necessity to establish and maintain order were paramount'.[48] The second issue concerns the extent to which mentally ill people who had been involved in 'petty offences' were criminalised.

In order to substantiate the extent, if any, to which Ranchi was used to lock away political dissidents, the legal proceedings for particular patients would need to be assessed. Unfortunately, the available records lack relevant detail. However, there is some indication that, at least occasionally, people were confined at Ranchi who had attracted attention on account of some action that could well have been politically motivated rather than solely the result of mental delusion. For example, the report for the period 1933–35 referred to two patients whose crime was identified as 'disobeying orders of Government' and 'waging war against the King' respectively.[49] Without further details, it is of course difficult to ascertain if these 'criminal patients' were in fact suffering from mental illness as well as having been involved in the offences they were charged with. This is also the case in relation to another male patient who was admitted in 1939, under section 126 of the Indian Railways Act of 1890 (amended in 1930). Reference to this section of the act was also used to press criminal charges against independence fighters who damaged train tracks and caused 'untoward incidents'.[50]

Given the acute pressures on hospital accommodation, it seems unlikely that confinement at Ranchi was considered preferable to the more straightforward and less costly incarceration in a jail. However, this cannot be said with any certainty. What is more, sending political activists to a 'madhouse' rather than a prison might have been considered as a way to humiliate and discredit them. It may well have been the case that politically motivated actions and alleged crimes linked with these were subsumed, and therefore made invisible, under the remaining main categories. It needs to be remembered though that a separate category for 'political prisoners' allowed for the identification of those who had committed politically motivated crimes. How the various categories (criminal, civil, political, diseased and insane, juvenile, female, under trial) were employed, was from the mid-1930s onwards left to provincial authorities.

Petty crimes and the criminalisation of the mentally ill

While the main criminal categories received but rare comment, minor offences drew superintendents' continued attention throughout. A major concern was that local police officers presented mentally ill people who had committed minor offences to magistrates who would charge and send them on to Ranchi as 'criminal lunatics'. Looking back on the period 1927–29, Dhunjibhoy's locum, P. C. Das, noted: 'It is a matter of regret that the tendency on the part of the Committing Magistrates to send such patients as criminal patients instead of as non-criminal patients has not yet ceased.'[51]

Dhunjibhoy had previously brought the subject to the attention of the Government of Bengal during his tenure of office as superintendent at the old Berhampore Mental Hospital. He induced the authorities 'to issue a circular letter' in July 1924, 'requesting all District Magistrates, Judges and Presidency Magistrates of that Province to treat such so called "offences" as possible symptoms of lunacy'.[52] Two years later, in 1926, it was still the case that mentally ill people were sent to the mental hospital with a criminal charge for minor matters. Dhunjibhoy fully outlined his continued objection to this practice when he asked that a 'similar circular' to the one previously issued for Bengal should be distributed in Bihar and Orissa, and that 'the Government of Bengal be requested to once again draw the attention of the committing Magistrates' to the earlier guidelines.[53]

Outlining his concerns, Dhunjibhoy provided details of such petty offences:

> It may be out of place to mention here that in several cases persons committed petty offences *while insane* such as indecent exposure, committing nuisance, disorderly conduct, house trespass and lurking, petty theft, etc., etc., and these offences have been treated as criminal acts and dealt with under the provisions of Criminal Procedure Code. As a result of these patients being classed as 'Criminal Lunatics' they often suffer long detention in jails awaiting legal proceedings. This is detrimental to their mental condition. Moreover, the discharge of these patients from this hospital after their recovery is delayed for the compliance of certain legal formalities and a considerable extra expenditure is incurred by Government in sending them under police escorts to the courts concerned to stand their trial. During this period they have again to stay in the district and sub-jail as the case may be. They are ultimately released and never convicted on the strength of the evidence of insanity.[54]

Despite several superintendents' efforts, these suggestions, based on medical and pragmatic considerations, remained unheeded. Some fifteen years later, four out of nine people admitted as 'criminal patients' had been charged with 'housebreaking, theft and other petty offences'.[55] Clearly, medical and penal priorities clashed, and local certifying officials did not adjust their certification habits to those considered at Ranchi and in some Western countries as appropriate practice. However, we need to consider that not all Western institutions made an effort to avoid the criminalisation of the mentally ill. In five out of the eight hospitals for the 'criminal insanes' in the US, for example, those who had committed 'minor crimes' constituted a significant number of patients confined alongside murderers.[56]

Certification was a problem not only in regard to those labelled as 'criminal lunatics'. In 1930, for example, Dhunjibhoy noted that 'in 19 cases papers were found to be defective on admission'.[57] There were also cases 'in which the gravest irregularities were committed', which were 'brought to the notice of the local Government'. Dhunjibhoy pointed out that

> still little attention is paid by most of the Committing Magistrates in complying with the provision of the Indian Lunacy Act in making Reception Orders for the admission of

patients, as a result of which a great deal of inconvenience is caused, specially to this office, for entering into enormous correspondence.

Dhunjibhoy did not reveal details of these irregularities, but it appears that they related to lack of information on patients' circumstances and administrative coordination rather than wrongful confinement:

> The descriptive rolls of the patients are very carelessly filled up and they practically contain no useful information for which they are meant.
> In some cases no previous enquiry was made by the Committing Magistrates to ascertain whether accommodation was available or not in this hospital.[58]

Intellectual Disability and Patients' Ages

While those who had attracted police attention on account of criminal, violent and dangerous behaviour constituted the single largest group among hospital inmates, those classified as suffering from 'idiocy' or 'imbecility' – later subsumed under 'mental deficiency' – were a clear minority (between three and five per cent only). Nowadays these patients would be referred to by the term 'intellectual disability'. The selective admission criteria required 'danger to the public', 'violence' or 'criminality' as essential features. Those who presented as harmless and nonviolent were excluded, and the tractable among the intellectually disabled would therefore rarely have made it to Ranchi.[59] This could account for the low numbers of intellectually disabled people in the institution. However, while the docile among them are likely to have been under-represented, a proportion of the 'criminal patients' would probably have been intellectually disabled. Dhunjibhoy made this point in 1938, arguing that

> today it is generally recognised that conduct, which was formerly attributed to evil intentions and spiritual wickedness, is often due to pathological causes. Besides the usual cases of mental defectiveness and psychosis, the jail population of India is practically teeming with the following groups of offenders:
>
> (1) Subnormal group.
> (2) Mentally inefficient group.
> (3) Constitutional psychic inferiors.
> (4) Unstable adolescents.
> (5) Temperamentally unstable adults.[60]

He added: 'No reliable statistics are available as to the number of such individuals in our Indian Jails but if such figures were available they would indeed be very large.' Despite the profuse reflections on 'mental defectives in India' in his report of 1938, Dhunjibhoy conveyed only a vague idea of how many of his patients belonged to this category. He merely noted in regard to the mental status of criminals confined at Ranchi: 'On thorough investigation, I find that [the] majority of them are mental defectives of various grades.'[61]

Hospital statistics for the period 1927 to 1939 do however show a steady rise in the number of patients classified as 'idiots' and 'imbeciles'. In relation to overall inmate numbers, however, this trend is not particularly remarkable, amounting to only three per cent in 1927 and five per cent in 1939. The number of newly admitted intellectually disabled patients varied considerably and apparently randomly from year to year, from as low as zero per cent for 'idiots' and one per cent for 'imbeciles' in 1929, for example, to only 0.79 per cent in 1934 and 10 per cent in 1939 for both. On Dhunjibhoy's part, a greater sensitivity towards the postulated link between intellectual disability and criminal behaviour towards the 1930s may have been reflected in the increased ratio among those confined at Ranchi.

Dhunjibhoy's attention was drawn to the issue of 'mental deficiency' during his overseas visits, at a time when psychiatrists as well as health and political campaigners in Western countries debated the value of specialist institutions for the confinement of the intellectually disabled. In the 1920s and 1930s, debates on 'mental deficiency' figured prominently all over the world. Eugenics and mental-hygiene campaigners focused on how reproduction among the intellectually disabled could be curtailed by means of compulsory sterilisation, with Nazi Germany going as far as exterminating them. The extent to which these highly fraught initiatives and the introduction of the Mental Deficiency Act of 1927 in England and Wales had an impact on institutional trends in British India has not yet been discussed in historical literature. On the basis of the available material it can only be suggested that the patient population at Ranchi was clearly skewed towards the admission and confinement of the dangerous and violent, and that the various groups among its inmates were representative neither of the general population nor of the mentally ill and intellectually disabled at large. Any colloquial reference to Indian mental hospitals as places designed for 'village idiots' and 'dimwits' is not only imbued with derogatory mockery of the intellectually disabled, but it also misconstrues the institutions' contemporary purpose and limitations.

In 1938, the government of Bihar set up a committee to investigate the scope for prison reforms in that province. Dr P. K. Sen, acclaimed author of *Penology Old and New*,[62] accompanied by the secretary to the government of Bihar, Mr K. B. Sahay, visited Ranchi and discussed 'fully' with the superintendent 'the psychological treatment of insane criminals and criminal insanes [*sic*] of which we [at Ranchi] have a large proportion'.[63] Although Dhunjibhoy considered psychotherapy to be 'unsuitable in cases of mental defectiveness', during the late 1930s his mind was clearly focused more than it had previously been on the needs of the intellectually disabled. In 1937, shortly after an extended overseas visit, he suggested:

> Since the true indictment of mental deficiency as a social evil of tremendous proportions has been found by Commissions appointed by civilised countries like England, America and Germany, we in India should take advantage of their findings which is offered to us free of cost and should start reform in this direction without any further delay.[64]

His proposal focused on a number of disturbing measures, some of which, such as the 'eugenic sterilization of all known adult defectives of both sexes', were controversial even at the time.[65]

Another matter of concern had been the approach to children. The Mental Deficiency Act, put in place in England and Wales in 1927, was not introduced to British India. Dhunjibhoy pointed out that it was 'very clear that some measure of reform is badly needed in this direction and the sooner it is taken up the better'.[66] In the absence of wider state provision for intellectually disabled children, he suggested 'a very inexpensive scheme for the conversion of one of the existing spare occupational therapy buildings in the Female Section into a children's ward', which was duly sanctioned. The necessity of a children's ward was overdue, he argued, as the 'number of mentally defective children is steadily going up'.[67]

Dhunjibhoy's observation of increased admissions of intellectually disabled children does not imply an overall rise in the number of those aged below 20. In comparison to admission practices at the old institutions at Berhampore, Dacca and Patna, Ranchi clearly tended to admit a higher percentage of younger people. However, from 1927 onwards, Ranchi's patient intake had developed its own momentum. There is much variation on a yearly basis in the ratio of younger to older people, with 17 per cent of those under the age of 20 in both 1927 and 1939, a minimum of 11 per cent in 1933 and a maximum of 32 per cent in 1937. There is no indication of the younger age cohort overall enjoying a greater share of the admissions over the years. It is not clear why the number of 'mentally defective children' among the younger-age cohort had increased, but it is likely that the greater attention paid to the issue of 'mental deficiency' during the 1930s had led Dhunjibhoy to focus more on this particular category of patients. The increased ratio may be an artefact of classification rather than a reflection of the admission of a larger number of intellectually disabled children.

There is however a gendered trend. Consistently at least twice as many young girls and women were admitted during the period 1927 to 1939. The average ratio of males under 20 years of age was about six per cent, while the equivalent for females was 14 per cent. This is an intriguing trend, as the reverse, namely male predominance, has been reported for recent institutional and general practitioner data in England and Wales as well as the United States.[68] However, like the pattern of female predominance in age groups from 35 years and above in Western institutions during the second half of the twentieth century, the trend at Ranchi is most probably a result of changing policies over the use of psychiatric beds.[69] This requires further research and comparison with 1920s and 1930s statistics from other institutions in Western countries. Unfortunately, with few exceptions, most historical work has focused on the pre-twentieth-century period.

The pattern of female preponderance also characterises the minimum and maximum ratios for males and females in this age cohort, namely 3 and 4 per cent for the former, and 10 and 23 per cent for the latter. The reasons for this are not commented on by the superintendents. It is possible that social tolerance towards the behaviour of young women was less than in the case of young men and that a good proportion of the females were devoid of family support on account of being intellectually disabled, unable to help with family chores and difficult to marry off. This has been observed in regard to current gender-specific social attitudes too, and it is not unreasonable to assume that a similar discriminatory pattern prevailed in the 1930s. In-depth assessment of the situation would however be necessary to substantiate the circumstances surrounding the observed gender bias. The relationship between gender differences in susceptibility to mental disorders (and assigned diagnoses) at different stages of the life cycle and hospital admission ratios also needs to be considered. As Busfield has pointed out in regard to age data from the 1980s, it is 'essential to examine the pattern of diagnosed disorders when analysing gender differences', as changing emphases in psychiatric theory and diagnostic practices have a bearing on the 'spectrum of complaints that receive attention, which could well, in turn, modify the extent and even direction of the gender imbalance in identified childhood disorders'.[70]

Figure 2.2. Age groups of patients admitted to Ranchi, by gender, as percentage of total male and female admissions, 1927–1939

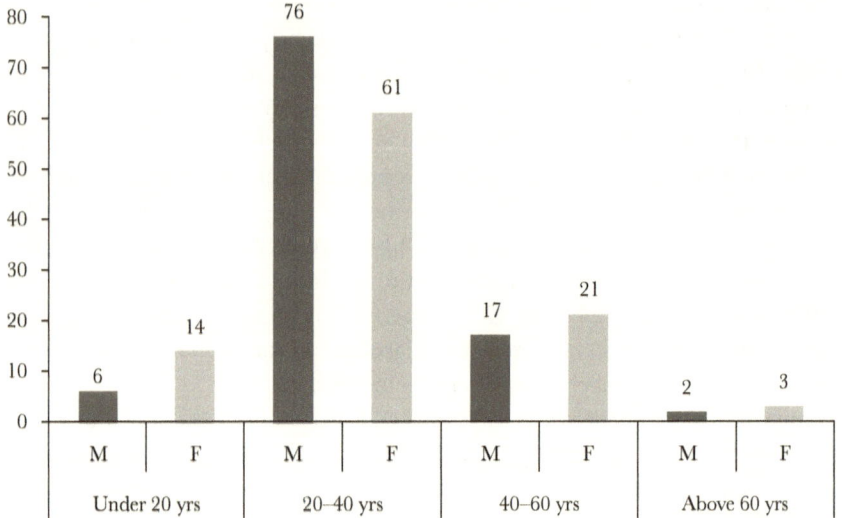

One clear feature of the data relating to age groups at Ranchi pertains to the 20–40 cohort (see Figure 2.2). The majority of patients belonged to this cohort, namely about 69 per cent on average. This differs considerably from the trend observed at St Andrews Hospital in England, for example, where until 1935 each age cohort (above 25 years) comprised about 17 to 19 per cent of total admissions.[71] What is more, from 1935 onwards, 40 per cent of admissions at St Andrews were aged 55 years old and more, compared with 34 per cent in the early 1920s.[72] The preponderance at Ranchi of the younger, 20–40 age group, at a time when in Norfolk increasing numbers of people from the older age groups were admitted, is even more distinct in the case of male patients (their average ratio was 76 per cent, whilst it was only 61 per cent in the case of females). This is in contrast to the second-largest age group from which patients at Ranchi were drawn (40–60). Here women figured slightly more prominently (21 per cent on average, compared to only 17 per cent for men). The numbers of people over 60 years on admission were too small to allow for sensible statistical comparison.

The tendency of gender differences to vary over the life cycle has been reported also in regard to institutions in Western countries. Age was after all a defining characteristic of senile dementia, for example. Age was also part of the construction of particular categories such as dementia praecox (now schizophrenia), which is still regarded as a disorder of adolescence or early adulthood. The aggregate data on patients' ages are unfortunately not refined enough to permit a more nuanced assessment, being based on crude 20-year periods. It is also questionable whether it makes sense to compare Ranchi to other institutions, such as St Andrews, as the patient profile and categorisations clearly depended on individual institutions' admission practices and government policies towards the mentally ill. It is however clear that they were not congruent with the demographic profile of the wider population in Bengal, Bihar and Orissa.

As shown in Figure 2.3 the highest percentage of the population was under the age of 20 and gender differences were not as distinct as at Ranchi. Apart from the under-20s however, the Ranchi cohort did disproportionately mirror the prevalence of the 20–40 age group in the census.

Figure 2.3. Age distribution of population in Bengal, Bihar and Orissa, by gender, census 1931[73]

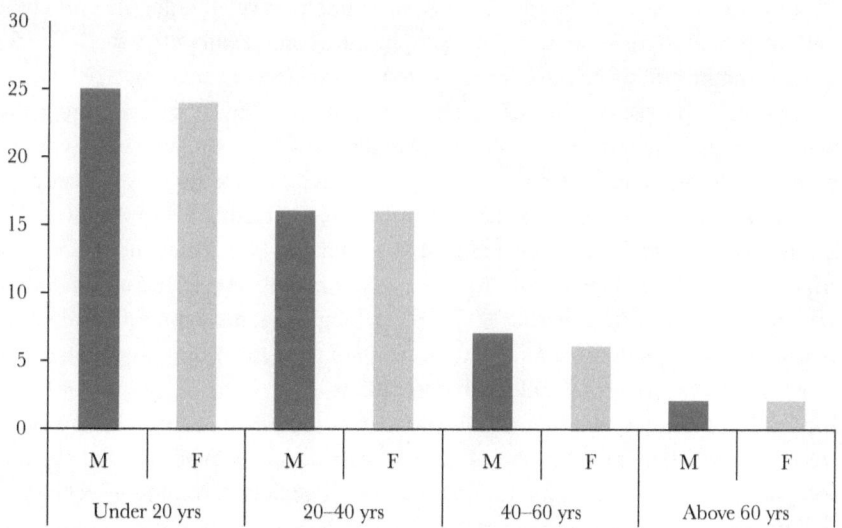

The gender-specific trends among Ranchi patients are distinct, if difficult to interpret, as so many factors are implicated in their generation. We can only state that the 20–40 cohort emerges as the foremost group more distinctly in relation to male patients, while a somewhat wider age distribution characterises the female patients admitted to Ranchi.

Occupational Background and Caste

Patients at Ranchi were drawn from the three large provinces of Bengal, Bihar and Orissa, which encompassed an extraordinary variety of rural environments and socio-cultural communities. These ranged from alluvial plains, tea plantations, mountainous areas and highland plateaus to coalfields, coastal areas and rice-, wheat- and pulse-farming areas, inhabited by varied peoples, from hill tribes to peasants, fishermen, merchants and labourers. The varied communities practised Islam, different branches of Hinduism, 'Paganism' (as the British characterised tribal belief systems) and Christianity. Such diversity could be expected to have been reflected among hospital inmates. However, the institutional records do not reflect a particularly high degree of diversity – particularly in relation to female patients. One reason for this is, of course, that – as Dhunjibhoy pointed out repeatedly – police and magistrates did not take the trouble to provide, or were unable to ascertain, background information on the patients they sent to Ranchi.[74] There is also the general problem of obtaining from mentally disturbed people an accurate account of themselves, when no relatives are forthcoming to provide relevant details. In the case of women, cultural prohibitions would have affected the ease with which (male) officials were able to identify female patients' occupations and social backgrounds. British officers' (restricted) knowledge of and sensitivity to Indian perceptions of what counts as an 'occupation' rather than caste or community affiliation would have complicated things further.

There exists a wealth of literature on how contemporary ethnologists and colonial officials attempted to make sense of, and simplify, the complexities of caste.[75] The focus by colonial administrators on the caste cluster or *jati* level of caste may have facilitated the categorisation of people for the census and other statistical purposes by homogenising particular groups – but it did not reflect social reality. As Cohn pointed out, *jati* categories have 'no structural reality in terms of corporate activities', nor do they 'directly affect the behavior of those who are classified' in a particular category.[76] For example, when a patient was categorised by a colonial official as a 'milkmaid', this may indeed have been descriptive of the work done by her. Alternatively, it may have referred to a member of the *goala* or *gwala* caste ('cattle herder').[77] People belonging to this community were known to have occupations relating to cattle, but this was not necessarily the case for all of them. Caste is not always interchangeable with occupation.

For census statistics more generally, the problem of identifying occupational groupings has received much attention in literature.[78] Census officials pointed out that the return of occupations was 'subject to several limitations'.[79] The figures commonly related 'only to the principal occupation, and persons who combine several means of livelihood were entered under the main one only'. As 'division of labour' (as understood in Western countries) was held to have 'not yet proceeded very far in India, and the same man often combines several pursuits which in Europe would be quite distinct', this was considered a 'serious defect'. 'The fisher-man, for instance, is often a boatman, the money-lender a land-owner, the shepherd a blanket-weaver, and the maker of most articles of common use is also the seller of the same.' Moreover, as one official noted:

> The entries were often (1) vague, so that it was impossible to say definitely what form of employment was referred to; or (2) incorrect, either intentionally, as when occupations which are held to be more reputable were returned instead of others of a meaner nature, or accidentally, owing to confusion of thought and the failure to distinguish clearly

between a man's traditional occupation, as indicated by his caste, and the actual pursuit by means of which he earns his living.

To map caste and/or occupation onto patients' standing in the social hierarchy and their socio-economic position, is clearly a highly fraught undertaking.[80] This makes it difficult to ascertain the social background or social class of the people who ended up at Ranchi. The issue of how social class can be extrapolated from caste assignations has been debated since the 1950s and 1960s, the heyday for historians', sociologists' and anthropologists' engagement with caste and social class.[81] The general consensus since has been that issues of caste and class are complex and subject to change over time, and that caste identities vary according to the specific socio-economic circumstances in particular localities – hence undermining attempts by colonial officials, anthropologists and sociologists to clearly circumscribe, hierarchise and 'fix' particular communities in an ahistorical and indiscriminate way.[82] When we rely on officials' occupational categorisations, we need to keep in mind that it may not be 'the "facts" of the case that allow for their classification but rather the availability of a scheme of classification that often determines how a "fact" is presented'.[83]

Another complication concerns the high percentage for whom previous occupation was entered into the registers as 'not known'. For women, this figure fluctuated between 22 and 34 per cent from 1925 to 1932. This at least conveys the clear message that staff in the hospital did not know much of up to one-third of their female patients' previous background. This is not only a problem for historical analysis. It would also have constituted an acute disadvantage for the treatment of the mentally ill, as empathy for patients and understanding of their previous circumstances and life experiences are important factors in beneficial and supportive staff–patient interaction, especially within institutional settings that rely, for a good proportion of the inmates, on 'maintenance' and 'management'.

It is also clear from the statistics that at Ranchi women's occupational background was known significantly less often than men's.[84] At the old institutions the difference in the ratio of 'unknowns' among men and women was less accentuated.[85] It is difficult to account for these differences. They may have been due to the tendency common also in Western institutions to classify women on the basis of their husband's or father's occupation. Or they may signal greater familiarity with patients' local circumstances among certifying staff in a particular locality. However, even from 1925, once patients were referred exclusively to Ranchi, it was still local officials in the various districts who provided the relevant background information on them in the referral report.

What is more, the three older institutions had admitted a smaller proportion of women than was the case at Ranchi,[86] making generalisations based on statistical trends more problematic. They also had made use of fewer occupational categories for females – namely between only one at Dacca (unhelpfully, 'no occupation') and nine in Berhampore (ranging from 'not known' and 'no occupation' to 'beggar', 'cooly', 'cultivator', 'labourer', 'prostitute', 'maidservant' and 'teacher').[87]

At Ranchi, in contrast, between 11 and 17 categories were in use for female patients from 1925 until 1932. For men, too, the old institutions used fewer occupational categories during the years prior to their closure, namely between 3 and 15. At Ranchi the number fluctuated between a low of 20 in 1930 and a high of 59 in 1927, with an average of 30 categories from 1926 to 1932. Consequently, different levels of detail are available on the occupational and caste background of the hospital population in the various institutions – particularly for the women. This cautions us further against sweeping generalisation.

The extent to which the occupational categories employed in the different institutions in regard to male and female patients did *not* overlap is intriguing. When staff at Ranchi devised the first triennial report, covering the period from 1924 to 1926, it had a total of 109 different occupational categories on its books, most of which it had inherited from Patna, Berhampore and Dacca. Less than half of these (only 42) were used at Ranchi in the 1920s. The important question emerges as to whether this variation was due to different kinds of classification, or if it is in fact indicative of varied hospital populations, in congruence with their particular socio-cultural catchment areas. It is difficult to decide which was the case, although it seems likely that we are dealing with a bit of both: an artefact of categorisation, as well as diverse locality- and culture-specific patient populations.

We certainly know more clearly how much we do *not* know about patients' backgrounds. For the period from 1925 to 1932 there is no information on women's pursuits for between one- and two-thirds of them, if the number of those categorised as 'unknown' and 'no occupation' are combined. The situation is somewhat less drastic in the case of male patients, for whom no information is available for between one-quarter and one-third. It therefore seems that the official decision to do away with statistics on patients' occupational background from 1934 onwards was appropriate and in tune with the vagaries of patients' classification on admission. Although it is often thought that occupational statistics became more detailed and sophisticated with provincial autonomy in the late 1930s, the statistics at Ranchi did not reflect this. This is also in stark contrast to practices reported for other institutions, such as leprosy hospitals, where significant detail was provided on occupations.[88] However, it is in line with the tendency noted in relation to the census of 1931, when W. G. Lacey, the official overseeing census operations in Bihar and Orissa, pointed out that for 'reasons of economy the tabulation of caste was restricted at this [1931] census, and several of the communities for which figures were shown in 1921 do not appear'.[89] It is of course problematic to conflate 'caste' and 'occupation'. As we have seen, there is a complex overlap between these categories. Above all, the lack of details on occupation may well reflect financially motivated omissions by census officials.

Some of the occupational descriptions that *are* available for between one- and two-thirds of women and two-thirds and three-quarters of men deserve further probing. In relation to 'dependents', for example, one census official pointed out in 1901:

> It is very difficult, in India, to distinguish between workers and dependents; but so far as the figures collected at the Census can be relied on, 47 percent. of the population work for their living and 53 percent. are dependent on others.[90]

On an all-India basis, of the males 'two-thirds were returned as actual workers, and of the females only one-third'. This is a startlingly low percentage for women, if the observation of census officials at the time was correct: 'In many classes of the community the wife takes a large share of bread-winning labour, besides being the domestic drudge.'[91]

At Ranchi, a decreasing percentage of women admitted to the institution were designated as 'dependent', namely 37 per cent in 1926, 18 per cent during 1927–29, and 9 per cent in 1930–32. This could be interpreted as a tendency towards greater refinement of categorisation on admission. We might conclude that, for example, from the 1930s, 'dependent' came to be reserved for children and unmarried women, whilst previously it may also have been used for married women ('housewife' first appears around 1930–32, with 11 per cent of women being described as such). However, this seems unlikely, as from 1926 onwards only females were labelled 'dependent', even though male children too were confined at Ranchi during this period.

The category 'dependent' is particularly sensitive to gender issues. It is consistently and significantly lower for men, ranging from 14 per cent in 1926 and five per cent in 1927–29, to zero per cent in 1930–32. As in the case of women, such 'dependants' would not necessarily have been young children. Older people, too, who had suffered from mental illness and were dependent on their relatives for long periods, would have qualified. The significantly higher rate for 'dependent' female patients may be indicative of a greater inclination among families to provide for and keep at home mentally ill men, rather than young females (who could be married off only with difficulty) and married women (who might not have been tolerated as easily by their husbands and in-laws as married men might have been who were looked after by their wives and relatives within their families of origin).

During the early 1930s, there were also important changes made centrally to the classification in census statistics of 'dependants', in contrast to 'actual workers'.[92] It is difficult to ascertain whether these were implemented by the local officials who filled in patients' certification documents prior to admission to Ranchi. It is likely that practices varied. Clearly, what social scientists refer to as the criteria of 'reliability' and 'validity' are not met, namely the consistency with which a label is applied, its accuracy and the extent to which it adequately captures the patient's situation. These problems affect all historical analyses of hospital statistics, yet authors rarely comment on them. This is particularly acute in epidemiological studies. It undermines attempts at the translation of contemporary diagnostic categories into modern ones, as we will see in the chapter on medical categories.

Two of the other occupational categories specified in the hospital reports deserve attention, albeit for quite different reasons: 'cultivator' and 'cooly'. The infrequency with which they were used is interesting. After all, the perception of at least one of Ranchi's officiating superintendents, J. N. J. Pacheco, was that 'a large number of the patients are agriculturalists'.[93] Census officials, too, confirmed this observation in relation to British India generally:

> Nearly two-thirds of the population in 1901 relied on some form of agriculture as their principal means of subsistence: 52 percent. were either landlords or tenants, 12 percent. were field labourers, and about 1 percent. were growers of special products or engaged in estate management, &c. In addition to these, about 2½ percent., who mentioned

some other form of employment as the chief source of their livelihood, were also partially agriculturists; and another 6 percent., who were shown as 'general labourers', were doubtless in the main supported by work in the fields.[94]

Contrary to Pacheco's perception and the officials' observations, female cultivators did not figure quite as highly in the Ranchi statistics. Only between zero and five per cent of women admitted between 1925 and 1932 were designated as 'cultivators'. For men, the numbers were considerably higher (between 15 and 22 per cent), but not to the extent suggested by Pacheco. It is therefore important to avoid relying only on medical officers' and other officials' general observations – as is so often the case in existing work on the history of psychiatry.[95]

In contrast to 'cultivators', the number of women labelled as 'coolies' was slightly higher, with percentages ranging from four to seven per cent. The term 'cooly' was used for plantation workers, who laboured under invariably appalling conditions in the tea gardens of Assam, for example.[96] This group could thus be considered to have engaged in agricultural activity in the wider sense. Southern Bihar or Chota Nagpur (present-day Jharkhand), where Ranchi is located, and the neighbouring districts were the main catchment areas for recruiting such labour, in particular people from Santhal tribal groups.[97]

'Cooly' was a label also applied to Indian indentured labourers sent abroad to work under equally inhumane conditions in places such as Mauritius, southern Africa and British Guiana.[98] However, it would not necessarily have been the case that 'coolies' were sent to work in plantations or agriculture, as many of those ending up in southern Africa, for example, built the railroads. 'Coolies' therefore cannot necessarily be seen as people solely engaged in agricultural work. What is more, a distinction was also made between 'cooly' and 'day labourer' (of which there were but few mentioned among female patients), perhaps indicating that these two classifications did not relate so much to the type of work (that is, construction worker or plantation worker) but its location in relation to the labourer's original home region.[99] The defining parameters for 'cooly' and 'day labourer' may also have changed from the 1920s to the 1930s, as the latter category seems to have disappeared from the hospital records from the late 1920s for women and from 1930 onwards also for men.

Recruitment of 'coolies' was dependent on fluctuations in the plantation business and overseas large-scale construction and agricultural projects. They were drawn predominantly from particular areas in India, whenever Indian and overseas economic developments created a demand for cheap labour. There was therefore considerable fluctuation in the number of recruits that might have been reflected in the statistics of mental hospitals in particular localities. For example, no patients, male or female, were designated as 'coolies' in the old Dacca Mental Hospital in 1924 and 1925, while in 1924, seven per cent of men in Berhampore and in 1925, three per cent in both Patna and Berhampore were classified as such. Similarly, there was a sudden spike in the number of 'coolies' admitted to Ranchi during the early 1930s when the Great Depression affected work opportunities, leading to additional economic hardship and, arguably, as will be discussed in the next chapter, mental problems.[100] The wider economic context within which occupational labels were applied is clearly relevant, if complex, in terms of its impact.

The remaining occupational labels that were applied to female patients encompassed between 4 and 23 per cent of women admitted between 1925 and 1932.[101] They consisted of a mixed and colourful array of categories: 15 maidservants; 5 *ayahs* (nursemaids); 3 milkmaids; 1 *dhai* (midwife); 8 nurses; 10 teachers; 1 assistant inspector of school; 4 students; 1 fisherwoman; 5 sellers of sweetmeats, eggs or vegetables; 1 cowherd and 2 pilferers.[102] Even if we take the various problems of categorisation into account, the range of occupations referred to does not suggest a bias towards the confinement of the lowest orders of society. A similar picture prevails among male patients.

In the case of men, too, the categories 'not known' and 'no occupation' were the ones most frequently employed. Percentages for these fluctuated, from 1926 to 1932, between 9 and 20 per cent for 'unknowns' and 7 and 10 per cent for those assigned the label 'no occupation' (see Figure 2.4).

Figure 2.4. Main male occupational categories assigned as percentage of average total admissions, 1929–1932

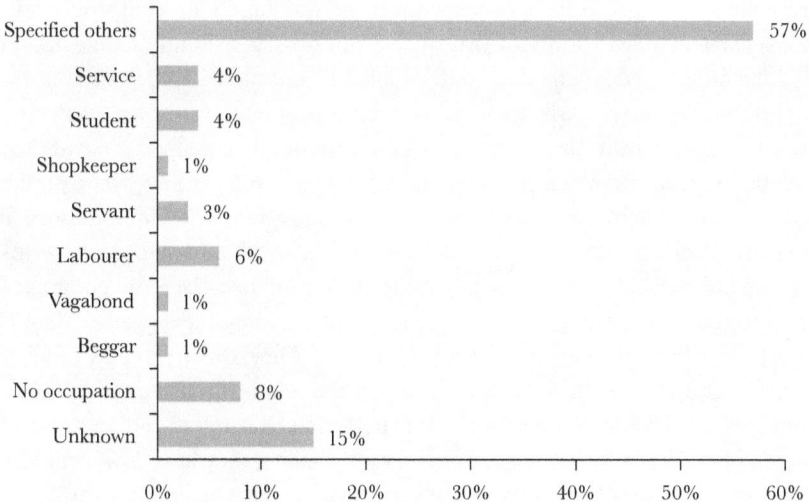

We do not know for sure what 'no occupation' meant in this context. It is unlikely that down and outs, beggars and vagrants were subsumed under this category, as they were specified separately (amounting to a rather low percentage of the overall hospital admissions, between a fraction of one per cent in 1926 and three per cent in 1927–29 in the case of 'beggars', and for 'vagabonds' zero per cent and two per cent in 1926 and 1930–32 respectively).

The only other categories used for men that were above the 1 per cent threshold of total admissions were those of 'labourer', 'servant', 'shopkeeper', 'student' and 'service'. The percentage of 'shopkeepers' remained at a relatively low and stable level, hovering around the one per cent mark (with the exception of 1926, when zero per cent was reported). It is not possible to ascertain if the patients so designated, owned just a little market stall, scraping an existence at the margins of economic viability, or if they ran a bigger, well-established shop and hence were better off economically and status wise.

An intriguing phenomenon is the discontinuation of the 'labourer' designation from 1930 onwards – despite the fact that quite a substantial proportion of patients had previously been designated as such (10 per cent in 1926 and 7 per cent in 1927–29). The trend is reversed in the case of 'service', which was not applied to any patients in 1926, then to only about 0.5 per cent in 1927–29, and a startling 11 per cent in 1930–32. It is difficult to speculate on why no 'labourers' were identified in 1930–32. This may well have been a one-off outlier. The same may have been the case for the 'service' group, although the quite sudden rise in the early 1930s does fit in with the move in colonial administration towards increased local self-government, which was fully implemented after the Government of India Act (1935) and the local elections in 1937. This development implied an increased need for low-level clerks.

Much has been written on 'service' people who came from a wide range of backgrounds but had to be literate and hence belonged to what could be described as the lower-middle classes of Indian communities.[103] Although the position of clerk in government offices and British commercial firms was highly coveted, the work itself implied a considerable measure of drudgery if not misery, as Sumit Sarkar has pointed out.[104] Like other occupations that were detailed in the statistics, such as *chaprassi* who performed menial office tasks such as carrying documents from one clerk's desk to another and hence were drawn from social backgrounds equally varied (though not equivalent to those from which the 'service' people came), clerks were particularly vulnerable to the whims, arrogance and racist humiliations of their superiors. In the eighteenth and nineteenth centuries they had been referred to in derogatory terms such as 'crannies' or 'scribblers'.[105] Although the term 'kerani' became more common in the twentieth century, and clerks were increasingly supervised by Indian rather than British officials, a flippant attitude against them continued.[106] They were frequently despised and continually reminded of their lowly position on the administrative treadmill. In socio-economic terms they did however not belong to the lowest rungs of Indian society. Being literate and benefiting, increasingly, from a regular salary, they led a lower-middle-class life, aspiring to what is known in Bengal as *bhadralok* status, assumed by a new group of middle- to upper-middle-class people who emerged during the colonial period. This would have been the case too for those classified as 'students'. Their numbers increased steadily (from one per cent in 1925 to five per cent in the early 1930s). As in the case of those in 'service', their higher numbers mirror the wider changes in colonial society, with an increasing proportion of Indians becoming educated in the Western idiom.

Given the wider context of political and social change, it is not surprising to find 'teachers' and even an 'assistant inspector of school' as well as a 'professor' and a 'scholar (research)' among the patients at Ranchi. Ranchi was located in Chota Nagpur (Jharkhand), where the Jesuits and other missions developed a basic educational structure. This included '"central schools" (often one each for boys and girls), which were of middle vernacular level, a seminary for theological training – all at Ranchi – and a string of village schools in the inner mission field'.[107] The disproportionate prevalence of students and teachers among hospital patients clearly reflects specific developments in the vicinity of the institution as well as wider socio-demographic trends.

On the basis of an assessment of occupational categories, it therefore appears that patients from the lower strata of Indian society were under- rather than over-represented. This has also been observed in relation to patients admitted to Ranchi during the postcolonial period. S. Rao, a psychologist based at Ranchi University, investigated the socio-economic and educational characteristics of 2,310 patients admitted in 1958–60 to 'Ranchi Mansik Aryogyashala', as the Indian Mental Hospital was called after Independence.[108] He found that higher castes from Bihar, from where patients were then drawn, were over-represented, concluding that while admissions in the West were generally higher from the lower social classes, the reverse was true for the caste groups he studied. This finding may not be true for all institutions in India during the colonial and postcolonial period. It is likely though that it applied, at least during the early twentieth century. This would however require further detailed research on patient populations in other mental institutions in India. Existing work on the colonial period is unfortunately still based only on under-evidenced guesswork.[109]

The categories discussed so far in relation to male patients covered between 55 and 90 per cent of the total admitted to Ranchi in the period from 1926 to 1932. The remaining 10 to 45 per cent were made up of a variety of categories, of which some relate to caste affiliation (such as *dome* and *mochi*) while others designate a specific type of work (such as pleader or assistant ticket collector). Patients were clearly identified in terms both of Western occupational categories and caste assignments. This was, and is, not uncommon. Census officials too had observed people fluctuating between caste and job categories, and even reporting more 'reputable' occupations or failing to distinguish between their caste group and the work they pursued.[110] This may have been particularly acute when a person had previously been employed by, or been known to, the British in some particular capacity as, for example, a watchman, servant or teacher. However, as Muslims and Christians, too, were admitted, caste terms would not always have been applicable to all patients.[111]

Although they appear to have been under-represented at Ranchi, the most easily identified social groups in this context are of course those belonging to the lower spectrum of the caste hierarchy (such as *dome-chamar*,[112] *dhobi*, *charmakar* and *mochi*) and the lower socio-economic groups (for example, *nayee*, vegetable seller, barber).[113] The term *dome-chamar* is still today used in the region as a pejorative term for those perceived as unclean or uncouth. It is more difficult to ascertain how patients labelled as *mazdoor* (mill hand), sepoy or musician for example could be classified in socio-economic terms as they could have been members of a variety of social communities or, in the case of brahmans, for example, might have benefited from a relatively elevated social status, but could have been either more or less well off in economic terms. In addition, as noted, not all patients were Hindu, and caste was not the only criterion for social classification.

A good number of patients came from Muslim communities and different levels of fluidity between castes and other social communities prevailed in the three provinces from which patients were admitted to Ranchi. Caste barriers in Bengal are usually considered to have been less stringent than in Bihar, for example.[114] However even such regional tendencies are not altogether clear-cut. If we look at the socio-economic position of particular communities, a more complex pattern emerges. For example, while due to the absence of clearly defined Kshatriya or Rajput castes in Bengal other groups such as the *kayasthas* claimed this more elevated 'upper caste' status from the nineteenth century onwards, *kayasthas* in Bihar could be considered as a mid-level caste.[115] On the other hand, *goalas* (*yadav* in Bihar), in the twentieth century, would increasingly emerge as better off in Bihar than in Bengal. However, *goalas* in neither region would have been a homogenous group. For example, in Bengal the 'Bengali *goalas*' were differentiated from 'up-country *goalas*' in district gazetteers; the latter were referred to as *ahirs*. Yet, the two groups might well have lived alongside each other, as they did in Howrah, for example. To what extent differences between them, in terms of life experience, social outlook and aspirations, were more marked than their commonalities, is a complicated issue.

Whatever insight we may derive from an analysis of hospital statistics, it is important to keep in mind that particular caste and other categories hide more heterogeneous cultural 'lifeworlds', social experiences and identity formations.[116] Social descriptors, such as occupational background, that were commonly used to ascertain the social background from which patients were drawn, clearly need to be viewed with much caution; particularly within a colonial situation where administrative practices of categorisation and labelling were politically fraught and would not necessarily be congruent with communities' and individuals' social identity formation.

A wide range of positions in the caste hierarchy and various occupational pursuits are covered in the institutional statistics, from the lowest to the highest strata of Hindu, Muslim and Indian Christian society. Although definitive information is not available, it seems that the more specific categories may also be indicative of a tendency to admit a disproportionate number of patients from the lower-middle-class groups upwards. It therefore seems likely that a good proportion of patients at Ranchi did *not* belong to the lowest social groups.

If Ranchi did not tend to disproportionately incarcerate patients from the lowest strata, it did not particularly suit the upper echelons of Indian society either. The superintendent commented on the latter in one of his first reports, as an omission that required attention. He pointed out the 'lack of special facilities and suitable arrangements' for treating upper-class patients, noting that he had been 'obliged to refuse many applications' from this group.[117] He argued for 'facilities consistent with their classes', outlining to government that in his opinion superior 'paying patients' blocks should be practically self-supporting and not a burden on the State', as their 'guardians will willingly subscribe towards maintenance in the shape of fees etc.' In contrast to developments in Britain, superior facilities for mentally ill people from the higher classes were not available in the region. Dhunjibhoy noted: 'At present there exists no such accommodation in the provinces of Bengal and Bihar and Orissa for treatment of mentally afflicted upper class people.'

Ranchi was not crowded with 'undesirables' (down and outs, prostitutes and beggars), as has been alleged in regard to institutions in Western countries. What about the institution being filled with what appears to the Western eye as 'exotic' characters such as *hijras* (members of the 'third sex'), *bauls* (minstrels), *faquirs* and *sanyasins*, whose presence in public places was not always appreciated by the British? It is quite clear that no evidence is available in the institutional records – apart from a few individual cases – that the patient population at Ranchi was disproportionately drawn from these more 'colourful' sections of Indian society. There is reference in the report covering the period 1930–32 of one fakir, two musicians and one sanyasi being admitted. Only between one and seven per cent of women admitted between 1925 and 1932, for example, were beggars, and between zero and three per cent were prostitutes. Without doubt, these are surprisingly low numbers and unrepresentative, if fascinating, cases. But, we might do well to note that among the admissions during this period, there were also rather 'respectable' types, namely one allopathic practitioner, one chemist, two constables and one laboratory assistant. Similarly, in 1925, the most 'colourful' job description surely belonged to the four 'professional thieves', who were admitted alongside one assistant of a mercantile firm, one compounder, one physician, three schoolmasters, two steno typists and many others.

Historians of medicine intent on suggesting that the colonial state aimed at colonising the body and the mind of the 'natives', and set out to clear the streets of the socially undesirable and those considered a nuisance by the European public would be unable to find clear evidence of these alleged trends at Ranchi. It could of course be argued that the high rate of 'unknowns' and patients of 'no occupation', may hide those who colonial society wished to 'make invisible' through incarceration. However, the fact that the high cost involved in maintaining patients in closed institutions encouraged authorities to restrict eligibility for admission to the violent and dangerous, mitigates against such an interpretation.

Religion

Ranchi's catchment area encompassed a region populated by people of varied religious backgrounds, with particular localities showing a preponderance of specific denominations. For example, Hinduism was by far the most widespread religion in Orissa and in Bihar, where census officials applied it to about 90 and 80 per cent of the population respectively. In the eastern part of Bengal, about two-thirds of people were Muslims. In contrast, in Chota Nagpur and in Orissa Muslims constituted but a minority, with only low single-figure percentage rates. 'Animists' – or 'tribals', as they were referred to by the British from the 1931 census onwards – were prominent in two districts of Chota Nagpur, where one in two belonged to this group, while they constituted only a fraction of 1 per cent of Bengal's population.[118] The regional population distribution pattern for 'native Christians' was similar to that of 'tribals', with about half of them being found in just one district of Chota Nagpur, namely in Ranchi, 'where Lutheran, Roman Catholic, and Anglican missions [were] busily engaged among the aboriginal tribes'.[119]

In addition to such locality-specific demarcations, it was also, as census officials pointed out, 'very difficult in practice to distinguish between Hinduism and some of the other indigenous religions of India'.[120] One example pertained to the perennial bugbear of colonial administrators' attempts at clear-cut classifications, namely 'aboriginal tribes', of whom there were a significant number in the Ranchi district. On an all-India basis, it was understood in 1941 that of 100 Indians, '66 are Hindus, 24 Muslims and 6 of tribal origins'.[121] However, particularly when 'tribals' were, as Meyer put it perceptively, 'hovering on the outskirts of Hinduism', it was 'impossible to define at what precise point a member of one of these tribes should be classed as a Hindu'.[122] What is more, although the censuses – and the mental-hospital statistics – provided seemingly clearly delineated categories, it was acknowledged that, in fact, classification often 'depended on the personal predilections of the enumerators'.[123] Greater reliability was alleged by census officials in relation to non-Hindu groups. It was suggested that there was 'no reason to doubt the accuracy of the return for Muhammadans and Christians', as in their case there was 'little room for doubt or misdescription'.[124] This conception disregarded the wide variety of beliefs subsumed under these denominations, not to speak of the varied social groups subscribing to them. However, the British clearly had more problems in making sense of, and pigeonholing, the various branches of Hindu religious beliefs, except in the case of its more easily demarcated monotheistic, and relatively recent, manifestations, such as the Brahmo Samaj and Arya Samaj.[125]

By 1940, census officials approached another problem of classification: the fraught equation of 'religious affiliation' with 'community' by the wider population and census enumerators alike. As a result, the headings of earlier tables were changed from 'religion' to 'community'. Yet this act of re-labelling did not really deal with the many problems it was supposed to solve; in fact, it aggravated communalism on religious lines. It was argued by census officials that the statistics supposed to pinpoint community affiliation had been 'based on the returns to the question "religion" but the results were interpreted as if the question had been community'.[126] M. W. M. Yeatts, the census commissioner for India in 1941, observed in relation to the earlier censuses,

> The religion question itself was unsatisfactory. If the results of the question had been used only as indicating the elements in the population professing a particular approach to unseen things the unsatisfactory nature of parts of the record would not have mattered so much. Unfortunately however […] the answers given or attributed to a question on religion were being used unconsciously as the answers to a question on community or origin, a most unscientific position which it was desirable to end.[127]

Colonial administrators and Indian reformers were both very much aware of the problem of jumping to conclusions about a person's community identity and social (and political) inclination on the basis of their religion. This issue is problematic also in relation to any attempt to judge patients' previous community affiliation or social background on the basis of census and institutional statistics that classify people on the basis of religion and community or occupation and caste. Despite these problems, colonial officials at the time considered the change of the statistical headings from 'religion' to 'community' appropriate. It was noted though that there prevailed 'much misunderstanding of the change […] and what it implies', and that part of it was 'of that kind which does not wish to be dispelled'.[128]

The most problematic aspect in all this was the religification of community and the politicisation of religious and communal identity within the wider context of anticolonial agitation during the 1920s and 1930s. Yeatts pointed out that peculiar problems had 'presented themselves 10 years ago' (from 1930), even 'in the main communities': 'Hindus or Muslims who particularly wished to be dissociated from Hinduism or Islam as an expression of religion' also wanted 'their membership of the Hindu or Muslim communities ("sub-nationality" was the word used to me by one person) to be recorded'.[129] Yeatts highlighted the problem succinctly, namely 'that a religion return was being used as a community one'. The response of simply re-labelling the tables, however, did not solve it. As in previous years, denoting people's religion had been particularly difficult in relation to 'tribals' because,

> to the ordinary member of a tribe, the word religion has no meaning and is not explainable to him by any enumerator. And that same enumerator, while he can appreciate the fact that a tribesman may be Christian or Muslim cannot grasp the peculiar manner in which this rather artificial concept of religion presents itself to the tribesman.[130]

As in many parts of the world, the British, as well as Indian, officials had a problem with nomadic and tribal people that were out of proportion to the minor fraction of the overall population of the subcontinent they constituted. Nomads and tribes crossed the borders of neatly settled lands and the conceptual boundaries of demographers' and tax officials' categories alike. They were not easy to pin down into the clearly circumscribed administrative pigeonholes established by colonial surveyors and census officials on the lands and, increasingly, in the minds of settled Indian people. It is quite clear that census and institutional statistics on religion, occupation and caste do not tell us much about communal identity in its many manifestations, nor are they necessarily indicative of people's social standing or cultural preferences. As is the case with other social categories, such as race, for example, they conceal internal heterogeneity, even if differences between people thrown together under one label might be as significant, if not more so, than those between people from different groups or 'races'.[131]

The information provided by Dhunjibhoy on his patients' religious backgrounds will therefore need to be considered with as much caution as any other census statistics. Bearing these caveats in mind, we can discern from the annual reports for the Ranchi Mental Hospital some clear statistical patterns in regard to the religious affiliations attributed to patients. To what extent these can be taken as indicators of the social, cultural and mental characteristics of the communities from which they were most likely to have been drawn is an entirely different matter.

According to the available statistics, Hindus constituted the clear majority of inmates, with an average of 63 per cent of admissions to Ranchi from 1927 to 1939. The rate was somewhat lower on average from 1928 to 1931, but, amounting to about 58 per cent, it was still well above the next most frequently admitted group, the 'Muhammedans'. The number of people from Muslim communities was low, at about 26 per cent or a quarter of admissions, and their admission figures over the years fluctuated, from a maximum of 32 per cent in 1929 to only 20 per cent in 1930. The third major group in the hospital statistics was referred to as 'native Christians'. They made up about eight per cent of admissions on average, with a minimum of five per cent in 1936 and a maximum of 15 per cent in 1930. No particular trend over the period is discernible for the three main religious denominations.

How do these numbers compare to overall population trends in the three provinces? If we compare Ranchi's data with the aggregate figures of the census of 1941 for the provinces of Bengal, Bihar and Orissa, it is clear that only the ratio for Hindus among the patients at Ranchi (63 per cent) mirrors the wider demographic patterns, as Hindus constituted about 60 per cent of the overall population in the region (see Figure 2.5).

Figure 2.5. Religious affiliation of patients at Ranchi (average percentage 1927–1939), and in population of Bengal, Bihar and Orissa as a whole (census of 1941)

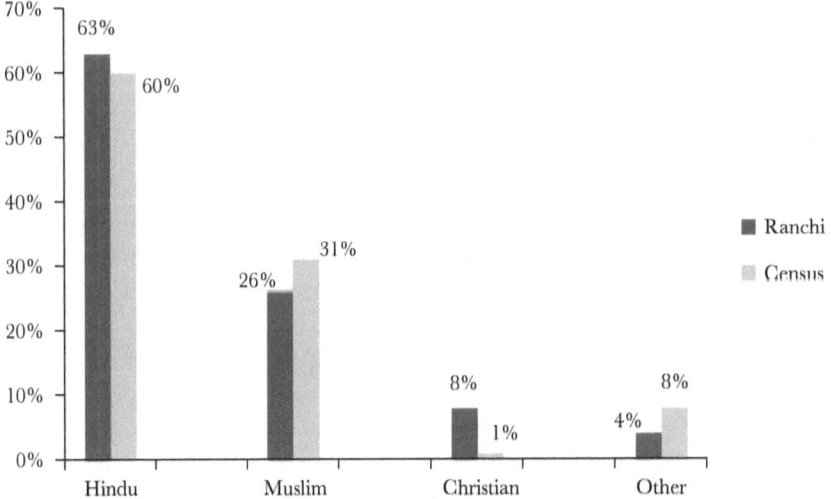

Muslims in contrast are somewhat under-represented and Christians are clearly over-represented at Ranchi. The former constituted 31 per cent in the census (in comparison to 26 per cent at Ranchi) and the latter only a fraction of one per cent (in contrast to eight per cent at Ranchi). This pattern for Muslims and Christians becomes even more pronounced when it is noted that 75 per cent of beds at Ranchi had to be reserved for patients from Bengal, where Muslims were in the majority (55 per cent, in contrast to only 42 per cent Hindus, according to the census of 1941). Admittedly, the Hindu–Muslim ratio was drastically reversed in Orissa, where about 78 per cent belonged to the former and Muslims made up only two per cent of the population. However, only five per cent of the beds were earmarked for patients from that province. As in Orissa, the Hindu–Muslim ratio in Bihar, too, was in favour of Hindus, although here the contrast was less accentuated (76 to 13 per cent). Yet Bihar too had a considerably smaller bed allocation than Bengal (20 per cent, in contrast to Bengal's 75 per cent). The prevalence of Hindu patients was therefore not in line with the wider demographic features in the three provinces. Patients from Muslim communities were clearly less likely to be admitted to the hospital.

It is difficult to ascertain whether this indicates a lower susceptibility to mental problems among Muslims or different levels of tolerance towards the mentally ill among Hindus and Muslims; or whether the fewer admissions from Muslim groups are due to peculiarities of the certification procedures in place at various localities. The situation in regard to Indian Christians is similarly hard to interpret. In contrast to the (moderately) under-represented Muslims, this group was significantly over-represented among patients.

There are also clear contrasting trends in regard to the likelihood of people from the main religious communities ending up in a mental hospital, when Ranchi is compared to the older institutions. The Dacca Hospital, having been located in *eastern* Bengal, had admitted a majority of Muslims. However, the Muslim to Hindu admission rates (53 to 46 per cent in 1924, and 57 to 40 per cent in 1925) reflected more closely population trends in the *whole* of Bengal (55 to 42 per cent for Bengal overall, according to the 1941 census ratio).[132] The hospital rate for Muslims was lower than their actual presence in eastern Bengal, or 'Bengal proper', where the institution was located, would suggest. Dacca admitted hardly any Christians and neither did the old hospital in Berhampore, which was also located in Bengal, but towards the west of that province. Patna in contrast admitted an unrepresentatively high proportion of Indian Christians, which, as in the case of the significantly increased ratio of Christians at the Ranchi Hospital, may have been due to its proximity to missionary ventures.

As noted above, it is difficult to determine whether the Muslim under-representation and Christian over-representation at Ranchi was due to differential cultural propensities to develop mental illness or behavioural tolerance levels, provincial officials' discriminative (positive as well as negative) certification practices, or the superintendents' preferential admission policy. It would also have been difficult for provincial officials and the superintendent at Ranchi to allocate any of the scarce free beds at the hospital according to the proscribed provincial formula of 75, 20 and 5 per cent for patients from Bengal, Bihar and Orissa respectively. To keep track of whether the varied religious groups in these provinces were treated equitably in terms of access to the hospital would have complicated the situation further. At any rate, religious affiliation was not an issue that received any attention in regard to eligibility for admission and it is debatable if it should have been. What is more, the high percentage of 'criminal patients', whose admission to Ranchi was more or less mandatory on account of lack of suitable alternative accommodation, would have made any screening for additional criteria, such as religious background, difficult.

The assessment of gendered patterns in regard to patients' religious affiliation reveals some significant trends. If we compare the 1941 census data for religious affiliation by gender with the gender ratio of people from different denominations admitted to Ranchi, it becomes very clear that patients' profiles did not reflect the pattern that characterised population trends in the provinces of Bengal, Bihar and Orissa. On the basis of the census – and taking into account the 75, 20 and 5 per cent distribution for bed allocation for patients from these three areas – we would expect the gender ratio by religion to be almost equal, as was the case for the population at large.[133] However, the actual average percentages for Hindu, Muslim and Christian men and women admitted to Ranchi deviated considerably from the census baselines (see Figure 2.6).[134]

Figure 2.6. Average gender ratio by religion (patients admitted, 1927–1939)

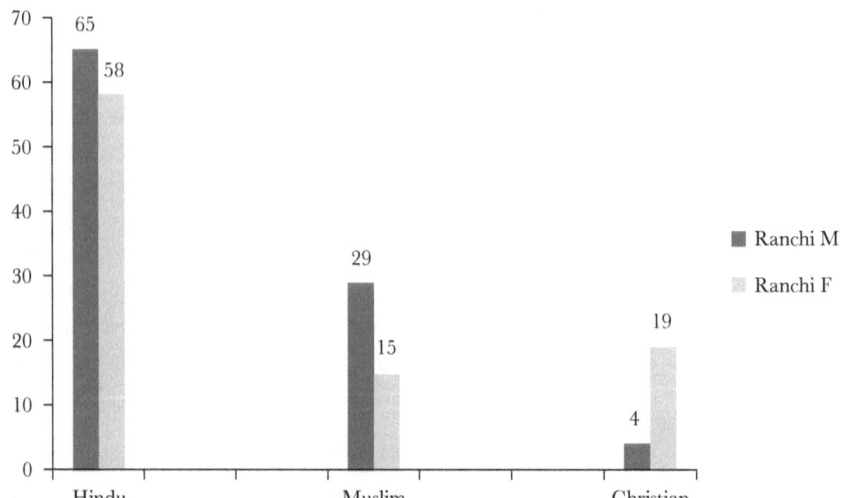

Both Hindu and Muslim women were clearly less likely than Hindu and Muslim men to be admitted to Ranchi. Women's under-representation is particularly accentuated for Muslims, with women being just under half as likely as their male counterparts to be sent to Ranchi. However, the trend of under-representation is reversed for Christian women who are nearly five times as likely as Christian men to find themselves in the mental hospital. The overall pattern at Ranchi of Muslim under-representation and Christian over-representation was therefore particularly stark in relation to the women in these two groups. How can these differences be accounted for?

Colonial officials at the time commented on gender-specific trends for Hindu and Muslim communities in relation to census statistics. The 'deficiency of females' in male to female population rates in 'the greater part of India' was not attributed to women's 'concealment at the Census', nor to the impact of 'climate, season of gestation, food, consanguineous marriages, and the like', and female infanticide, which the British claimed to have 'put down'.[135] Rather, it was suggested that,

> there is no doubt that female children receive far less care than those of the other sex. It follows that, in comparison with males, fewer survive the diseases of infancy than in Europe, where the number of males at birth exceeds that of females to almost the same extent as it does in India, but where their excess mortality is so great as to reduce them to a minority before the close of the first year of life.[136]

It was also suggested that females were disadvantaged further, by 'the danger of functional derangement due to premature cohabitation and child-bearing, unskilful midwifery, exposure, and hard labour'.[137] These kinds of speculation by British colonial administrators have rightly received critical attention by postcolonial historians as they were frequently used to justify the British colonial presence in South Asia. However the preferential treatment of males and abuse of and disregard for females has also been observed in relation to current social trends among particular communities.[138] The varied extent to which females were (and are) disadvantaged has been seen to be dependent on their socio-cultural background. During the colonial period, race, caste and religion were identified as influential factors. For example, it was suggested in relation to the census report of 1901, that among 'the Dravidians, females are distinctly more numerous than among the castes of Aryan or semi-Aryan descent'.[139] In regard to 'Mongoloid races' the situation was considered 'less uniform'. Regional differences were also observed. In Bengal 'the sexes [were] on a par', whilst a 'superfluity of females' prevailed in Bihar, Orissa and Chota Nagpur'. However, in the eastern part of Bengal, or 'Bengal proper', a 'marked deficiency' of females existed.[140]

As the data for the census of 1941 show (see Figure 2.7), the situation in the provinces of Bengal, Bihar and Orissa deviated from the all-India average.

Figure 2.7. Ratio of females to males, India overall, Bengal, Bihar and Orissa (census 1941)[141]

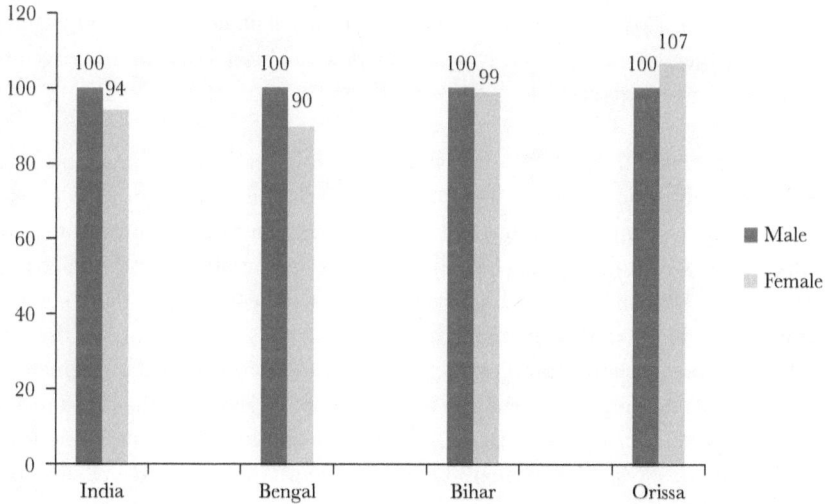

Towards the end of the colonial period, census officials were decreasingly inclined to put forward speculations on the causes of these trends. This is illustrated by Yeatts's comment in the 1941 census, when he noted: 'I have no time to add to the volume of speculation on the causes of [a deficiency of women] which would merit a monograph in itself.'[142] His predecessors had mused, in relation to the 1901 report, for example, that it was due to the better care bestowed on Muslim women in contrast to 'their Hindu neighbours'.[143] Muslim girls, so it was thought,

> are given in wedlock at a later age, and their widows are allowed to remarry, so that a larger proportion of their females of the child-bearing ages are married; their dietary is more nourishing; and in the absence of the various marriage difficulties which so often

embarrass the Hindu father of a large family of girls, their female children are taken better care of than is often the case with the Hindus.[144]

The fact that the male–female ratio in 1941 was most weighted against females in the very province (Bengal) that had a majority of Muslims (55 per cent) and should, according to earlier official speculations, have constituted the most favourable place for women, highlights how problematic British preconceptions about communities' predilections were. In Orissa, where Muslims made up only two per cent of the population, females outnumbered males most. And in Bihar, where the gender ratio was more or less equal, Muslims were in the minority (13 per cent), while Hindus accounted for 76 per cent of the population. Reflections on the alleged causes of the all-India under-representation of women clearly tells us more about certain colonial administrators' prejudices than actual social trends.

Even Yeatts, in 1941, could not resist some speculation on the matter. He noted:

> There is much more to this question than merely the actual count. Nothing is ever single in the world of human causation and this matter of female defect is not sep[a]rable from a wide range of considerations, which begin in public health and end in social custom, covering, for example, such features as maternal mortality, early marriage and prohibition of widow remarriage.[145]

It is difficult to ascertain which factors may have been implicated in Hindu and Muslim women's lower admission rates at Ranchi. Certification and admission procedures will certainly have had an impact. Muslim and Hindu women, particularly those from middle- and upper-class backgrounds, may have been less visible in public places on account of socio-cultural restrictions, such as the practice of *purdah* (seclusion) or the confinement of women to the home. But even among those communities that did not practise formal seclusion of women, socio-cultural restrictions on women's freedom of movement were in place. It could therefore be argued that women would be less likely than men to attract adverse police attention and be referred to a mental hospital. However, if the level of social tolerance was lower for women's behaviour, then those who did not shun public exposure would have been more likely than men to receive adverse attention. On the other hand, as exhibition of dangerous and violent behaviour was the major criterion for transfer to Ranchi, minor transgressions of public peace and order would not have qualified women for admission, and, given that gender-specific socialisation and child-rearing behaviour might have made the display of violent and risky behaviour less likely for females, major transgressions would have been rarer than for males. Given the patriarchal male-focused family structures, it is likely that deranged women who were kept at home, faced hostility and lack of tolerance if not ill treatment from their in-laws or families of origin once they lost their capacity to contribute to the family's wellbeing.

Whichever of the above arguments we adduce to explain Hindu and Muslim women's under-representation among patients at Ranchi, is easily countered or at least complicated by other, equally plausible, suggestions. This conundrum is not solved even by looking at the issue of differential admission patterns the other way round, namely by focusing on the men, asking why Hindu and Muslim men were more likely than women to end up in a mental hospital. Either side of the gender divide, we must proceed from generalised assumptions about particular groups' assumed socio-cultural customs that are difficult to substantiate by any specific evidence available to us in relation to patients at Ranchi. Cultural, religious and sexual stereotyping or 'essentializing' of Indian communities' alleged characteristics has been rightly criticised by postcolonial scholars. In order to avoid it and allow instead for a more complex assessment, we would need to examine individual cases of women and men – both those kept at home and those admitted to Ranchi. Furthermore, we should not lose sight of the fact that the numbers of women and men admitted to the mental hospital every year was minute in relation to overall population numbers. This is best illustrated by contrasting male and female admissions to Ranchi and the overall patient numbers in 1939 with overall population statistics from the census of 1941 (see Table 2.3).[146]

Table 2.3. Number of patients admitted to and confined at Ranchi, 1939, and overall population numbers in Bengal, Bihar and Orissa, 1941 (male, female, total)

	Male	Female	*Total*
Admitted to Ranchi, 1939	84	36	*120*
Confined in Ranchi, 1939	1,096	262	*1,358*
Population of Bengal, 1941	31,747,395	28,559,130	*60,306,525*
Population of Bihar, 1941	18,224,428	18,115,723	*36,340,151*
Population of Orissa, 1941	4,218,121	4,510,423	*8,728,544*

However, despite the enormous discrepancy between patient numbers and overall population figures, some questions need to be raised in regard to the over-representation of Christian women at Ranchi. For example, did conversion to Christianity lead to social and psychological pressures and hence an increased likelihood for women in particular to exhibit potentially dangerous, mentally unstable behaviour? Or were Christian families, clerics and missionaries less tolerant of deviant female behaviour, or – to put a different, benevolent construction on it – more inclined to seek out care and treatment for them? On the basis of the available background information on patients and their family circumstances, these questions cannot be answered. We do however have some details on inmates' places of birth, which we owe mainly to colonial officials' eagerness to charge incurred expenses to patients' relatives or their local authorities.

Among Christian women, the largest number by far came from Chota Nagpur, an area in Bihar that had a large tribal population. Missionaries were particularly active here and the one district of Chota Nagpur that predominated in terms of tribal presence and missionary endeavour, as well as female admissions to the mental hospital, was Ranchi. 23 of the 29 Christian women admitted from 1928 to 1939 were from this district (a further six patients came from other nearby districts in Bihar, namely Patna (five) and Saran (one).[147]) If the admitted women were mainly from recently Christianised tribal groups, access to an institution such as Ranchi in the middle of the tribal area may well have been a factor. Colonial officials considered 'tribals' particularly sensitive to being away from their home region. There were many instances when those who had been sent to work as coolies in Assam and further afield overseas were reported as homesick and prone to return to their native tracts of land as soon as they could. Psychological pressures caused by missionary fervour and spiritual dis- or reorientation, missionaries' zeal in getting intractable women incarcerated or looked after, and/or the effect an amenity has to encourage usage among patients, their relatives and police and district officials in its vicinity, might have been implicated.

However, any speculation regarding admissions from the tribal tracts in Chota Nagpur needs to be considered alongside the fact that the next-largest group of female Christians came from Bengal (25), with 13 of these from Calcutta alone.[148] Although missionaries had been active in Calcutta too, the impact on the population in this conurbation was different from the situation in tribal Chota Nagpur. It seems probable that the Christian women admitted from the former area had more diverse (and probably non-tribal) backgrounds than those drawn from the latter. The Bengali women may even have come from the lower- to upper-middle classes, as Christianity, at least in Calcutta, went along with some degree of linguistic facility in English and hence opened doors for regular employment and a certain degree of social status.

There were only two Christian women who had been admitted from Orissa, one from Samalpur and another from Cuttack. The actual admission numbers in the case of Christian women were therefore not in line with the administrative allocation of beds on the basis of provincial origin (75, 20 and 5 per cent for Bengal, Bihar and Orissa, respectively). If we disregard admissions from other Indian provinces (such as one each from the Central Provinces and the Princely State of Sikkim), and cases in which women's place of birth was unknown (five) or where they were classified as 'homeless' (three), then the actual admission ratio for Christian women would be 40:56:3 for Bengal, Bihar (including Chota Nagpur) and Orissa respectively. While Orissa would nearly have got its projected share of the allocation, the actual ratio was reversed for Bengal and Bihar – at least in relation to one particular group of inmates. Local factors, such as the accessibility of the mental hospital to specific communities, were clearly important. Why particular groups among them were more highly represented in the institution remains subject to speculation on the basis of the available evidence.

What kind of people ended up at the mental hospital? Despite the caveats regarding the accuracy and validity of contemporary statistics, some clear trends emerge from them. Most importantly, patients were not a representative sample of the population in Bengal, Bihar and Orissa, in terms either of sex, age, socio-economic background or the kind of behavioural symptoms commonly displayed by the mentally ill. Mainly the violent and those perceived as dangerous among the mentally ill at large qualified for institutional treatment. The single most prevalent group were those who had been convicted of serious crimes or of repeated violent offences. Those considered socially harmless were rarely present at Ranchi, and only a negligible number of the intellectually disabled were catered for. Given the absence in British India of institutional and public services dedicated to the care of the intellectually disabled, the mental hospital would have constituted, rightly or wrongly, the only institutional option for this group of people. Women were greatly under-represented at Ranchi, particularly among the public patients. Well-to-do families were keen to use the mental hospital for the (mainly shorter-term) treatment of relatives. However, the demand for treatment as a 'private patient' consistently outstripped the availability of facilities. The governments of Bengal, Bihar and Orissa were not inclined to extend hospital provision to enable more privately financed people, nor a wider range, and hence a more representative sample, of the Indian population to be institutionalised. Austerity measures in the wake of World War I and during the lead up to World War II provided provincial governments with the impetus as well as the legitimation to restrict access to mental hospitals.

The majority of patients were drawn from the lower-middle to middle range of socio-economic groups, with those who were employed in the 'modern' sector (as educational professionals and low-level bureaucrats, for example) constituting a significant minority. Even among 'criminal patients', those who were educated and 'accustomed to a superior mode of living' tended to outnumber people drawn from classes lacking any such special status. The lower strata of Indian communities, generally well removed from the kind of modern, largely urban-based, privileged life that was pursued by both the British colonial administration and English-educated Indian groups, was rarely present in the hospital; nor were members of the upper echelons of Indian society, who found the available facilities unsuitable. Dhunjibhoy considered Ranchi a 'modern' institution. It clearly was, in several respects; not least in catering disproportionately for the needs and purposes of the relatively well-educated, lower-to-middle levels of Indian colonial society.

Chapter 3

INSTITUTIONAL TRENDS AND STANDARDISATION: DEATHS, DISEASES AND CURES

The scientific purist, who will wait for medical statistics until they are nosologically exact, is no wiser than Horace's rustic waiting for the river to flow away [before he crosses].
—Major Greenwood, 1948

The rate and pattern of patients' mortality in mental institutions are important parameters in the assessment of clinical outcomes. They provide a way of measuring the effects of mental healthcare provision.[1] The study of death rates has been an important focus of analysis since the first half of the nineteenth century. Mortality is, of course, closely related not only to the care and attention an institution bestows on its inmates, but also its patient intake and their health status on admission. Recent research in Western countries has shown that mortality among psychiatric patients in both institutional and community-based care settings remains high. In Sweden the mortality rate for 12,103 patients in the late 1990s was three times that of the wider population;[2] a Norwegian study of psychiatric inpatients from 1980 to 1992 concluded that 'mortality of psychiatric patients is still unsatisfactorily high'[3]; and an assessment of data from seven German hospitals in the mid-1990s revealed that over six times more patients died than expected.[4] Furthermore, an Italian team of epidemiologists concluded in 1997 that:

> longer periods of hospitalization and non-discharge from hospital are the main risk factors for death in psychiatric patients, who globally experience higher death rates than the general population for a wide spectrum of causes of death, whatever their diagnosis or gender.[5]

Mortality statistics for institutions in the early twentieth century need to be considered with these issues in mind. Caution is however necessary as neither the figures for Ranchi nor those for other hospitals in British India were adjusted for age, gender and patient intake (nor were their equivalents in Britain). Ranchi's patient intake does not appear to have been more – or less – selective or reliable than any of the other institutions in British India. In contrast to Western institutions, however, the criminal element in Indian mental hospitals was more prominent; a specialist facility such as Broadmoor in England was lacking.[6] One mental institution in India that cannot by any means be compared to Ranchi, or indeed to any of the others in India, was the small European Mental

Hospital, just down the road from Dhunjibhoy's institution. Employing a very different, racially selective and class-specific admission policy, it restricted its intake to Europeans and more privileged patients of Eurasian background. Given the colonial context and the structures of power, we would expect quite different and superior conditions to have prevailed at this institution.

Mortality

In comparing various institutions' statistics with one another, as Dhunjibhoy did in 1932, a startling trend emerges. Mortality in the Ranchi Indian Mental Hospital was consistently lower, not only in contrast to a number of other institutions for Indians in northern India, but even in relation to its European counterpart. This is shown clearly in the average percentage of death from 1930 to 1932 (see Figure 3.1).

Figure 3.1. Average percentage of death to daily average of patients in different mental hospitals in British India, 1930–1932[7]

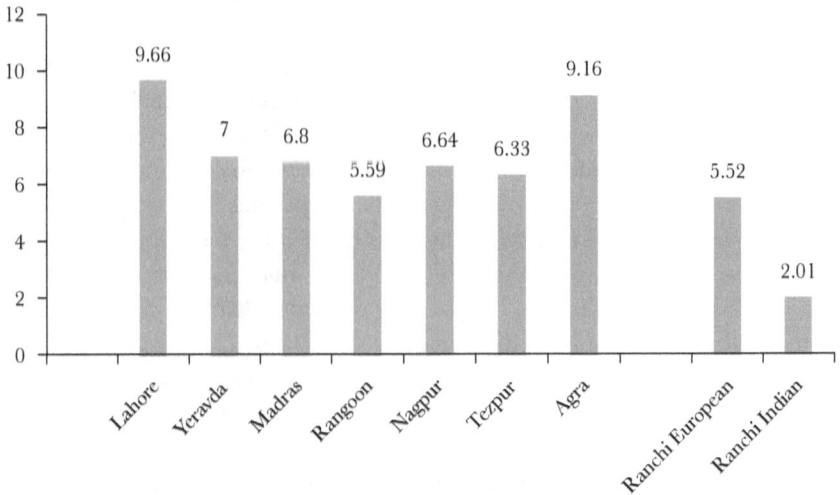

An average figure of about two per cent mortality is a great achievement – not only compared to the higher rates prevalent at other institutions, but also taking into account that mortality levels were high among the wider population. Reported and estimated rates for Bengal could amount to anything between 1.9 and 4.5 per cent.[8] A rate that is equal to or even below the one of the population at large, and less than half of the one achieved at the neighbouring European institution put the Ranchi Indian Mental Hospital into a league of its own. This was the case not only during the early 1930s, but also for the whole period that Dhunjibhoy was in charge of the hospital. The trend for Ranchi was also favourably out of step with the pattern reported for Western mental hospitals, where institutional death rates were consistently well above those in the wider population. From 1930 to 1932, the percentage of deaths in mental institutions in England and Wales was 6.76 per cent – over three times the Ranchi figure.[9]

In Western countries variable and unstable mortality rates have been observed within and between mental hospitals, in contrast to more stable rates of the general population.[10] This was evidently different in British India, where a high degree of volatility generally prevailed in both institutional data and census statistics. Census officials in India reported that provincial mortality statistics revealed 'great variation' over place and time.[11] For example, in 1909 it was noted that,

> [rates] vary greatly in different areas during the same period, and in the same areas from year to year; and while this is characteristic of the figures at all times, we have to distinguish the exaggerating effects of special morbific [*sic*] influences, such as famine.[12]

In the period from 1881 to 1900 for example, the mortality rate per 1,000 of the general population of British India fluctuated between 18.8 and 36.6. With deaths being under-reported, the recorded details were considered unreliable. A 'probable true normal rate' was therefore estimated: it amounted to an extraordinary rate of 44.8 per 1,000.[13] This was, as noted at the time, 'much above the European standards if Austria-Hungary and Italy be excluded'.[14] Mortality statistics continued to pose a challenge in subsequent censuses, not least because age-specific details were difficult to obtain. The census report for 1941 still lacked reliable data on age cohorts, which made the calculation of age-specific mortality a matter of speculation.[15]

Figures at Ranchi did of course vary over time. The annual number of deaths fluctuated between a low of 1.65 per cent in 1932 and a high of 3.49 per cent in 1935 when a locum was assigned to Ranchi while Dhunjibhoy was abroad. During the very early years of the institution, the figures were also higher. At that time, the patient profile still more closely reflected the intake and previous health status of inmates transferred from the old institutions at Dacca, Berhampore and Patna, where the combined average figure had been 4.01 per cent in 1925 and 5.06 per cent in 1925.[16] It is likely that it took Dhunjibhoy and his staff a couple of years to establish the best clinical and managerial practice to ensure a lower mortality rate in the newly founded hospital. An average rate of about 2.5 per cent from 1927 to 1939 is particularly striking in an institution that had to deal not only with the debilitating consequences of endemic malaria and the enduring prevalence of infectious respiratory diseases such as TB and pneumonia, but also, more significantly, with the sudden effects of waterborne diseases as well as sporadic influenza outbreaks. Arguably, these conditions are better dealt with in an institutional setting – provided it is set up to do so effectively. This seems to have been the case at Ranchi. Despite the statistical peaks in 1928 and 1935, Dhunjibhoy was able to happily report in 1939, just before being sent to Karachi to take up military medical duties, that his institution had 'continued the reputation of maintaining the lowest death-rate since its inception [in 1925] amongst the Indian Mental Hospitals in India'.[17] This was indeed an extraordinary achievement.

Death and Illness by Gender

No particularly strong gendered pattern emerges from disaggregating the mortality figures for Ranchi. Again this contrasts favourably with trends in Western institutions – as well as some Indian ones – where mortality rates for females were frequently higher. At the old institutions of Dacca and Berhampore, for example, figures in 1924 and 1925 were three and six per cent for men and 10 and 8 per cent for women respectively.[18] However, as rates tended to fluctuate considerably at institutions, any generalisations on gender-specific rates of death are problematic. At Ranchi, too, the number of male and female deaths varied from year to year. The trend for men remained relatively stable.[19] In contrast, the female death rate followed a slight upward trend from 1927 to 1939, which may have been due to increased overcrowding. The major exception occurred again in 1935, when the mortality rate among males and females was considerably higher, and significantly so in the case of the women.

This apparent irregularity may not necessarily be indicative of any failures on the part of the locum, J. N. J. Pacheco, who was in charge during that year. The total numbers involved were still comparatively low, with female fatalities amounting to 11 out of a total of 239 women present in the hospital during the year. The provincial health authorities did not comment on the distinct spike in mortality that was revealed in the annual report. However, they tended to ask for explanations only if a trend had emerged in an institution that consistently deviated from patterns in other places. As mentioned above, Indian doctors and authorities were used to considerable fluctuations in people's health status as an outbreak of smallpox, influenza and cholera, or drought and famine conditions, for example, could lead to sudden increases in mortality rates. Whether the raised mortality rates in 1935 are to be accounted for by epidemiological factors, random statistical variation or mismanagement on the part of the acting superintendent is difficult to ascertain.

Some suspicions remain regarding whether or not the superintendent's management of patients and staff could have been a factor in an inmate's likelihood of dying, particularly in relation to female patients. After all, Pacheco had mentioned that the general physical health of patients had been 'good', despite the hot weather of 1935 that caused cases of diarrhoea and dysentery.[20] He did report 'an increase of flies', in spite of 'all precautions taken'. He also pointed out the risk of 'infection' when patients 'irrigate the sullage water from one of the septic tank outflows'. However, first on his list of 'chief causes of deaths' were pneumonia, TB and heart failure, rather than waterborne diseases. Even the 'severe epidemic of cholera in the village of Sukurhutu behind the hospital' did not appear to have affected patients.[21] Did Pacheco fail to manage staff and patients properly? We do not know. The fact is that on Dhunjibhoy's return in 1936, mortality among men and women returned to its previous level (2.56 and 2.38 per cent respectively). This was despite a mild influenza epidemic in the male compound that put about 300 patients into the infirmary, as well as the appearance of small pox and chicken pox in 'mild epidemic form', which was 'almost endemic amongst staff children in the staff line'.[22] More importantly perhaps, Dhunjibhoy had imposed 'stringent sanitary measures with timely vaccination and segregation of contacts' that 'just enabled' him to keep the infection 'away from the patients as well as the staff'.[23] In the absence of more information, it is only possible to speculate that Pacheco may not have taken similarly effective precautionary measures to ensure patient and staff wellbeing.

The fact that Pacheco related a highly objectionable episode of racial prejudice and cruelty in an obituary in 1961 makes it difficult to put an entirely positive construction on his management of an institution dedicated to the care of 'natives'. Narrating the lucky escape of highly decorated medical officer J. J. Harper Nelson, CIE, OBE, MC, MD, FRCSEd, MRCPEd onto a life boat when the P&O ship he was sailing on was sunk by a U-boat in the English Channel, Pacheco told the readers of the *BMJ* that, 'One of the ship's officers tried to push him off with an oar, thinking he was a khalasi [a South Asian manual worker or sailor], as Nelson was black all over from oil and soot, and there was little room in the crowded boat'. Harper Nelson 'shouted out', and was 'at last recognized and taken in'. Being oblivious to the important questions raised by the British officer's attitude towards the *khalasi*, Pacheco mused instead: 'Was it coincidence, was it chance or fate, that came to his help in an impossible and extraordinary situation? I prefer to think it was the hand of Providence that mercifully extricated him from certain death.' Pacheco seems to come to an astounding conclusion as it was the British officer who decided who was to survive the ordeal; he would not have rescued a *khalasi*.

In contrast to the discriminatory attitude displayed by the British officer, Dhunjibhoy was particularly successful at keeping both male and female patients alive, more so than any of his colleagues at other institutions for Indians and at the European Mental Hospital. But even his record was not always successful. Prior to his assignment to Ranchi in 1925 Dhunjibhoy had been made superintendent at Berhampore in 1923. Mortality the next year was high, with rates of six per cent for men and eight per cent for women in 1924. Although these figures were still in line with those achieved at other institutions in India, they were considerably above those Dhunjibhoy could boast of at Ranchi once he had established stable clinical and managerial momentum there. A doctor's experience is clearly an important factor driving institutional outcomes. What is more, Berhampore was, like many of the other mental hospitals, in a severe state of dilapidation, with unsanitary and rundown facilities. Brand-new premises like those provided at Ranchi would no doubt have helped Dhunjibhoy to keep his patients in good physical condition, even during periods of austerity such as the 1920s and 1930s.

Given that the European Mental Hospital next door was only seven years older and according to one of its superintendents, Owen Berkeley-Hill, '[v]ast sums of money had been expended in erecting this fantastic asylum', buildings alone clearly cannot account for patients' chances of survival.[24] An in-depth assessment of individual institutions and of the varied factors that had a bearing on their statistics are required to enable an accurate comparison.

In contrast to the overall mortality rates, gender-specific trends emerge in relation to patients' length of confinement prior to death. A large number of those who died did so within five years of admission. This was the case in 27 per cent of men and in 36 per cent of women. We might consider the difference an indication of a more precarious health status among mentally ill women or even as evidence of inferior treatment at the institution. However, the disaggregated figures reveal that men were more likely to die within the first year of admission. This may suggest that more men than women tended to suffer from the last stages of a life-threatening disease on admission. Taking these two patterns together, it is difficult to assess whether they were indicative of gender discrimination or of gender specificity in mortality trends during the first one to five years of institutionalisation. It is also difficult to discern if parameters prior to hospital admission or inner-institutional factors are implicated. In relation to longer-term confinement trends (specifically death after five years' stay in Ranchi), women's average period of hospitalisation tended to be almost equal to men's (22 and 21 years respectively). This means that there was no gender-specific pattern once patients had survived the first five years after admission to the hospital.[25]

In regard to morbidity, the prevalent gender-specific pattern for the incidence of reported sickness can more easily be accounted for. As Figure 3.2 indicates, it varied considerably by gender.

Figure 3.2. Average percentage of sick patients admitted to the infirmary, for males (mainly upper graph) and females (mainly lower graph), for all diseases, 1927–1939

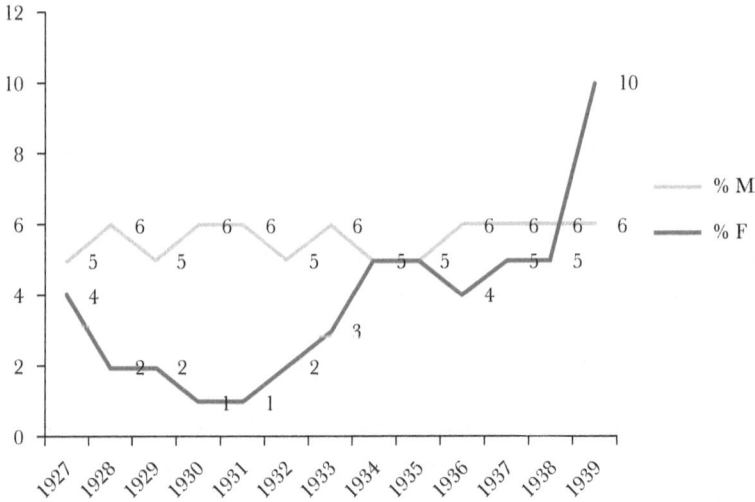

The figures for men remained relatively stable over the period, fluctuating only between five and six per cent. In contrast, those for women rose from an average of about half the male rate during 1928 to 1933 to a rate of the same order as men from 1933 and 1934 onwards. The year-to-year fluctuation among sick men is fairly negligible during most of the period. Variations can be accounted for in most cases by particular events and circumstances. The discharge or transfer to other institutions of groups of chronic patients and/or lepers in some years, for example, affected the numbers of those confined in the infirmary. This occurred in 1928 and 1931, for instance, with a dip in the number of infirmary patients reported the following year. The lower figures in 1934 might have been due to the rectification of an unsanitary enclosure the year before and the consequent impact this would have had on the prevalence of waterborne afflictions.

It is peculiar however, that sickness rates were at the lower five per cent level during the year when a sullage and drainage problem in the male compound had emerged while Dhunjibhoy was abroad in 1935. Potential sanitary hazards are therefore not necessarily always reflected in statistical trends. Other factors may have been implicated. Dhunjibhoy's locum, Dr Pacheco, had provided 'improved accommodation' for first-class paying patients by 'removing them from the dormitory they shared with those paying less, giving them each a well furnished single room in the Infirmary Block'.[26] It is possible that this restriction of accommodation in the infirmary led to the considerably lower number of patients being treated there during that particular year. This might have led to the increased number of admissions once Dhunjibhoy returned in 1936, as he seems to have been highly dedicated to the preservation of the health of his patients.

Still other factors may have been implicated in the tendency for the male sickness rate to remain at the slightly higher level of six per cent from 1936 onwards. The continued extension of cultivation and the rise in the number of patients who were employed in the paddy fields and in garden work may have been one of them. Increased irrigation presented a breeding ground for mosquitoes.[27] In addition, although the 'outfalls from the septic tanks, especially that which flows through the vegetable garden', were being treated with phenyle and kerosene oil, a 'fly nuisance' was reported during the hot season and an 'increase of mosquitoes during the rainy season' in 1935 for example.[28] Given these various changes in the wider ecology of disease, it is important to acknowledge that Dhunjibhoy and his staff managed to keep the numbers of male patients treated in the infirmary at a comparatively stable level. Of course, spatial restrictions in the infirmary would have constituted a limitation in regard to the number of patients that could be accommodated.

On the female side across the road from the male compound, the situation was less stable. Quite different circumstances prevailed here during the period. Ward occupation did not reach full capacity until 1938; any illnesses influenced by overcrowding would therefore not have had a strong effect on women until the mid-1930s. This may explain the steady increase in the number of females admitted to the infirmary from 1933 and 1934 onwards, when – apart from a one-off decrease from five to four per cent in 1936 – the female sick rate began to equal and, in 1939, surpass that on the male wards. The slight decrease in the number of sick women treated in 1936 may have been due to adjustments made by Dhunjibhoy on his return, as the considerably increased female death rate during his absence might have alerted him to take prompt action to improve conditions. Judging from the tenor of his reports, Dhunjibhoy was justly proud of his institution's reputation as the mental hospital with the most favourable patient statistics in India. Unusually high mortality and morbidity rates would certainly have led him to focus his efforts accordingly.

It seems that overcrowding was an important factor adversely affecting overall morbidity rates among both men and women. The male enclosure was congested throughout the period; the male sick rate remained at a stable level. In contrast, the female part of the institution was under-occupied during the first seven to eight years, with a correspondingly low morbidity rate. Once overcrowding began to become a feature on the female side, sickness levels among the women reached those prevalent among the men.

It is not clear what caused the very sudden rise in the female rate of illness during the last year of the period depicted in Figure 3.2, prior to Dhunjibhoy being recalled for war duty. It may be a random statistical 'blip' or it may have been related to the influenza epidemic during that year. However influenza affected both males and females on the then equally overcrowded wards; yet rates for men did not follow a similarly distinct rise in the incidence of reported illness. Dhunjibhoy did not comment on the situation, but whatever may have been the matter, it is likely that the increased pressure on accommodation for women would not have helped. Dhunjibhoy hinted at this in his report of 1938, when he noted that 'a scheme to increase the accommodation of [the female] Section by 48 beds without prejudice to the health of the inmates' was required and being considered by government.[29] The impending war made such measures unlikely.

Causes of Death

The types of diseases from which patients were reported to have died in this period varied. It is perhaps surprising that much-feared killers such as small pox, cholera and plague were rarely among them. As was the case in the Western institutions, at Ranchi the most significant causes of death prevalent in most years appear to have been respiratory diseases (TB and pneumonia), gastrointestinal conditions (dysentery and diarrhoea), debility of various kinds and unspecified other general diseases.[30]

Among these illnesses TB and pneumonia were the most commonly specified.[31] These are conditions that tend to affect particular patients who already suffer from a fragile state of health due to pre-existing illnesses. They are also highly infectious and easily transmitted in closed institutional settings, even to those of a healthy physical condition. Lacking details from individual patients' medical case notes, it is not possible to discern if these sicknesses developed on top of other conditions or constituted the immediate causes of death. It is also difficult to judge if these particular diseases were contracted inside the hospital or if they were already present when the patient was admitted. Medical practitioners suggested that the latter was the case in mental hospitals in Britain.[32] Dhunjibhoy for his part, referred to observations from England that focused on the importance of dealing with patients' physical conditions on admission, such as those expressed by 'His Majesty the King Emperor, while opening the Shenley Mental Hospital in England on 31st May 1934'.[33] Indeed, he emphasised that at Ranchi 40 per cent of 'so-called new admissions were not only suffering from chronic mental diseases but were equally bad in their physical health'.[34] In nearly every year's report, he kept reiterating that 'many were admitted in a very low state of health, markedly anaemic with consequent debility'.[35] However, the incidence of TB among new admissions may have been low, as Dhunjibhoy noted in 1934 that 'tubercle bacilli' were detected in the sputum of only two newly admitted cases out of a total of 126 that year.

In Western institutions high death rates from pneumonia and TB were frequently reported, with slow downward trends towards the late 1930s. The surgeon in charge of the female section at St Andrew's Mental Hospital in Norwich from 1922 to 1935, A. W. B. Livesay, for example, held that the steadily decreasing general mortality rate during this period correlated with the fall in deaths from phthisis or pulmonary tuberculosis. 'Two-fifths of the reduction in the death rate', he argued in an article in the *BMJ* in 1936, 'was attributed to the lessening of this disease'.[36] Dr Percy Stokes of the Department of Applied Statistics at University College London had earlier noted 'much higher mortality from tuberculosis' in mental hospitals. He alerted medical practitioners in a letter published in the *BMJ* in 1924 that this made comparisons between hospital statistics and those pertaining to the wider population problematic as inpatients tended to die from TB before they had a chance to develop any of the other diseases that affected those living outside institutions.[37] Figures for Western institutions are inconclusive though as they vary greatly. Michael, for example, refers to the steady rise of death from TB at the Denbigh Mental Hospital in North Wales during the First World War, with an average death rate of 20 per cent.[38] For the inter-war years she notes that the disease still 'presented a problem of considerable proportion'.[39] At Ranchi, 15 per cent of deaths were attributed to TB between 1926 and 1933.

The problem of death from respiratory diseases persisted well into the post–World War II period in Western countries. In the early 1950s, sex and age adjusted mortality rates (SMR) in the state mental hospitals in Michigan revealed that even in this period, death from pneumonia and tuberculosis among patients was about 30 and 13 times respectively as high as in the general population.[40] Death from tuberculosis among mental patients has become rare in modern institutions. Pneumonia, however, still figures highly, alongside cardiovascular disorders. Hewer et al., for example, have shown in 1995 that in seven psychiatric hospitals in Germany roughly one half of deaths were due to these two conditions.[41]

The Ranchi data appear to roughly chime with mortality trends prevalent in Western institutions in regard to TB and pneumonia. These diseases were assigned as causes of death in a significant number of cases, namely 41 and 21 respectively (out of a total of 272 deaths during the period from 1926 to 1933). Together with other illnesses of the respiratory system, the number amounted to 69 (or 25 per cent) of all classified causes of death (see 'airborne' in Figure 3.3). This is in contrast to 26 deaths (or 10 per cent) caused by a variety of parasitic and waterborne illnesses.

Figure 3.3. Mortality: Aggregate disease categories and diseases assigned to those who died, in per cent, 1926–1933

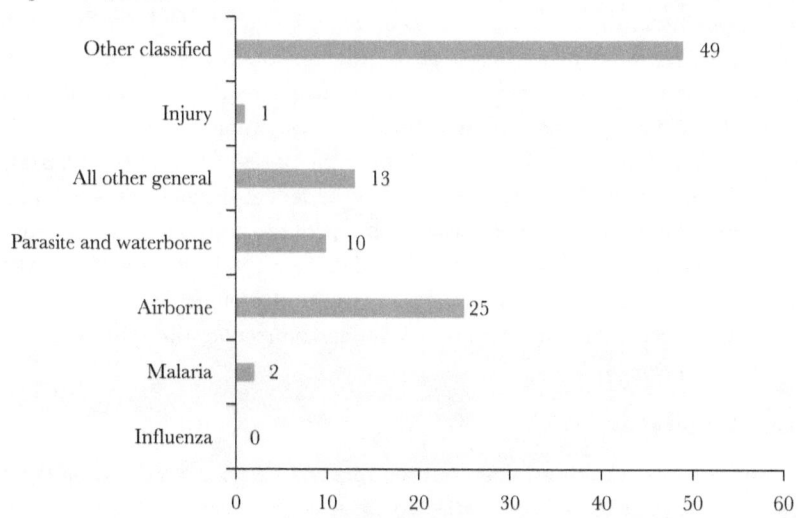

The high number and great variety of the remaining causes of death and their variability from year to year make comparisons between institutions more difficult. Nearly half (49 per cent) of all deaths were due to other causes than those specified in the table above. In other institutions the data were no less diverse. This may have been due partly to epidemiological factors as well as variation in classification within and between institutions. Despite worldwide attempts to make mortality diagnostics more uniform, at least some of the disease categories were used inconsistently such as in the case of General Paralysis of the Insane (GPI), the occurrence of which among Indians Dhunjibhoy had first denied and later confirmed. The contemporary system of listing specific conditions such as encephalitis lethargica, kala-azar and leprosy alongside wide-ranging ones, such as general debility and senility, as well as basing some categories on the symptoms observed (diarrhoea) and others on the identification of the location of disease (diseases of the circulatory system, for example), does not in itself constitute a barrier to inter-institutional or longitudinal comparisons. However, as we cannot ascertain their consistent use by practitioners, it is difficult to determine with confidence any differential mortality patterns and changes over time.

There is however evidence of attempts at a greater degree of precision in the identification of the causes of death as the residual category 'all other general diseases' was no longer a category that figured prominently in the designation of the main causes of death towards the late 1930s. Whether developments in laboratory diagnostics and post-mortem techniques during the 1930s had an impact on this trend or whether it was due to a more diligent application of a wider range of disease categories suggested in the various versions of the International List of Causes of Death (ICD) is again difficult to judge on the basis of currently available historical data. Dhunjibhoy does not comment on these aspects either.

The gradual disappearance of anaemia, for example, as a main cause of death indicates the recognition of the varied causes underlying it. Increased diagnostic precision and better use of laboratory testing prior to a patient's death may have also been factors. In addition, Dhunjibhoy's attention to patients' diet may have eliminated anaemia caused by deficient nutrition, which was particularly common among those whose staple food prior to hospital admission consisted of not much else but polished rice. The focus on the treatment of parasitic worms that patients presented on admission and the increasing use of ankylostomiasis (hookworm) as a separate category, for example, would have also contributed to the disappearance of anaemia as a cause of death.

The less frequent use of debility as one of the main causes of death from 1928 onwards raises further important issues. As in the case of anaemia, debility described a general condition or weakness that could be caused by many things and could be concomitant on a person's advanced age. Prior to the mid-twentieth century the term asthenia was used in similarly inconclusive ways. Cases of debility were still identified in relation to elderly patients, as when general debility was referred to in connection with senility.

Towards Standardisation

It is necessary to keep in mind that considerable changes occurred during the 1920s and 1930s in regard to the categories to be used for the registration of deaths.

Not all clinicians may have been up to date with these.[42] The debate on taxonomies of causes of death can be traced back to Francois Bossier de Sauvages de Lacroix's (1706–1777) *Nosologia Methodica*, Linnaeus's (1707–1778) *Genera Morborum* and William Cullen's (1710–1790) *Synopsis Nosologiae Methodicae*, if not John Graunt's (1620–1674) work on the 'Bills of Mortality'. Drawing mainly on Cullen's categories, William Farr (1807–1883), statistician in the General Register Office of England and Wales, developed a classification for the International Statistical Congress (1853 in Brussels, 1855 in Paris). His nomenclature of the Causes of Death was arranged into five groups:

(1) Epidemic
(2) Constitutional (general)
(3) Local (by anatomical site)
(4) Developmental
(5) Result of violence

This system, however incongruous it may appear to us now, constituted an important step towards standardisation. It eventually informed – alongside French, German and Swiss nomenclature – the development under Jacques Bertillon (1851–1922), of the Statistical Services of Paris, of the International List of Causes of Death. This list was to result in the modern International Classification of Diseases (ICD), a standardised and regularly revised classification system that now encompasses not only causes of death (mortality) but also diseases and injuries (morbidity).[43] The process of standardisation – however conceptually fraught and contested its various metamorphoses may have been (and are still considered to be) – dealt with the even more unsatisfactory situation prior to 1893, before Bertillon's system was adopted by some countries. A commentator in the *BMJ* remarked in 1927: 'As late as 1893 no two countries in the world used exactly the same forms and methods for the statistical classification of the causes of death.'[44]

The shortcomings of the system, clearly detectable also in the Ranchi data, were widely acknowledged. It was argued that it did 'not pose as an academic or scientific classification or proper nomenclature of *diseases*, but is intended to be a practical working list whereby the compilers of statistics can correctly tabulate the causes of death'.[45] Bertillon's system was the best that was available at the time and it constituted an improvement on previous practices. His manual was adapted for use in England and Wales in 1911 and for Scotland and Northern Ireland in 1926.[46] Absolute uniformity was not guaranteed as each country exercised a 'certain amount of latitude in adapting to its own special requirements the model of an abridged list' provided by Bertillon.[47] It is difficult to construct 'a satisfactory classification of diseases on the ever-shifting sands of medical knowledge', as a commentator in the *BMJ* put it. For our insight into morbidity and mortality patterns prevalent at Ranchi, too, considerable problems arise as 'there is a considerable difference between a nomenclature of diseases classified as far as may be possible on a scientific basis and a list of causes of death'.[48]

Nosologies, diagnostics and medical statistics have improved but are still far from perfect. However, as White has pointed out:

> If some clinicians have come to think that 'making a diagnosis' is more important than helping the patient to ameliorate or resolve his problems, so some epidemiologists may have been unduly concerned with descriptive and observational precision. Both mistake ends for means.[49]

Historians of medicine may also wish to heed White's contention, especially in view of the fact that Major Greenwood's important comment of 1948 continues to be referred to by modern medical epidemiologists, medical statisticians and clinicians.[50] Greenwood's statement serves well as a preface for this chapter as a whole and particularly for the examination of Dhunjibhoy's data from Ranchi.

Mortality and Morbidity

As the health researcher and medical historian Guenther Risse noted, diseases are never 'static' but subject to a 'shifting ecology of disease', whereby 'sickness shifts constantly in specific ecological settings', influenced by physical and social agents.[51] If we follow this biosocial and ecological proposition, we need to place any particular disease and its reported incidence into the context of all the others that 'form part of a specific panorama of diseases'.[52] Risse refers to the case of plague in fourteenth-century Europe as a disease with an increased incidence, juxtaposed to others that apparently diminished as 'individuals died of the plague before they could die of leprosy', for instance.[53] On the other hand, lower mortality rates from infectious diseases may lead to a higher number of people surviving and becoming afflicted with chronic problems and common endemic or sporadic ailments. A comparison of the various illnesses implicated in mortality and morbidity figures at Ranchi is therefore important. Of course, we need to be mindful of caveats, such as changing meanings and definitions of particular disease categories and the vagaries of record keeping. A comparison is however still bound to generate, at the very least, some guiding questions for future in-depth analysis of patients' case files and potentially further more nuanced statistical assessment.

In the following analysis the terms 'other classified diseases', 'airborne' and 'parasite/waterborne' will be used as descriptors to assess particular institutional disease trends in relation to their mode of transmission and the adequacy of the measures taken to deal with them (see Figure 3.4). These terms were not employed in the mental hospital reports. 'Airborne diseases' encompass TB, pneumonia, and all other general respiratory diseases, while the 'parasite/waterborne' label refers to dysentery, diarrhoea, all other diseases of the digestive system, all other diseases of the intestinal system, and ankylostomiasis (hookworm). These aggregate categories and the contemporary disease designations subsumed under them are of course highly selective, as they include only a few of the diseases explicated in Dhunjibhoy's reports. Their selection is informed by modern debates sparked by McKeown in the 1950s regarding the causes of the decline of mortality in Britain.[54] During the 1980s in particular, these debates focused on the role that public health measures played in the rise of population in European countries during the modern period, with emphasis on the mode of disease transmission and incidence and related mortality patterns of airborne in contrast to waterborne illnesses. However, the specific diseases included in McKeown's categorisation are not identical with those selected here for the analysis of trends in the Ranchi mental hospital.

Figure 3.4. Morbidity: Aggregate disease categories and diseases assigned to those admitted to the infirmary, in per cent, 1926–1933

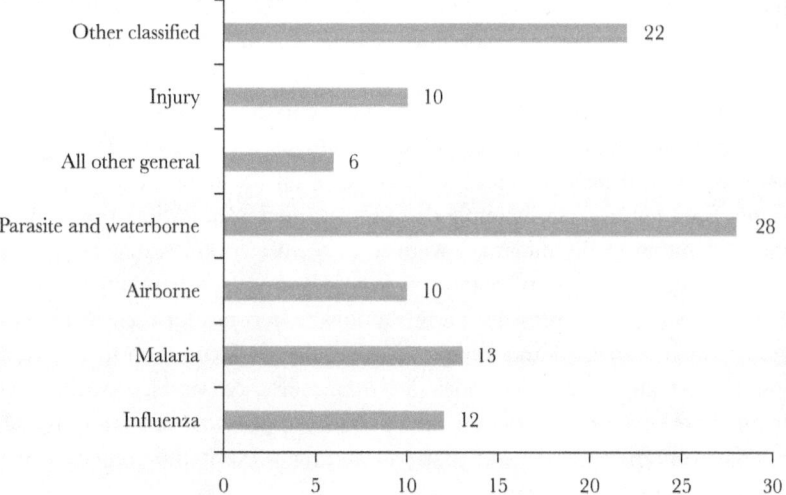

The attempt to fit some of the diseases from Dhunjibhoy's reports into labels used by modern historians and epidemiologists may be considered anachronistic. The debates on these labels were at the time politically sensitive in the UK, as they related to controversies surrounding the role of the state in the provision of public health measures during Margaret Thatcher's period as prime minister (1979–90). However, the airborne versus waterborne discussion also mirrors earlier concerns. In Britain the response to Chadwick's report of 1842 on *The Sanitary Conditions of the Labouring Population*, during a period of political upheaval, for example, was no less politically heated. The debates preceding the transfer of responsibility for public health and welfare from central to local governments in British India in the 1930s provided the context for further engagement with the priorities to be set by authorities. Furthermore, in India the paradigm of airborne contagion among medical professionals persisted well into the early twentieth century, longer than it did in Britain. The analytical juxtaposition of 'airborne' and 'parasite/waterborne' diseases therefore seems justified on account of a number of historical, historiographical and methodological reasons. Focusing on the mode of transmission of particular diseases enables us to assess if the preventative and curative measures taken at the time were likely to have been successful.

In contrast to 'other classified diseases', which is used as a descriptive umbrella term here, the category of 'all other general disease' was one specified in the International List of Causes of Death (1909, 1938)[55] and employed in Ranchi's reports in relation to causes of both death and sickness. It figures much less prominently in regard to illnesses than deaths, namely in only six per cent of cases of illness, in contrast to 13 per cent of cases of death. While this residual category was employed throughout the period in regard to mortality, it was not used in relation to sickness until 1930. We are therefore dealing with an artefact of categorisation rather than any difference in reported incidence. This imposes further restrictions on the analysis of this as well as the remaining categories used at different times between 1926 and 1933.

The spectrum of diseases people die from does not necessarily reflect the afflictions they may suffer from. Not surprisingly, the incidence of some illnesses at Ranchi differed considerably from the causes of death in the mortality statistics. In addition, as shown in Figures 3.3 and 3.4, a smaller range of reported diseases led to treatment in the infirmary than to death, that is, the individual diseases reported in the sick lists are fewer in number. This is indicated in the tables by the percentage rate for 'other classified diseases', which is 22 per cent for infirmary patients but 49 per cent for attributed causes of death. The discrepancy does not necessarily imply that patients died from a wider range of illnesses than those admitted to the infirmary were seen to suffer from. It may simply indicate that post-mortem assessments were more precise and varied, perhaps not least due to the fact that there was greater pressure on institutions to account for their dead. With two exceptions ('other classified' and 'airborne'), the illnesses focused on in Figure 3.4 are clearly more relevant to reported morbidity than mortality (see Figure 3.3). Given the greater variety of assigned causes of death, it is more appropriate to focus our analysis of Ranchi's data on reported morbidity patterns and the preventative and curative actions taken by staff to ameliorate them.

In regard to some of the diseases subsumed under the descriptive labels of 'airborne' and 'parasite and waterborne' diseases respectively, the pattern is reversed in relation to their significance in the death and morbidity statistics. Twenty-five per cent of those who died had been diagnosed as having been afflicted by airborne illnesses. Yet only 10 per cent of individuals on the sick list were reported to have suffered from these. In contrast, only 10 per cent were reported to have died from parasitic and waterborne illnesses, while 28 per cent of those sent to the infirmary were treated for these. This supports the suggestion that the diseases people are reported to have died from may be different from those commonly diagnosed in patients admitted to the hospital for treatment.

Another distinct difference of incidence patterns in the mortality and morbidity figures relates to influenza, malaria, and injury. These were not prominent among those who died. Influenza was particularly notable among patients in the infirmary (12 per cent); yet no patient was reported to have died from it. The recurrent, nearly annual bouts of influenza appear to have been benign in contrast to the strains that caused such extraordinarily high fatality rates around the globe in 1918–19. There were similar trends for malaria, as only around two per cent of deaths were directly attributed to it, while 13 per cent of those diagnosed as ill suffered from this affliction, which was endemic in Ranchi's vicinity and great parts of its patient catchment area. In both cases, the conditions may have caused further complications and secondary afflictions, leading to different causes of death being assigned.

Disease Prevalence

Three major trends in relation to morbidity can be discerned from the annual hospital reports. One relates to the impact of influenza epidemics and malaria; the second to the correlation between these two trends and overcrowding; and the third to the link between the extension of agricultural activity and particular diseases, such as malaria and parasitic/water-borne illnesses.

Influenza and malaria

As Figure 3.5 shows, influenza had a prominent presence at Ranchi. This may come as a surprise as places like India were, and to a certain extent still are, considered to be breeding grounds for allegedly 'typically tropical' illnesses such as cholera, smallpox, malaria and a range of waterborne diseases. What is more, influenza had in its pandemic form been considered to have originated in Spain and was, in its annual non-pandemic manifestation, part of the usual range of infections such as measles, chickenpox and scarlet fever, contracted by people in Western, temperate climates. Influenza epidemics were reported at Ranchi in 1931, 1936 and 1939, when about a quarter of patients (that is, 27, 23 and 22 per cent respectively) in the infirmary suffered from it. It was however also present during most years from 1925 to 1940 apart from 1926 and 1934, when only few cases were reported.

Figure 3.5. Percentage of patients admitted to the infirmary for influenza, by gender, 1927–1935

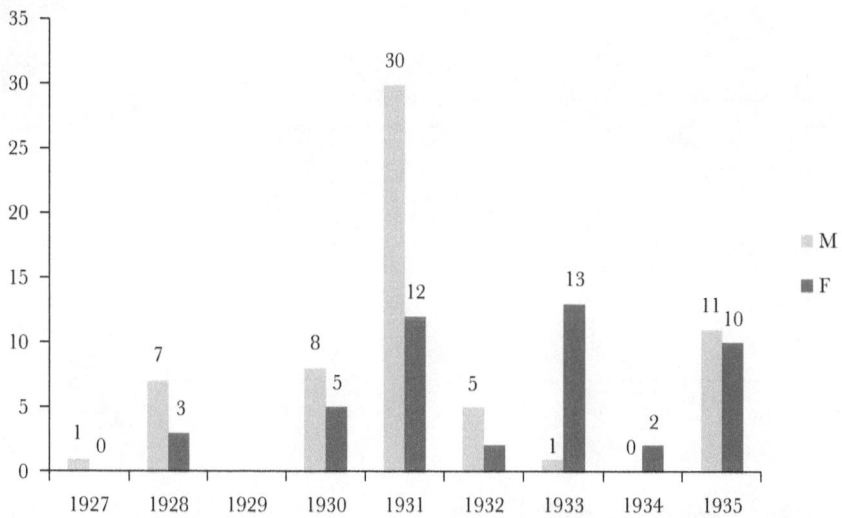

Note: No separate data for male and female patients for 1929 was available. The percentage for men and women combined is four per cent.

Influenza thrives in overcrowded surroundings. The gender-specific data confirm the correlation between overcrowding on the wards and higher prevalence of infectious disease requiring admission to the infirmary. Although there is a lack of gender-specific data for 1929 and the late 1930s, Figure 3.5 indicates that until 1933 the incidence of hospital admissions on account of influenza was consistently lower for women. Subsequently overcrowding became an increasingly severe problem on the female wards.

As previously noted, other factors such as drainage and water supply problems had an impact on overall disease rates on a year by year basis as part of the 'ecological panorama' within which a highly infectious disease such as influenza and other illnesses were thriving. It is difficult to pinpoint the role of any one particular illness or environmental factor in admissions to the infirmary. Patients may have suffered from 'co-infection' of a variety of illnesses, while only the seemingly most prevalent one would have been entered in the records. Dhunjibhoy himself hinted at this in regard to influenza and malaria in 1939. Referring to it as a 'slight rise in sickness' that year, (indicated by the six per cent illness rate in Figure 3.6), Dhunjibhoy attributed the increase to the outbreak of malaria and influenza in what he considered a 'mild epidemic form'. He made a 'very interesting clinical observation', namely that 'those patients with latent malaria in them also suffered from Malaria during the Influenza attack showing that the latent malaria was actually lighted up in those cases by Influenza'.[56]

Figure 3.6. Percentage of sick treated in the infirmary out of total number of both male and female patients at Ranchi, based on average daily number, 1927–1939

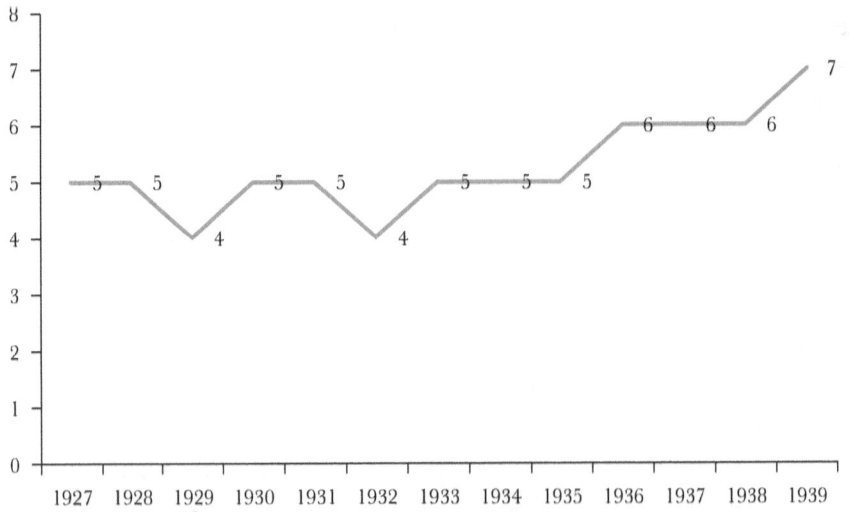

Malaria was endemic not only in Ranchi but also in most of its catchment area. A high prevalence of the disease among in-patients is therefore not surprising. The overall incidence of this condition among all mental hospital patients is of course likely to have been much more significant than the infirmary admission numbers suggest. Only the most severe cases were admitted to the infirmary. Unfortunately no details were provided in the reports on the average incidence rates of conditions among the wider hospital population. As far as infirmary patients were concerned, malaria rates began to stabilise briefly around four to five per cent before rising steadily to 14 per cent in 1935 (see Figure 3.7). Given the considerable extension of agriculture from that year onwards, it is likely that the figures would have risen further towards the late 1930s.

Figure 3.7. Percentage of infirmary patients admitted on account of malaria, 1927–1935

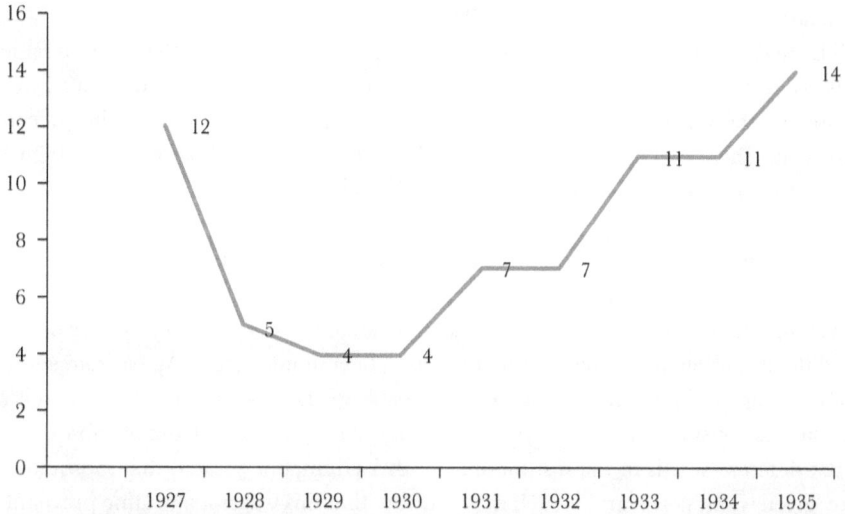

The relationship between agriculture and malaria was discussed extensively by Dhunjibhoy in his report of 1933. Referring to the increased number of patients who had contracted malaria in 1931, 1932 and 1933, he noted that '[a]ll practical measures were adopted to prevent the breeding of mosquitoes inside as well as outside the hospital area by the sanitary squads of the hospital under the direct supervision of the Second Assistant Superintendent and myself'.[57] However, he had to concede that:

> In spite of all stringent sanitary measures to prevent the breeding of mosquitoes, no satisfactory results were achieved on account of the vastness of the breeding grounds (paddy-fields) in the immediate vicinity of the hospital, which always remained a source of danger.[58]

Dhunjibhoy continued to explain that the situation was made worse due to:

> a small area within the male enclosure [that] also proved a great menace to the health of the patients of the blocks situated in close proximity of this insanitary area. On account of the deficient drainage in this area, the water stagnates and it helps the breeding of mosquitoes.

Dhunjibhoy appears to have kept track of the situation, contending that 'Statistics show that nearly 50 per cent of the positive Malaria cases […] were contributed by this insanitary area in the male enclosure'.[59]

In view of these circumstances, the mental hospital management committee recommended to government that work should be undertaken at a cost of Rs.1,180, so that 'adequate drainage in this area' could be provided.[60] The incidence rate for malaria could consequently be contained – but only for a year. The continued extension of agricultural work at Ranchi was too great during the late 1930s to prevent the occurrence of malaria among patients above the 10 per cent level.

The high malaria rate prior to 1928 appears to have been due to the fact that patients transferred from the old institutions suffered disproportionately from malaria as well as diseases of the digestive system. This was revealed in the reports from the preceding years, when these two categories accounted between them for 52 per cent of all illnesses leading to admission to the infirmary in 1926.[61] Dhunjibhoy pointed out that those who had arrived from Berhampore were 'heavily infected' with malaria, while the inspector-general of civil hospitals, H. Ainsworth, referred to a 'certain amount of malaria chiefly among patients transferred from Berhampur and Dacca'.[62]

Malaria rates varied according to gender and fluctuated considerably from year to year. It is difficult to speculate what factors may have been implicated.[63] Apart from sporadic local drainage problems and the impact of possible gender-specific co-infections, it is also necessary to consider day-to-day preventative measures, such as the use of mosquito nets on the different wards in the institution. In 1925 Dhunjibhoy stated that mosquito nets were 'given when necessary', which may indicate that this was not a routine preventative measure – at least not during the early years of his superintendence.[64] Practical problems with compliance may have also arisen, especially in the case of highly disturbed, paranoid or violent patients who might have experienced sleeping under netting as fearsome and restrictive.[65]

Airborne diseases

Among the other illnesses that are assumed to thrive in overcrowded environments are airborne diseases (such as pneumonia, TB, and other respiratory infections). Given the severe space limitations on the male wards throughout the period and on the female side increasingly from 1933–34 onwards, we would expect that this would have had an impact on the number of patients being treated in the infirmary. However, the airborne diseases accounted for only 10 per cent of all cases requiring treatment from 1927 and 1939. Their individual incidence among all inmates between 1927 and 1935 did not reach more than about one per cent each in the case of TB and pneumonia; no data is available for the late 1930s. It might well be that the individual figures increased during this period due to overcrowding on the women's wards. However, any rise due to accommodation problems is likely to have not been more than around a one per cent increase, given that continual overcrowding in the male section did not cause the incidence rates of pneumonia and TB to rise above the one per cent level. The available data for TB and pneumonia are in fact so negligible that no sensible gender-specific comparison can be made.

At three per cent, the reported incidence of 'all other diseases of the respiratory system' among infirmary patients was however somewhat higher and clear gender-specific differences are evident.[66] Alas, accommodation-related patterns can be identified on the basis of these figures for neither males nor females. The rate for men fluctuated more, between a maximum of eight per cent and a minimum of one per cent. In contrast, the likelihood of women being admitted to the infirmary remained at a relatively consistent level of three per cent, excluding 1927 (when the morbidity pattern was still influenced by the patient intake from the old institutions) and 1931 (when the influenza epidemic may have led to a decrease in the number of other airborne illnesses). This highlights the importance of assessing any one disease in relation to all others. The reported incidence of other respiratory diseases between 1927 and 1935 consistently correlated inversely with pneumonia. In 1928, when no case of pneumonia required treatment in the infirmary, 80 patients were admitted with severe respiratory problems. The following year there were six pneumonia patients and only 35 with other respiratory diseases. Conversely, the incidence of respiratory diseases peaked in 1930, with 96 patients, while there were only three pneumonia cases. The staggered year by year pattern of these two conditions suggests that at least some of those patients diagnosed with other respiratory diseases might have come down with pneumonia in the following year.

As pointed out earlier, mortality and morbidity rates need to be assessed in tandem. Deaths from pneumonia for example, reached a peak of six cases in 1928 (in contrast to a yearly average of three from 1927 to 1933). No cases of pneumonia were reported, but 80 patients suffered from other respiratory diseases. To complicate the situation further, different diagnostic practices may also have had an impact, as the incidence of pneumonia increased rapidly in 1935 to a hitherto unprecedented level of 13 reported cases (and just six cases of other respiratory diseases), when Dhunjibhoy's locum, Pacheco, was in charge. And in 1930, the year when the number of respiratory cases peaked and a lower incidence of pneumonia was reported, another locum (P. C. Das) managed the institution.

If 1928 was a bad year for fatalities from pneumonia and TB, 1929 was the year in which an increased number of patients, 6 and 19 respectively, were sent to the infirmary for these conditions. Significantly, it was also in 1928 and 1929 when Dhunjibhoy reported a severe shortage of accommodation.[67] Consequently, fewer patients were admitted to the institution.[68] It may well be that the provision of 50 emergency beds freed up space on the wards, leading to a decrease of male patients suffering from airborne diseases in the subsequent two years, 1930 and 1931.[69] The number of TB and pneumonia patients decreased to one quarter and one third respectively of the numbers reported in 1929. This was only a temporary reprieve though, as figures began to rise again from 1933 onwards. This increase may have been due to accommodation problems re-surfacing on the male wards and becoming pressing concerns also among women.

It might be considered ill-conceived to linger on the assessment of a group of diseases that figured comparatively little among the others in the statistics, affecting only 10 per cent of infirmary patients and around one per cent of all patients at Ranchi in the case of pneumonia and TB and around three per cent in relation to other respiratory diseases. However, pneumonia and TB were at the time the single most commented on diseases among psychiatrists in Western institutions. Dhunjibhoy too must have been influenced by this preoccupation with particular airborne diseases in medical literature, as he commented on these disproportionately to their actual occurrence at Ranchi. A cursory reading of the reports could cause us to assume that the two diseases constituted a major problem in India also. However, in 1934, for example, 'tuberculosis of the lungs' totalled only 13 cases (eight being bacteriologically and the rest clinically positive) while the three most prevalent categories of disease were 'all other diseases of the digestive system' (178), malaria (140) and ankylostomiasis (90), alongside 105 injuries that required treatment.[70] Despite its low incidence, TB was the only disease Dhunjibhoy singled out for specific comment, noting that among the newly admitted patients 'some were treated as suspected cases of Tuberculosis of the Lungs'.[71] In fact, part of the rationale for explaining the prominence of TB and pneumonia in the mortality statistics was that newly admitted patients suffered from 'poor physical health'. During the 1920s this poor health was apparently due to anaemia and debility, both considered by Dhunjibhoy to be 'the result of chronic malaria'. During the 1930s it was primarily related to TB and pneumonia. Indeed, a substantial number of patients died from these afflictions soon after admission to Ranchi.[72]

The higher prevalence of TB and pneumonia in Ranchi's mortality in contrast to its morbidity may have influenced Dhunjibhoy's perception of the relative importance of different diseases. Airborne diseases such as pneumonia, TB and general diseases of the respiratory system were responsible for one quarter of deaths. Alongside cure-rates, mortality statistics were the single most important way in which an institution's efficacy was assessed. Like other superintendents, Dhunjibhoy's mind, too, would have been focused not only on keeping mortality low but also on providing a rationale for the prevalence of the diseases most likely leading to patients' death.

The prolonged persistence of the medical paradigm concerning the airborne mode of disease causation among medical practitioners in India, in contrast to those in Western countries, may have been another important factor. Medical professionals with long-standing colonial experience as well as the wider European public in India considered the free circulation of fresh air and maintaining distance from crowded and foul-smelling unsanitary places vital to the preservation of good bodily and psychological health. Issues of race and the British upper- and middle-class ambition to ensure social, and hence spatial, distance from the living spaces of those considered to be inferior constituted the wider context within which the airborne transmission paradigm flourished.

Dhunjibhoy was also familiar with the global situation. The hierarchy of the colonial medical service may have had an impact here too. The inspectors general of civil hospitals, who scrutinised the annual reports before referring them to the attention of the secretary to the government, were always high-ranking British medical officers, such as Lt. Col. H. Stott, OBE, MD, FRCP, DPH, IMS in 1936. Stott may not have had an intimate expert knowledge of all branches of medicine, but he would at least have been familiar with persistent trends and debates in Western psychiatric institutions and other specialist hospitals. Given that promotion prospects depended on one's superiors' goodwill and positive evaluation, Dhunjibhoy would have been wise to act in accordance with what he thought they might have wanted to hear. Considering that concerns about TB and pneumonia in psychiatric hospitals figured highly in the medical literature,

Stott might well have expected superintendents to comment on these particular diseases. The establishment of a TB sanatorium in the vicinity of Ranchi would no doubt also have focused local medical practitioners' attention on this condition. In 1936, Dhunjibhoy even acknowledged the 'valuable advice and help in some intricate cases of tuberculosis' by Dr D. G. Muthu of the TB Sanatorium at Ranchi.[73]

Given their prominence in Western countries and within an administrative setting that focused on the reduction of death rates, the tendency to comment on airborne diseases may be understandable. To a certain extent this masked the much higher, yet not quite as fatal, incidence of waterborne diseases in the institution that affected 28 per cent of those admitted to the infirmary.

Waterborne and parasitic diseases

It could be argued that it was easier to prevent waterborne diseases than it was to keep those suffering from TB and pneumonia alive during a period when no effective drugs were available for them. TB and pneumonia constituted a greater potential threat to patients' lives and a bigger challenge for superintendents than those diseases that could be prevented through means of careful management of water supply, drainage and hygiene, and, if all else failed, treatment in the infirmary. This is not to say that parasites and waterborne diseases were not a major threat to Indian patients' and Europeans' health in India. They were highly prominent in institutional morbidity statistics and *Raj* folklore, and they still figure in modern tourists' accounts of episodes of 'Delhi belly', for example. Some of these diseases such as dysentery and ankylostomiasis (not to speak of cholera), can result in long-term deterioration of health and eventual death. Dhunjibhoy did not manage to bring down their high incidence rates, let alone eradicate them, but kept them sufficiently under control by means of attention to food and water safety, and drainage measures, which prevented the high morbidity figures from translating into increased death rates. Sanitation, drainage and water supply problems were mentioned in the reports – most frequently in relation to requests for funding of measures required to deal with them. It seems, however, that there existed a tacit understanding that dysentery, bowel complaints and worms were common problems in India that required sanitary attention, but not much epidemiological explanation.

As much as sanitary and hygiene measures may have been considered a basic necessity that did not require any particular medical discussion and justification, their implementation on the ground was time-consuming and highly dependent on the people skills of the officer in charge. It required a good working relationship with those members of staff who were entrusted with coordinating and supervising the groups of cleaning and sewage disposal workers who lived with their families in the 'sweeper lines' adjacent to the institution. Furthermore, because of the proximity of the servants' quarters to the patients' enclosures it was just as important to control hygiene measures among employees. This required considerable delicacy of judgement to ensure compliance and avoid resistance to what could be construed as interference in private family matters. Dhunjibhoy was highly successful in managing these aspects via his subordinate staff, as is attested by the low mortality rates at Ranchi. He was also well aware of the importance of a good relationship with and support by subordinate staff, making a point of frequently praising them in his reports.

The diseases subsumed here for ease of analysis under the label of 'waterborne and parasitic diseases' accounted for nearly one third of the cases admitted to the infirmary. There was, however, considerable variation in the incidence of the individual conditions. Dysentery, for example, was reported as rarely as some of the airborne diseases, amounting to not quite two per cent on average from 1927 to 1935, with the maximum number of cases in 1927, when patients had recently been transferred from the old institutions. This compares to the figure from Denbigh Mental Hospital, where periodical outbreaks of dysentery were observed to be at a rate of 3.8 per cent in 1931. However, reported rates were lower by a factor of ten in all mental hospitals in England and Wales combined, namely 0.35 per cent in 1931.[74]

In contrast, the incidence of all other diseases of the digestive system was more substantial, with an average of six per cent. Here a pronounced rise occurred from 1934 onwards, when the rates reached 14 and 13 per cent in 1934 and 1935 respectively. Like the Denbigh Mental Hospital, Ranchi suffered badly from sanitary and hygiene problems – although bad at Ranchi, they compared relatively well with other institutions. Men were more affected during these years than women, as 16 per cent of males in contrast to only six per cent of females were treated in the infirmary for severe digestive problems in 1934. Dhunjibhoy did not comment on the reasons for the rise during the mid-1930s. The rectification of the 'unsanitary area in the male enclosure' in 1933 clearly did not have a positive effect on the waterborne diseases (and only temporarily on malaria cases as the breeding ground of mosquitoes was restricted).[75] Pressures on accommodation and spatial limitations could not have been responsible for the higher incidence of dysentery cases either, as conditions here remained as congested as ever. It is likely that the extension of patients' engagement in agriculture along with the sullage overflow into the vegetable garden reported by Pacheco in 1935 were major factors.[76] In fact, the incidence of ankylostomiasis and intestinal conditions also rapidly increased in 1934.

Clearly, drainage, hygiene and water problems, and increased agricultural activity had an immediate impact on the health of patients, leading to sudden rises in disease incidence. Pacheco had referred to the 'probable source of infection' in the garden, where, he noted, 'patients irrigate the sullage water' from the septic tank outflow. To 'minimise' the danger of disease, 'precautions were taken to make all those working in the garden wash their hands and feet in a solution of phenyle at the conclusion of work'.[77] The septic tank outflows, 'especially that which flows through the vegetable garden, were constantly treated with a solution of phenyle [disinfectant] and kerosene oil [insecticide]'.[78] Pacheco noted in 1930 that he 'now' made this 'a routine measure'; it seems to have had a positive effect on hookworm and intestinal disease, but not on dysentery, digestive problems or malaria.[79]

Three categories among the waterborne and parasitic diseases, namely diarrhoea, ankylostomiasis and intestinal disease, show perhaps the most intriguing patterns. The incidence for diarrhoea correlated inversely with those for all other intestinal diseases and ankylostomiasis. This is due to the fact that diarrhoea as a disease category was no longer being used from 1931 onwards. In that same year hookworm appears for the first time as a classification in the sickness reports (although it had been known prior to this date – in 1928 a female patient was reported to have died from it).[80] Similarly, the category of 'all other diseases of the intestinal system' began to appear in the reports from 1931. In this case, it had previously been referred to in relation to patients transferred from the old institutions, but not from 1928 to 1930. This is not to suggest that the new ankylostomiasis and intestinal diseases took over from the old diarrhoea category. In fact, those diseases in which diarrhoea constituted the main symptom, such as dysentery, would have been more likely candidates. However, the dysentery pattern does not show an inverse correlation with the discontinued diarrhoea classification. Other diseases may have been implicated in the change from a category based on symptomatic description (diarrhoea) to aetiologically and anatomically based designations (such as hookworm and intestinal diseases). It seems however justified to suggest that towards the later 1930s more precision was employed in the diagnosis of particular conditions. The fact that from 1933 onwards hookworm and roundworm were listed separately under the new rubric of animal parasites is yet another indication of this process.[81]

The increased diversification and greater precision of the disease labels used is mirrored in and, to an extent, caused by the greater emphasis on laboratory testing from 1930 onwards. The number of blood, urine, stool and sputum samples examined in the hospital laboratory was diligently recorded in the annual reports. In 1930, for example, 319, 328, 141 and 109 samples respectively of these bodily fluids were investigated. From 1931 Dhunjibhoy provided specific details in relation to malaria and TB, as to whether the reported cases were bacteriologically or clinically positive. During that year, out of the 85 malaria cases 19 were the former and 66 the latter; while for the five TB patients the figures were four and one respectively.[82] In 1934, dysentery began to be differentiated into amoebic and bacillary. It is at this stage that the number of cases of dysentery, hookworm, and intestinal and digestive diseases increased significantly. While the sullage problems reported in 1935 and more extensive agriculture may have been partly responsible for the highly increased numbers, the attention paid to laboratory testing during the same period may have also facilitated the identification of the actual incidence of particular diseases. Changes in the number of reported cases may therefore reveal modifications in medical technology rather than variations in disease patterns.

It may also be of significance that major changes in disease classifications occurred in 1931, the year that Dhunjibhoy returned from an extended overseas visit. Engagement with practices abroad may have encouraged him to adopt them back home in Ranchi. During this period the ICD classifications and their local adaptations changed also, so that it is not clear which factor was more decisive in bringing about greater precision of medical nomenclature. It is likely that both were influential.

Given that Dhunjibhoy was so determined to implement the latest insights and techniques at Ranchi, it is puzzling that he did not identify ankylostomiasis among his ill patients until 1931. Hookworm was very common in tropical countries, having been identified as early as 1838 (then referred to as chlorosis by Theodor Bilharz in 1852), and was linked with severe anaemia. It had also received much attention in the medical literature when Italian workmen suffered from 'pernicious anaemia' during the building of the St Gotthard Tunnel in Switzerland during the 1880s, resulting in newspaper reports on this 'mysterious', new 'miners' disease'.[83] A similar mystery was reported in the early 1900s, leading to a home office inquiry in 1903, when cases of anaemia had been detected in Dolcoath Mine in Cornwall. It was found that these were due to 'an outbreak of ankylostomiasis', possibly caused by a miner who had previously contracted it at Mysore.[84] But even if Dhunjibhoy had not heard of these widely discussed cases, he would not have been able to avoid exposure to the frequent reports in the medical literature on hookworm in a range of tropical locations – India included – during the early part of the twentieth century. Ankylostomiasis was discussed, alongside typhoid fever and dysentery, for example, as diseases of tropical areas that required hygiene and sanitary measures. Hookworm was therefore a disease regularly encountered and discussed in India. What is more, the Rockefeller Foundation had launched a hookworm programme in the southern states of America at the beginning of the twentieth century, which proved highly successful.[85] Given Dhunjibhoy's interest in international developments, he must have been aware of these reports and initiatives.

Admittedly, the clinical diagnosis of hookworm is difficult because it does not present specific symptoms. Anaemia is the most prevalent result of hookworm infestation. However, anaemia is implicated also in malaria. Dhunjibhoy may well have attributed patients' anaemia to malaria. What is more, as both malaria and hookworm were endemic in this part of the world, it is likely that patients may have suffered from both simultaneously. Malaria was diagnosed clinically, by observation of prevalent symptoms (such as periodic fever and anaemia) and only from 1931 onwards on a regular basis through means of laboratory examination of blood specimens for the presence of the protozoan parasite, *Plasmodium falciparum*. The only way to diagnose ankylostomiasis was by faecal sample in order to identify the presence of hookworm eggs by microscopic examination. Laboratory tests were focused on at Ranchi from 1930 and it is from the following year onwards that ankylostomiasis suddenly appears as a regular disease category.

The introduction of routine laboratory examination may also account to a large extent for the fluctuation of the reported incidence rate for ankylostomiasis. The use of laboratory tests increased gradually from 1931 onwards, being applied in the first instance to newly admitted patients. There was a noteworthy spike of reported cases of ankylostomiasis in 1934 (90 cases), followed by a decrease in 1935 to the average during the previous three years (29 cases). This sudden rise and then decrease could well have been due to the tendency for the incidence to level out following a concerted effort in one particular year of disease detection among a numerically limited group of patients in a closed institution. It may have also been influenced by different practitioners' individual diagnostic styles, especially in regard to a disease in which the clinical presentation consists of no specific symptoms, the range of symptoms are present in other endemic diseases, and within an environment where co-infection is highly likely. These may have been factors in 1935 when Pacheco's report showed a pattern of disease prevalence that differed from Dhunjibhoy's.

General paralysis of the insane (GPI) and syphilis

General paralysis of the insane (GPI) is another example of a condition in which individual doctors' diagnostic styles as well as wider social attitudes may have had a bearing on its profile in the reports. As with TB and pneumonia, GPI was seen as a major problem among patients admitted to mental hospitals in Europe and North America. Yet, the recorded incidence varied widely. For example, 20 per cent of all patients in mental hospitals in the US suffered from paresis during the 1930s.[86] By contrast, in North Wales 'there were never more than a few cases' during the interwar period'.[87] At Ranchi, Dhunjibhoy rarely mentioned GPI and syphilis until Pacheco set a temporary trend for it in 1935. The low incidence in North Wales was explained by the region's demographic characteristics as 'an agricultural district, with few large towns and without a floating population', while cities and in particular large ports were considered to account for higher rates of syphilis.[88] Ranchi's catchment areas, in contrast, were diverse and included both large cities and plantation and tribal areas. Dhunjibhoy, like many of his peers in India, also believed that GPI was intrinsically rare among Indians (see Chapter 4).

The hospital statistics appear to substantiate this contention, as those diseases considered to be sexually transmitted are mentioned neither in relation to mortality nor morbidity. Reference to syphilis is made in the records, but only under the rubric of 'treatment of special conditions', alongside 'Piles, Dental, Leprosy and Tuberculosis'.[89] It is however particularly interesting that of the 557 blood samples sent for Wassermann reaction testing between 1927 and 1930, 105 showed positive and 20 doubtful results.[90] This indicates that as many as one in five patients may have suffered from syphilis! It is surprising that a practitioner like Dhunjibhoy, who was tuned into the latest professional debates, would not have explored the situation further.

Accidents and Injuries

At 10 per cent, injury was nearly as frequent a cause for admission to the infirmary as influenza. Only two patients (one per cent) died from whatever wounds they had sustained during the eight-year period from 1926 to 1933. However, the high incidence of injury requiring treatment comes as somewhat of a surprise, especially as the reported 10 per cent may well have been an understatement. Injuries were not always listed in the records when Dhunjibhoy's locums were in charge of the institution. In 1929, for example, Das did not note a single injury during the year. This seems improbable given the high number of violent and highly disturbed patients in the institution, particularly on the overcrowded wards on the male side, and considering that a large number of patients were employed in manual labour. Forty-nine incidents of injury had been identified in the year before, and 63 during the subsequent year.

It is likely that Das failed to report injuries requiring hospitalisation, for whatever reason. It is generally difficult to assess how the majority of the injuries were caused, as little information is provided on whether they were the result of work-related activities (in the workshops, kitchens, dairy, fields and orchards) or due to violence inflicted by fellow inmates or, possibly, staff. In 1931, Dhunjibhoy merely referred to 'minor cases of accidents and injuries' and listed as examples 'falls, simple fractures, sprain of ankle joints, wrist joints and injury caused by foreign bodies etc.'.[91] The same year he also recounted the case of 'one epileptic patient who died from fracture of skull due to a fall during an epileptic fit'.[92] However, on all other occasions only the most serious cases were commented on in the main part of the reports. These involved mainly staff and sometimes also patients as victims of violent attacks by inmates. In 1928, for example, the following two cases were reported:

> A hitherto quiet patient suddenly struck an attendant on the head with a spade while working in the vegetable garden of the hospital. In another case a patient who had several previous convictions to his credit kept at bay 40 attendants by means of a *dao* (scythe) which he snatched away from a sane patient working in the garden, and he further declared that he wished to kill two attendants against whom he had some grudge and that he would kill any one who attempted to take away the *dao* from him. This matter was reported [to the superintendent] and I persuaded the patient to hand over the *dao* to me and a very unpleasant situation was relieved.[93]

The second case occurred in 1929 when 'one male patient very nearly throttled to death the *jamadar* [senior attendant] of his block under the mistaken idea that the latter was his father against whom he had a grudge'. In the same year, on the female side, a patient 'climbed up a tree and kept at bay a large number of staff with a stick in her hand. She was, however, brought down unhurt by a keeper who had received serious injuries from her on his head'.[94]

It was not only members of lower-grade staff who were reported to have been subject to patients' violence. More senior staff were also attacked. For example, Dhunjibhoy reported in 1934:

> A hitherto dependable hypochondriac patient who had borne some secret grudge against one of the Sub-Assistant Surgeons, a not very uncommon occurrence with this class of patients, suddenly got excited and attacked this Sub-Assistant Surgeon with a improvised knife made of tin and after inflicting a few injuries on his person with it he immediately ran after the Second Assistant Superintendent and also attacked him and assaulted him with the knife causing severe injury on his head before he could be caught and overpowered by the staff.[95]

This particular case raises different issues from the other reported incidents as the patient's attack was clearly premeditated. His targets were higher-grade yet still subordinate staff members who were comparable, in terms of position in the institutional hierarchy and tasks, to sergeants in the military. Sub-assistant surgeons were in charge of day-to-day management decisions and hence decided on inmates' privileges as well as sanctions and matters of treatment. Just like sergeants, they could be greatly loathed by the people under their charge if they were seen to display any unfairness or cruelty. Whether the grudge against the staff members in the case reported was unfounded or based on prior offensive behaviour by those in a position of power is difficult to ascertain. As is always the case when dealing with one-sided institutional evidence, the account of the patient is silenced.

Superintendents tended to stress that they only commented on the most serious cases, which they repeatedly asserted to be 'exceptions'. The majority of cases were, so it was noted, 'minor accidents and injuries',[96] not 'serious',[97] or 'not worthy of note'.[98] This is somewhat peculiar as an accident or injury that required admission to the infirmary would have surely not been simply a superficial wound. Clearly, judgement of what was to be considered either serious or noteworthy was made solely by the person in charge. Given the subjective nature of this assessment, it may well be that the recorded cases were highly selective as most of them involved attacks on staff members. The only patient-to-patient violence reported related to extreme cases such as when a 'very dependable patient suddenly struck another patient without any provocation with an axe while working in the garden'.[99] In 1933, another hitherto 'dependable patient', an epileptic, 'suddenly ran amok and caused serious injury on the head of the first patient he met before he could be caught and overpowered by the staff'.[100]

One of the key terms in all descriptions of injury by patients stressed their previously 'dependable' nature. Had injuries been afflicted by patients who had a known history of violence, concerns about the attention paid by the superintendent to safety would have been raised by the senior medical officers who scrutinised the reports. The tone of the cases reported and explanations provided seems to indicate that, unsurprisingly, Dhunjibhoy and his locums were determined to portray their efforts in regard to maintaining safety in the best light possible. Attacks that were selected for comment were annotated as unexpected and usually aimed at staff. The efficiency, devotion and precarious nature of work in the mental hospital were stressed. Das reported in 1929 that in 'a large Mental Hospital like this all the staff have had to run the risk of personal violence in some way or other in their attempts to avert sudden critical situations brought on by dangerous patients'.[101] In 1930 Dhunjibhoy pointed out that 'no case of serious accident or injury' occurred 'in spite of the fact that all patients admitted were sent here as definitely dangerous'. He contended that notwithstanding the 'few minor accidents and injuries', this 'can fairly be attributed to the kind treatment meted out to this class of patients in this hospital as already stated in my annual report of 1928'.[102] In 1937, when the rate of accidents and injuries increased, Dhunjibhoy repeated Das's earlier suggestion, apologetically emphasising the permissive regime prevalent at Ranchi that enabled many patients to move freely:

> That there should be a number of accidents in a Mental Hospital of the size of the Ranchi Indian Mental Hospital is inevitable where a large number of certified highly dangerous patients are treated and a maximum amount of freedom is allowed for therapeutic reasons.[103]

By this time, patients' engagement in labour pursuits had been greatly extended. This made work-related accidents more likely and presented more opportunities (and access to tools as potential weapons) for the commission of violent acts on the part of those latently inclined to them for whatever reasons. The pattern of violence inflicted during this period may have been different from ten years earlier, when a lower percentage of patients were employed in work. During this period, Dhunjibhoy had explained the incidence of injuries differently, focusing on the predilections of new patients and contrasting the kindness bestowed on them at Ranchi to the ways they had been treated previously. He stated that:

> assaults are more common with newly-admitted cases. In my opinion this is due to the fact that insane patients whether violent, aggressive or otherwise are often roughly handled by tactless, unsympathetic relatives and friends before admittance. The result is that they temporarily develop a wild temper due to continuous bad treatment and assault anyone with whom they come into contact. Such patients become docile, amiable and admirably adapt themselves with the disciplinary routine of the institution in a very short time under treatment which consists [...] of a mixture of tact, kindness, sympathy and liberty of speech and action. I take this opportunity of recording my grateful acknowledgment of the services of those attendant staff who suffered bodily ailments due to unprovoked assaults by patients during the year [...][104]

We should not read Dhunjibhoy's and his locum's statements simply as whitewash intended to account for and explain away the high numbers of accidents and injuries at Ranchi. Superintendents would of course have tried to put their management into the best possible light, selecting evidence that reflected positively on their procedures despite unfavourable statistics. It is also likely that at least some of the patients' accidents and injuries were due to inappropriate staff behaviour towards the people under their charge. Reports on particular incidents such as the one provided by Pacheco in 1935 raise more questions than they answer as to how exactly and under what circumstances some of the patients happened to sustain their injuries:

> In 1935 three elderly patients sustained a fracture of the leg as the result of accidental falls. In the case of one, a female suffering from a psychoses [*sic*] of the M.D. type of long standing, it resulted in a marked improvement in her mental condition. A male patient, whose general behaviour was exemplary, one day suddenly inflicted several wounds on his legs while working in the kitchen.[105]

However, staff at Ranchi worked under difficult circumstances, especially during the late 1930s when they were supposed to extend patients' engagement in profitable manual labour, despite the fact that a high percentage of inmates were 'criminal lunatics' and potentially dangerous. What is more, during a period when mental symptoms could not yet be controlled effectively except by sedative drugs, staff sailed between the Scylla of over-sedating patients to make them pliable and submissive – yet unable to work – and the Charybdis of keeping them at work and alert – yet liable to dangerous or careless behaviour with sudden outbursts of excitement and violence.

Suicide, Escapes and Patients' Freedom of Movement

The currently available literature on suicide is concerned mainly with its prevalence and its changing meanings within the wider population in different countries.[106] Very little has been written on suicide in early twentieth-century mental hospitals.[107] As with other topics in the history of psychiatry, authors still tend to focus on the nineteenth century. It is therefore difficult to compare the situation at Ranchi to mental institutions in the Western world during this period. In the case of England, there is some indication that the number of deaths by suicide declined towards the end of the nineteenth century and the first decade of the twentieth. Contrary to common belief that industrialisation and modern civilisation led to increased social evils such as crime, madness and suicide, Anderson's figures for England suggest otherwise. In 1867 the suicide rate was 0.63 per cent, in contrast to 0.14 per cent in 1911.[108] Shepherd and Wright provide data on the proportion of deaths listed as suicides in asylum statistics for England and Wales that fluctuate between about 0.5 per cent and 0.1 per cent (from 1862 to 1882), indicating a downward trend over the period.[109] It should not necessarily be assumed that the decreased incidence of accomplished self-destruction in mental hospitals was maintained during subsequent years, but it does seem likely, not least because the use of sedatives became more intensive over the decades, enabling staff to prevent suicidal activity by immobilising patients pharmacologically.

At Ranchi suicides were extremely rare. Only one case was reported from 1926 to 1940. Being so uncommon, this particular occurrence, in 1934, was extensively reflected on by Dhunjibhoy:

> I regret to have to report that a very dependable and well behaved patient, who had hitherto never shown any suicidal tendency, suddenly committed suicide by hanging [...]. The patient was perfectly sane and took part in a theatrical performance got up by patients and retired to his bed in a very jovial mood after the play was over, and committed suicide towards the latter part of the night in the night-latrine of the Dormitory in which he lived.[110]

Despite the excellent record of suicide prevention, Dhunjibhoy clearly felt it was necessary to explain the circumstances and justify staff's failure on this singular occasion. He noted that it was 'practically impossible for any human agency to prognosticate or prevent persons with such sudden impulse' and that some instances were 'beyond human control'.[111] Just a couple of years earlier, in 1932, he had reported proudly that suicide was 'practically unknown in this largest mental hospital of India'.[112] On both occasions he praised his staff for their 'unremitting zeal, care and supervision' (1932) and extended his 'deepest debt of gratitude to those attendants who guard the suicidal wards [...] day and night' (1934). The single tragic event had occurred on a regular ward, where surveillance was clearly not as strict as on the dedicated 'suicidal wards' where '82 potential suicides who often make attempts at suicide' were observed around the clock.[113] These wards where suicidal patients were segregated and 'kept under strictest vigilance and supervision' had been in place since 1926.[114] Even the otherwise ever-critical Pacheco corroborated Dhunjibhoy's appreciation of staff's efforts in 1935 stating that:

> The fact that there are many potential suicidal patients who were prevented from converting their intentions into overt action, in spite of the many opportunities that present themselves speaks much for the discipline and vigilance of the attendant staff.[115]

Up until 1938, the number of potentially suicidal patients was reported to have been about 80 (six per cent) of the daily average population at Ranchi.[116] However, in 1939 and 1940 the numbers rose suddenly to 'about 160' and 'more than 150' respectively.[117] No reason was provided for this extraordinary increase to 11 per cent. It is difficult to ascertain whether the change was related to superintendents' changing perspectives on indicators of suicidal behaviour, financial austerity measures having an impact on conditions or whether it was due to patients' increased suicidal inclinations during a period of increasing pre-war anxiety and political strife, resistance to the intensified labour regime or perhaps even the impending departure of Dhunjibhoy. It is also difficult to compare the Ranchi figures to any data currently available for Western institutions; Shepherd and Wright's and MacKenzie's calculations are based on suicidality on admission. These rates fluctuate between 10 and 15 per cent in private asylums and 5 and 30 per cent in public institutions during the Victorian and Edwardian periods.[118] Set against this background, the number of potentially suicidal patients at Ranchi must seem comparatively low.

As Shepherd and Wright pointed out in their work on suicide in two nineteenth-century county asylums in England, namely Surrey and Buckinghamshire, 'medical superintendents and staff [were] eager to avoid such occurrences within the walls of the asylum' on account of penalties imposed on the staff on duty and the ensuing bad publicity following coroners' reports.[119] Although there was only one case of an actual suicide to report at Ranchi, the tone of superintendents' statements on attempted suicides throughout the period suggests concerted efforts to thwart them. Senior staff depended in this respect on the vigilance of their subordinate employees. Dhunjibhoy, too, imposed penalties on staff in case of failures to ensure patients' safety and secure confinement – at least during the very early years of the hospital – when he also expressed more general displeasure about the calibre of the staff that had been recruited on opening the institution. On that occasion he also mentioned the penalty system in place at Ranchi. Fines and, most likely, dismissal, were implemented when 'five patients escaped during the year under review, out of which four were recaptured and brought back'.[120]

Only one other episode of punishment being inflicted on staff is reported. This occurred in 1935, when an escape happened under Pacheco. It involved a male 'criminal patient', a *Kabuli* (from Kabul, Afghanistan) who had 'absconded from the Refractory Ward'.[121] The fact that the escapee had been subject to criminal procedures required a 'full enquiry', which was duly held by Pacheco, and 'those of the attendant staff who were found guilty of neglect of duty were properly punished'. The specifics of the punishment are not recorded. This disciplinary action would have made Pacheco unpopular among staff members who were – in contrast to the early few years – steady, well settled and regularly praised by Dhunjibhoy. On the other hand, no escapes occurred in subsequent years, despite the 'considerable amount of freedom' that was 'allowed to the patients of all classes'.[122]

Dhunjibhoy and his locums went out of their way to praise staff continually for their efforts. In 1937 Dhunjibhoy elaborated at length the difficult circumstances under which his subordinates had to ensure that no suicides occurred, despite so 'many definite attempts'. He stated:

> The Attendant Staff of the Suicidal Wards of the hospital seldom appear in the limelight although on their shoulders rests the heavy responsibility of watching so many potential suicides day and night; to all of them I owe a deep debt of gratitude and I wish to record my appreciation and sincere thanks for their good work.[123]

Dhunjibhoy went on to describe cases that illustrated attendants' efforts to remain one vital step ahead of patients who 'are constantly on the watch for an opportunity as their life is devoted to courting death'.[124] It is worth quoting his account in full, as it also provides insights into the wider concerns of hospital management:

> The ingenuity of such patients at times is very great. One female potential suicide, who has apparently made up her mind to drown herself, twice jumped down the hospital well whilst employed on watering the plants in the garden and twice she was rescued by the staff on duty at the well at the risk of their lives. The third time she jumped down a cauldron full of water which was kept on one of the ovens of the kitchen for boiling but fortunately had not reached the boiling point. She was again rescued by the staff on duty. Another patient, a Marwari [business man][125] from Calcutta, has a strong desire to end his life but he wants someone to take his life. Ever since his admission he is asking whoever goes near him to kill him but his wish is not yet fulfilled. Finding that no one seems to oblige him in this direction he hit upon a novel way of killing himself by refusing food and drink, what is in present day known as 'hunger strike', until such time as he is fed by the Governor of Bengal. We induced some friends to impersonate His Excellency in order to make him eat but to no avail, and I am sure even if His Excellency the Governor of Bengal comes to feed him his request to him would be to kill him and he would refuse food. He has been fed nasally twice a day by the staff for the last five years to keep him alive. Many times we stopped his nasal feed for a day or two and induced him to take his food but he flatly refused and fervently requested us to allow him to die of starvation. He is a case of 'Involutional Melancholia' [depression][126] and most melancholics are potential suicides. These and other potential suicides of the hospital are watched day and night, yet they must be given certain facilities and freedom on humanitarian as well as therapeutic grounds. In a modern mental hospital where too much freedom is given to all patients the suicides also have their fair share of it and are not locked up day and night as was the case in the old asylums, and sometimes they take advantage of this and let down the administration of the hospital who are doing their best for them. But this should not deter a conscientious Medical Superintendent in discharging his duties to his unfortunate suicidal patients, for such accidents must happen even in the best regulated institutions.[127]

Dhunjibhoy's reflections highlight a number of issues that require further assessment. His first case shows that even suicidal patients were involved in work duties rather than being immobilised by means of shackles, full-length and armless tight cloaks or sedation with chloral hydrate, as had reportedly been the case in large asylums in England and Wales during the previous century. However, such engagement also put much responsibility on the attendants who had to be ever vigilant and prepared to take urgent action even to the extent of endangering their own lives, as Dhunjibhoy pointed out so graphically. Pulling a drowning patient out of a deep and narrow well is highly dangerous. Although physical activity in cases of depression may be advantageous, exposure of a persistently and 'ingeniously' suicidal woman, such as the one referred to by Dhunjibhoy, to activities that involved large vats of hot water and deep wells can be considered as an error on the part of the hospital staff.

Ranchi clearly put much emphasis on work therapy, particularly from the late 1930s. This harboured risks not only in the case of the potentially violent patients who might use tools as weapons, but also in regard to those with suicidal tendencies who could use them against themselves. In either case, the role of staff was vital. The high incidence of injuries and accidents that required attention in the infirmary may well be related to cases when staff members were not able to take swift preventive action. On the other hand, engagement in work duties implied that sedation was not a preferred method of institutional management at Ranchi. This could be considered preferable to the situation described in English lunatic asylums during the nineteenth century, in which 'medical staff relied on the use of sedatives and narcotics to control those at risk of killing themselves, ushering in an increasing reliance on pharmacological interventions'.[128] In order to weigh up the relative merits, disadvantages and potential cruelties of each approach, it would be necessary to find out patients' and their families' views on the matter.

The second case reported by Dhunjibhoy also raises issues of the propriety of restraint and force on the one hand and a patient's right to freedom of movement and self-expression on the other. At the time it was understood that suicide, including attempts at self-starvation, was to be thwarted, and Dhunjibhoy clearly adhered to this principle by keeping the patient alive by nasal feeding over a lengthy period. Refusal of food was not uncommon at Ranchi and it was always responded to by forced feeding. Cruel as this may sound to modern observers, it was a practice that was considered not only fully appropriate at the time but also a strictly medical procedure, just as bleeding or blistering had been in earlier periods. Patients' views on this would no doubt have been different. Dhunjibhoy's opinion was that 'too much freedom' had its cost, but that this should not induce staff to revert to the reputedly inhuman old days of locking patients up. As with so many practitioners who believe that they have the best interests of their patients at heart, Dhunjibhoy felt let down when they subverted or took advantage of his best intentions.

The 'considerable amount of freedom' that was 'afforded to the patients' within the mental hospital was commented on by Dhunjibhoy also in regard to escapes or 'absconding'.[129] Like suicides, escapes were extremely rare at Ranchi, despite patients' freedom of movement within the hospital compound and in the workshops, paddy fields and dairy, fruit and vegetable gardens. Five escapes occurred in 1926 when Dhunjibhoy was still trying to attract suitable staff to an institution opened the previous year. During the subsequent period, from 1927 to 1939, only seven successful escapes were reported and most of these occurred during the very early years (five between 1927 and1929). Following on from his reflections on suicidal patients in 1937, Dhunjibhoy proceeded to explain the alleged effect his approach to hospital management had on the inmates. He stated that:

> A feature of the modern mental hospital is the friendly and homely atmosphere and absence of any real evidence of the detention and this is the very reason why we have few escapes now a days from modern mental hospitals as compared to olden-days asylums. Often we come across patients who on discharge show great unwillingness to go home as they anticipate an unpleasant home situation. Such patients I have often noticed return very soon to the hospital as relapsed cases.

Again it is difficult to ascertain if the superintendent's perception of the matter would have agreed with that of patients' and their families. Other issues might have had a bearing on patients' inclination to seek out asylum in the mental hospital. For families under economic pressure, it would have been more difficult to take care of an additional family member, especially during times of famine or if he or she was not able to work. Finnane reports this to be the case for nineteenth-century Ireland, where families sought out lunatic asylums during periods of famine and economic hardship in order to increase the odds of the family unit surviving.[130] It is likely that in India, too, relatives attempted to make use of the institution in order to have their loved ones taken care of or to get rid of undesirable family members with whom they found it hard to cope under financial pressures. In fact, Dhunjibhoy referred to instances when chronic patients could not be discharged to their families as they were unable to take care of them. However, he did not suggest any general link between families' economic hardship during the 1930s and patients' disinclination to leave a place in which their next meal was guaranteed. The number of these kinds of patients may have been restricted as there was increasing emphasis on the selective admission of dangerous patients only. It may also have been the case that the reported unwillingness of some patients to be discharged was indeed due to preference for the more 'friendly and homely atmosphere' at Ranchi rather than any more basic economic need underlying it.[131] We simply do not know which motive may have been more prevalent. There is evidence however to suggest that Dhunjibhoy honestly believed that his patients were grateful for the atmosphere he tried to create at Ranchi.

He will have been aware of the more basic and material needs the institution catered for, but making too much of this in official reports might have distracted from his ambition to establish Ranchi's reputation as a specialist medical institution run on modern scientific principles. Furthermore, government accountants had a habit of keeping an ever-keen eye on costly services that could be cut. As long as Ranchi could prove itself as a place for the safe confinement of 'criminal lunatics' and a medical institution that also contributed to its own upkeep by means of patient labour, rather than serving as a poor house, the hospital's survival and Dhunjibhoy's position were secure.

Cures

Along with the mortality rate, the cure rate of an institution was a crucial parameter for measuring its efficacy. It also provided a rationale for its existence. Why maintain a costly place if it had no positive effect – especially at a time of austerity, such as during the 1930s and the lead-up to the Second World War? Like the superintendents of other institutions in India, Dhunjibhoy felt the need to justify continued government support for the institution (and for his post of senior medical officer responsible for its management). In not one single year did he fail to remind his superiors that 'so-called new admissions were not really new admissions in the true sense of that expression, but were cases of long standing mental disorder'(1933),[132] and that '40 per cent of this so-called new admissions were not only suffering from chronic mental diseases but were equally bad in their physical health' (1934).[133] Furthermore, Dhunjibhoy was evidently aware of the effect that any reference to one of the high-profile and much discussed diseases of the period would have in soliciting a more favourable assessment of the low cure rates as he stated that a 'good many [of the patients] were admitted in a very low state of health, markedly anaemic with consequent debility. Some were treated as suspected cases of tuberculosis of Lungs.'[134] Even without reference to TB, Dhunjibhoy's statements about the precarious physical state of those admitted to and confined at Ranchi were persuasive.

The term 'cure' is problematic within the context of mental illnesses. Unlike with many physical conditions, mental symptoms may temporarily subside, almost regardless of the treatment applied. Such spontaneous recoveries or remissions, whether these were persistent or short-lived, would have been subsumed under 'cures' in the institutional records. This applied to Ranchi as much as to any other mental institution during the period. Cure rates can therefore not be seen as indicative of permanent cures. This potentially contentious status of the term 'cure' was one that Dhunjibhoy was aware of. In 1936, the year following his return from extended overseas leave, he suggested a change in nomenclature on the basis of what he had observed in other countries. The format of and technical terms for the statistical tables and the rubrics to be discussed in the institutional reports were proscribed centrally by the provincial medical authorities, and it was not in the power of individual clinicians to revise them. Dhunjibhoy noted:

> In the statement no. 1, attached to this report the word 'cured' in columns 6A and 11 A, C should in my opinion be replaced by the word 'recovered' for obvious reasons. The word 'recovered' seems to be more appropriate and in fitness of things with mental disorders and all that it connotes, and is used in the mental hospital returns all over the United Kingdom, Europe and America.[135]

Although no such change to the report template was introduced by his superiors during Dhunjibhoy's time at Ranchi, he repeatedly referred to the 'recovery and the improved rates' from that year onwards in his clinical accounts.[136]

Two other issues concerning the cure or recovery rates achieved at Ranchi received continued attention by Dhunjibhoy and his locums. These were the accumulation of 'infirm, incurable and homeless cases' in the institutions as well as the poor state of health and 'chronic' condition of those newly admitted.[137] The same pattern prevailed in British institutions. The medical superintendent of Denbigh Hospital, for example, reported in 1937 that out of a total of 1,359 patients, he regarded 1,308 as incurable.[138] Trying to account for the significant decrease in cures at Ranchi in 1929, Das noted that the 'progressive fall in the percentage of cures to daily average strength is mainly due to fewer patients being admitted every year and then of those admissions most being chronic and incurable cases'.[139] His observation was valid because, as he explained, 'no restriction was imposed on the admission of patients in 1927', whereas in 1928 and 1929 admission was denied to all but dangerous patients 'for want of accommodation'.[140] Contrasting the favourable cure rates of 1927 with the lower ones of 1928 and 1929 would be 'no useful comparison'[141], he rightly suggested. In fact, from 1929 onwards the overall cure rate (calculated on the basis of the percentage cured of the daily average number of patients institutionalised), stabilised at a significantly lower level, namely an average of six per cent, as shown in Figure 3.8.

Figure 3.8. Percentage cured of daily average strength (lower line) and percentage cured of total admission during the year (upper line), 1927–1939

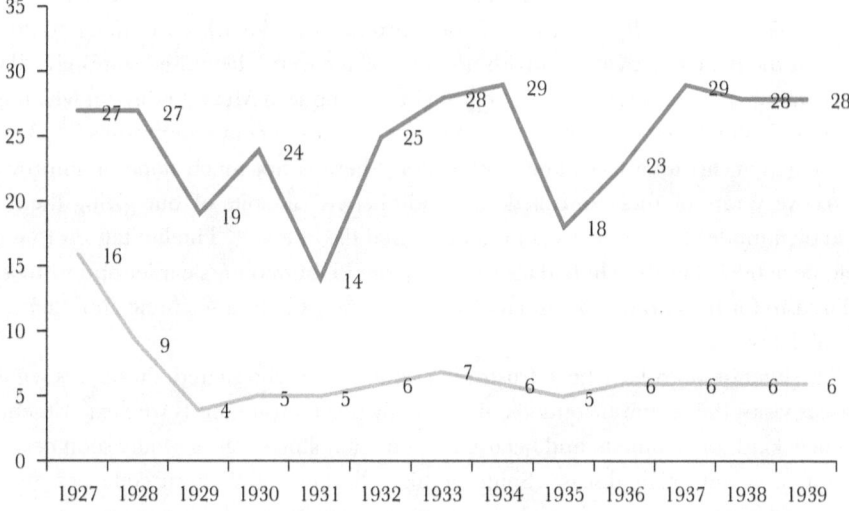

The cure rate calculated in relation to total admissions and re-admissions per year tended to be much higher, by an average factor of about four, with considerable fluctuation on a year by year basis. The variation of this rate over the years was due to a number of incidental factors related to admission restrictions resulting from congestion, as well as superintendents' different styles of medical management. In 1931, for example, when the cure rate among admissions fell by about 10 per cent, 'selected cases were only admitted to [the 50] emergency beds' on account of congestion in the male section of the institution'.[142] Overcrowding clearly took its toll, influencing admission patterns and hence cure rates. Dhunjibhoy responded to the pressures also by discharging 'incurable harmless insane patients'.[143] However, he noted that despite 'this progressive increase in discharges our ratio per cent of admissions of cures to total admissions is low compared to 1930 and 1929'. This, he contended, was due to the reception of a large number (123) of 'chronic insanes' who had been kept for a considerable time either at their homes or in jails 'for want of accommodation in this hospital'. He concluded: 'One, therefore, cannot expect cures from such chronic cases within a year, hence the low percentage of cures to total admissions.'[144]

Towards the second half of the 1930s, when Dhunjibhoy's ambition to excel in the treatment of the mentally ill on the most modern scientific lines had been refuelled by a recent overseas visit, his tone in regard to the low cure rates that continued to plague his institution became steadily more resigned. The focus of his comments shifted. Initially Dhunjobhoy had tried to accentuate the positive elements of a bad situation, pointing out that the cure rate in 1933, for example, was in fact 'extremely satisfactory and serves as a direct incitement to the staff who devote every possible care to the employment of the modern methods of treatment to the newly-admitted patients in the reception wards of this modern mental hospital of India'.[145] By 1938, the realities of over ten years at Ranchi appeared to have begun to gnaw away at his managerial enthusiasm and ambition to maintain the reputation for cutting-edge and advanced scientific treatments. Noting, as he had done in previous years, that the majority of 'new admissions' actually consisted of 'old chronic cases for whom nothing could be done but the palliative treatment with no hope of recovery', he mused sombrely: 'This has been our misfortune since the inception of this modern Mental Hospital which has immense facilities for the treatment of early cases with encouraging results.'[146] By the following year, his tone was almost mournful: 'there is not much hope of improving the recovery rate of these so-called "new admissions" in spite of our giving them all the known modern scientific treatment of mental disorders.'[147] The limitations to what could be achieved at Ranchi had clearly dampened Dhunjibhoy's earlier optimism and enthusiasm for the curative potential of the many new modern scientific approaches to mental illness.

The situation must have been frustrating for a doctor who shared, during his regular overseas visits, the optimistic outlook of the many psychiatric experts who experimented with new kinds of treatment and believed that mental illness was or would soon become as curable as any other disease. Some of his colleagues in Western countries greatly inflated their successes, implausibly boasting recovery rates of 80 per cent or so (for example, H. A. Cotton at New Jersey State Hospital from 1907 to 1930).[148] Nevertheless, rates at Ranchi were significantly below even the more realistic rates reported for the US and Britain.[149] In England, an average recovery rate on admission of 40 per cent was reported for St Andrew's Hospital, Norfolk, and for Denbigh Mental Hospital in North Wales, for example.[150] For all mental hospitals in England and Wales the mean cure rate was approximately 32 per cent during the interwar period. Comparisons are fraught, however, as the figures were based on different methods of calculation. The board of control of mental hospitals in England and Wales critically referred to some institutions' practice of calculating recoveries only on the basis of the number of 'recoverable' cases admitted.[151]

The other major problem for enthusiastic practitioners hoping to implement the latest cutting-edge procedures was that in public institutions such as Ranchi (and in county mental hospitals in England and Wales) many patients suffered severe, often untreated physical illnesses when admitted. This is an issue that has been ignored by historians of psychiatry. As shown above, Dhunjibhoy was acutely aware of the effect this had on what he could achieve at Ranchi. In some cases particular physical conditions may have caused patients' mental problems (for example, in malaria and GPI). Attention to the former could lead to relief from or remission of the latter. In other cases, when physical illnesses persisted alongside a mental affliction, treatment would have been needed for both ailments. In either case the superintendent's general medical skills were as vital as his expertise in psychiatry.

The contemporary focus on early treatment of mental illness, which still prevails among modern-day practitioners, was another issue that conflicted with the actual conditions at Ranchi. From 1928 onwards, admission was refused unless patients had become dangerous or unmanageable. In 1938, Dhunjibhoy still held, against all the odds, that mental illness was 'as much curable as any general disease', as long as it was treated 'in its early stage'. In a special section in his report that year titled 'Advantages of early mental treatment', he referred to successful treatment in 'hospitals in the West which are fortunate enough to receive early cases for treatment', where they achieved '70 per cent recovery'.[152] The focus on the need for early treatment may unwittingly have caused an over-optimistic tendency to discharge new patients on early signs of remission. This could account for the comparatively high readmission rate at Ranchi. On average readmissions accounted for about 10 per cent of all admissions from 1927 to 1939, with notably low readmission rates in 1930 and 1935 (one and three per cent respectively), when Dhunjibhoy's locums, Das and Pacheco, were in charge. Dhunjibhoy's enthusiasm and hopeful outlook may have inclined him towards a more lenient assessment of patients' state of mind on admission and discharge.

As was the case in Western institutions, gender was a differential factor also at Ranchi, in regard to both the readmission and the cure rates (calculated on the daily average number of patients resident). Both of these figures were higher for women, with some notable but predictable exceptions. In 1935, the year when Pacheco was at Ranchi, women experienced significantly lower readmission and cure rates (of both total hospital population and of admissions). This practitioner's style of management clearly affected patients very differently from that of Dhunjibhoy. In the period prior to 1931 no women at all were re-admitted. This might have been due to the fact that no overcrowding prevailed on the women's side of the institution during this period, easing the pressure on superintendents to discharge patients prematurely as cured. The cure rate of admissions seems to substantiate this, although it may also reflect a tendency for only very seriously ill women to be put forward for institutional confinement by authorities and families. The only other exception to the trend of women being more likely than men to be readmitted and discharged as cured, occurs during Dhunjibhoy's last year at Ranchi, in 1939. During this year the male rate of cure (of daily average strength) increased significantly from a mere six per cent in 1938 to a high 15 per cent. There is no indication of what had caused this sudden increase, but war conditions and staff's ambition to lower the number of inpatients may have had an impact.

It is clear that many factors have an influence on the 'cure' or recovery rates reported for an institution. Furthermore, it is necessary to keep in mind that 'cure' or recovery in a mental hospital may reflect an improvement of mental symptoms as a result of successful treatment of an underlying physical condition. On the basis of the available data, it is difficult to establish whether the recovery rates, low as they were at Ranchi, reflected successful treatment of mental illness. If we believe in the validity of retrospective diagnoses, an assessment of individual patients' case histories may enable us to disaggregate the reported figures to distinguish the percentages of those who had recovered from mental illness from those cured of physical conditions that were accompanied by mental symptoms.

Mortality, morbidity and cure rates are usually discussed together as vital criteria of the efficacy of an institution in providing a wholesome environment for its patients. However, while the alleviation or cure of any diseases of the body is no doubt an important and desirable factor to consider in any institutional setting, it does not exhaust the specific purpose for which a psychiatric hospital is designed, namely the diagnosis and treatment of mental illnesses. To these latter concerns we now turn.

Chapter 4

CLASSIFICATIONS, TYPES OF DISORDER AND AETIOLOGY

The word is the house of Being. In its home man dwells. Those who think and those who create with words are the guardians of this home.
—Martin Heidegger, 1947

The ambition to standardise the classification of different types of mental illness and to develop more sophisticated diagnostic categories during the early twentieth century has been well documented. The traditional nineteenth-century mode of diagnostics, with mania, melancholia, idiocy and dementia at its core, was, as historians of psychiatry have shown, reshaped by the adoption of more refined systems throughout the world during the early twentieth century. This general trend seems well established. What is less clear is how this process towards modern classification systems and standardisation manifested itself on the ground, in diagnostic practice in individual institutions. Historians have traced the varied conceptual developments of the main figures driving this process such as Bleuler, Kraepelin, Meyer and Leonhard.[1] But the ways in which changes in nomenclature induced and mapped on to conceptual changes in less prominent, individual psychiatrists' cognitive mind-sets and diagnostic practices have scarcely been considered.

Even institutional reports and statistics have not been evaluated to any great extent. With the exception of works by Andrews et al. (1997), Cherry (2003) Crammer (1990), Gardner (1999), Gittins (1998) and Michael (2003), the number of institutional histories of Britain with which case-studies from other localities could be compared is indeed restricted.[2] What is more, historians of psychiatry have only very recently begun to shift their focus from the nineteenth to the twentieth century and, as Hess and Majerus have argued, 'no narrative' is as yet in sight 'which can explain the psychiatry of the 20th century, comparable to the authoritative coherence achieved for the 19th century'.[3]

Judging from the material that is currently available, at least in some British institutions such as the Denbigh Mental Hospital in Wales, the 'range of illnesses diagnosed was much the same as before' the interwar period.[4] At Denbigh Mental Hospital, mania and melancholia topped the list of diagnoses with recorded levels of 30 and 23 per cent respectively. This pattern is at odds with the trends identified in historical research on the development of new disease categories during this period. Was the break with nineteenth-century terminology and, possibly, older understandings, less significant and widespread during the interwar period than indicated by historical accounts focused on changes in nomenclature and progress towards standardisation?

The assessment of the classification schemes used at Ranchi will provide some indication of how diagnostic patterns here fitted in with the well-documented trend towards new categories and attempted standardisation of nomenclature, on the one hand, and evidence of continuity, on the other. The case of Ranchi could of course neither prove any general trend nor validate any potential exceptionality. Nonetheless, like the few currently available case studies on British institutions, it will expand our understanding of how particular places worked within a wider context of classification schemes that were seemingly characterised by a break with earlier conventions.

Standardisation and Variation of Classifications

What patterns emerge from an assessment of the classifications at Ranchi between 1925 and 1940? As at Denbigh Mental Hospital, the types of disorders attributed to patients continued to privilege the three main categories of mania, melancholia and dementia. In 1930, for example, an overlap with what was happening at Denbigh can be discerned (see Table 4.1). Of course, discrepancies in the data between the two institutions may be due both to different classification practices and to dissimilar admission policies. The issue of context and locale specificity therefore requires attention.

Table 4.1. Particular types of disorders attributed on admission as a percentage of the total of conditions identified (male and female) at Ranchi and Denbigh mental hospitals, 1930[5]

	Ranchi	Denbigh
Mania	30%	30%
Melancholia	13%	23%
Confusional Insanity	11%	[not used]
Senile Dementia	1%	11%
Delusional Insanity	5%	7%
Dementia Praecox	7%	6%
Epilepsy	4%	6%
Imbecility	5%	[no data available]
GPI	[no cases recorded]	5%
Percentage of diagnoses identified above as a percentage of all types of disorder assigned:	76%	83%

The types of disorder attributed to patients admitted to both institutions share some features. Mania, for example, is by far the most frequent category, constituting 30 per cent of new admissions at Denbigh as well as Ranchi. Melancholia, too, is in a leading position, albeit more so in the case of Denbigh (23 per cent) than Ranchi (13 per cent). The 10 per cent difference may arguably have been due to different diagnostic styles. In the case of senile dementia (11 per cent at Denbigh but only one per cent at Ranchi), the Indian institution's exclusion from admission of harmless, chronically ill patients may account for the low reported incidence. In contrast, the absence of confusional insanity as a category in the Denbigh reports clearly attests to different diagnostic practices. While this diagnosis was added in Wales only in 1939 (then accounting for six per cent of admissions), it had been on the books at Ranchi continuously since the opening of the institution in 1925.[6] On the other hand, the officially documented reluctance of Dhunjibhoy to identify general paralysis of the insane (GPI) among Indians, may explain the lack of such cases recorded in 1930. Diagnosticians in Wales did not have any such qualms, as is attested by the five per cent rate for GPI.

A number of suggestions can be made on the basis of the above observations. Firstly, although the low frequency with which some categories are applied (for example, senile dementia) directly reflects particular admission policies and the diverse makeup of patient intake, in other cases (GPI, confusional insanity and melancholia), discrepancies are more likely to have been due to different diagnostic preferences on the part of the medical superintendent. Secondly, despite their overlap in regard to reported incidence of the main diagnoses, the classificatory schemes used at Ranchi and at Denbigh were not completely congruent. The omission of confusional insanity in North Wales is one example and the use of the India-specific category of cannabis insanity at Ranchi is another. (In 1930, the latter diagnosis was attributed to three per cent of patients on admission. About 10 per cent of the overall hospital population – all of them male – were assigned it.)

These points highlight the considerable degree of variety in classification practices despite the seemingly similar nomenclature used in the UK based schemes. Standardisation and conformity may have been ideals pursued by health policy makers, epidemiologists and professional associations. How this was implemented in individual institutions is a quite different matter. Lack of compliance by individual institutions and medical staff with official classification guidelines was one of many issues that raised concerns among medical professionals. The German-born American psychoanalyst Martin Grotjahn noted that the classification system that clinicians were supposed to follow in German institutions from 1901 onwards was woefully dated by the time new diagnostic entities such as schizophrenia emerged, eventually causing institutions to develop their own unofficial house style pending a new scheme eventually introduced in 1933.[7] The fact that diverse classifications and medical codes were championed in different parts of Europe and in the United States did not help to establish consensus across countries either. For example, while a certain degree of equivalence of codes for Austria, Switzerland, The Netherlands and Scandinavia was considered achievable, discussants involved in the development of the new German classification system during the early 1930s surmised that substantial synergy with other countries, especially in the English-speaking world, was nigh impossible.[8]

Given this wider context of failed attempts at conformity, neither Denbigh nor Ranchi could be considered representative of what was happening in other institutions. Widespread heterogeneity in official classifications, institutions' modified house styles and variation in their implementation notwithstanding, we might ask whether the discrepancies between the Indian and Welsh institutions, for example, could be accounted for by cultural factors. The case of cannabis insanity could, for example, be considered as such a culturally specific phenomenon. Alas, there is no further conclusive evidence for this. Difference can also be identified between Ranchi and other institutions in South Asia. At the Madras Mental Hospital in the south of India, for example, the most frequently assigned category on admission was dementia praecox (23 per cent), which is in striking contrast to Ranchi's seven per cent and Denbigh's six per cent.[9] What is more, mania and melancholia appeared with only 18 and 2 per cent respectively (30 and 13 per cent at Ranchi; 30 and 23 per cent at Denbigh). These are significant differences that can most likely be accounted for by the Madras superintendent's preference for dementia praecox as a diagnosis. There are other, less significant but still important, differences. Unlike Ranchi, at Madras syphilis is represented in the reports, with a rate of one per cent for GPI and four per cent for dementia from cerebral syphilis (similar to the five per cent for the latter condition diagnosed at Denbigh). The allegedly 'Indian' speciality of cannabis insanity is identified in eight per cent of admissions (only three per cent at Ranchi). There may well have been cultural differences. However, this is difficult to ascertain on the basis of the existing data.

On the evidence that is currently available, it can be suggested that variation in diagnostic styles prevailed across cultures and localities. These variations warn against over-confident assertions regarding the extent to which standardised psychiatric nomenclature may reflect actual classification practices during the interwar period. The diagnostic categories listed in the annual report forms of both Ranchi and Madras were identical, but the frequency with which they were used by staff in charge at these institutions differed considerably. These discrepancies cannot be considered to have been simply due to lack of expertise on the part of the Indian superintendents in contrast to their British colleagues. The Indian doctors were well qualified in the same mode of Western-style psychiatric practice. Nor could the Indian report forms and diagnostic practices based on them be considered to have been out-dated in contrast to those used in North Wales. In fact, given the recognition of confusional insanity at the Indian institutions and the frequent use of dementia praecox at Madras, we might even consider them as more up to date with the diagnostic trends discussed in the specialist literature. Confusional insanity had a firm place in UK psychiatric classifications and dementia praecox and schizophrenia were to emerge as the most frequently used categories in institutions across the globe by the late 1930s.[10]

Ruptures and Continuities

The analysis of diagnoses attributed to patients in 1930 provides only a snapshot of a wider picture of categorisation. There are two ways in which developments over time in Ranchi's mental hospital reports need to be assessed. The first concerns the incidence of specific disorders reported from 1925 to 1940. The second relates to the introduction of a new standard report form in mental hospitals in British India during the early 1930s and the impact this had on diagnoses. In Ranchi, the new classification system was adopted in 1934. The important question we must ask is to what extent these new categories created a new panorama of disorders and clinical perceptions of their causation. Alternatively, there is a possibility that we are merely dealing with a formal swapping of labels that has no real bearing on the frequency with which particular conditions are reported and on psychiatrists' understanding of them. In other words, it is necessary to explore the nexus between terms and concepts and, ultimately, therapeutic practices. These issues are important because in well-managed institutional settings, patients' treatment depends on the type of disorder they are believed to be suffering from and consequently, the causes attributed to it. Hence classifications, the causal explanations underpinning them and changes in diagnostic practices are not merely of academic interest but may also have a vital impact on treatment and hence patients' experiences.

In 1934 the new report form was used at Ranchi for the first time.[11] Instead of the earlier form's title of 'Types of Insanity', the new heading referred to 'Form of Mental Disorder'. This change of nomenclature had been mooted by psychiatrists for a long time and was finally enshrined in the Mental Treatment Act in Britain in 1930. In a merely formal sense the new classification scheme is particularly striking due to its tighter focus on a smaller range of conditions (22 only in contrast to the previous 33). In some cases, multiple categories are merged and subsumed into one heading, as in mental deficiency in lieu of the earlier idiocy and imbecility. In other cases they are expunged, as in acute delirium and stupor. The underlying rationale was to depart from the traditional focus on the most prominent symptom, towards identification of a mental disorder on the basis of the patients' history and age, and the pattern of a range of reported and clinically observable symptoms over time. It is debatable when exactly this break with earlier traditions occurred. At Ranchi, a range of single symptom-based diagnoses was phased out long before the new classification was introduced.[12] Rather than creating or enabling new practices, the new form merely caught up with what had already been happening in institutional practice for many years, echoing Grotjahn's earlier observation on the situation in Germany. However, the reduction in the number of categories was not necessarily characteristic of developments in other countries. In Germany, an earlier classification (in place from 1901) specified only eight entities, while the new one, introduced in 1933, was based on 21, with a number of further subcategories.[13] The official medical coding in mental institutions in England and Wales between 1907 until 1948 relied on 17 main diagnostic entities, with subcategories bringing the overall number up to 25.

It seems doubtful that much changed in terms of practice at Ranchi when the new report form was introduced. As well as continuity in the number of the main diagnoses actually made use of, the categories of melancholia and mania were also retained. Despite modifications in nomenclature, some conditions appear to have been reported in a relatively constant way, even if under different terms: mental deficiency (subsuming the previous idiocy and imbecility); schizophrenia including dementia praecox (previously referred to as dementia praecox only); paranoia and paranoid states (previously delusional insanity [acute or chronic paranoia]); manic depressive insanity (previously circular insanity/alternating insanity); acute confusional insanity (previously confusional insanity, associated with infective, toxic and other general conditions); and cannabis indica psychosis (previously insanity due to cannabis indica or its preparations or derivates).

It is however important to bear in mind that we cannot be certain of any potential synchrony between old and new categories or the extent to which the new terms may also have implied different concepts, meanings and understandings.[14] The apparent stability of a category over time, as manifested in institutional statistics, is no proof of conceptual equivalence or construct reliability even with no change in terminology. For Ranchi there is a lack in information on how individual patients were re-classified in the wake of the transition from old to new record forms in 1933–34. Furthermore, as ideas about specific mental disorders and their aetiology were undergoing rapid change, it is likely that Dhunjibhoy's cognitive mapping of patients' conditions adapted accordingly, as did the treatments he applied to patients. The record forms used by institutions created their own panorama of conditions, which may have been quite different from the one conceived of by particular superintendents in relation to their patients. In fact, there is evidence that Dhunjibhoy used his own system of classification alongside the official nomenclature. We will now turn our attention to this evidence.

Berrios, Luque and Villagran have pointed out that an analysis of diagnoses ought to concern itself with the 'history of the behaviours in question, whatever the names they have travelled under'.[15] This is a difficult undertaking for medical historians, who, lacking valid and reliable data on actual behaviours, may have to rely on institutional data. However, Berrios et al. concede that while nomenclature, whether 'coined anew (schizophrenia) or recycled (mania, melancholia)' is 'rarely informative', its study remains important, 'for like semantic ghosts, original meanings may linger on and influence later usage'.[16] The extent to which we will be able to gain insight into the 'semantics' of the particular terms used at Ranchi on the basis of trends in the official statistics is doubtful. It is more likely that we instead gain some understanding of the administrative constraints and the 'peer and medico-legal pressures'[17] that led to the use of particular terms, as well as the role of transnational networks that enabled the formulation and practice of alternative diagnostic schemes. It is within this wider context of professional and administrative concerns that the following discussion of classifications needs to be understood.

The formal change of nomenclature in 1934 did not entail a semantic rupture in regard to the main categories. The reported incidence of particular conditions that might be considered equivalents corresponded well to the old (up to 1933) and the new (from 1934) classification schemes. Dementia praecox/schizophrenia is a good example of this. The reported rates remained the same for an almost identical cohort of patients (assessed at the end of 1933 under the old system [with dementia praecox] and reclassified at the end of 1934 under the new one [schizophrenia, including dementia praecox]), namely 20 per cent in both 1933 and 1934. The term changed and the new label was applied to more or less the same patients. What requires assessment is the longer-term trend for individual categories to ascertain any potential changes in the conceptualisation of particular conditions. Two main trends can be discerned from the late 1920s to 1939. Firstly, the stability in the frequency with which dementia praecox/schizophrenia and melancholia was assigned and, secondly, the gradual decline for mania and secondary dementia on the one hand and the significant rise in circular/manic depressive insanity on the other.

Dhunjibhoy diagnosed dementia praecox/schizophrenia in a numerically consistent fashion from around 1927 onwards, with relatively stable figures, fluctuating from

19 to 22 per cent. This stability emerges even more clearly once the data are disaggregated for gender (see section below, on male and female maladies.) The figures for melancholia were approximately 10 percentage points below those of dementia praecox/schizophrenia for the majority of the period, but similarly stable. The question is of course whether this apparent statistical stability for melancholia before and after 1934 and for dementia praecox/schizophrenia from 1927 onwards also indicates the stability of the constructs during those periods – regardless of the names used for them.

'On the omnibus': Dementia praecox and schizophrenia

In contrast to many other terms of early twentieth-century nomenclature, schizophrenia has survived well. As Berrios et al. have pointed out, this is not due to it having remained unchanged as a reliable and valid category since Bleuler coined the term in 1907, but rather to its intrinsic vagueness[18] and the extent to which it lent itself to various scientific, professional and social interests. Its more recent relevance to genetics and the financial interests of the pharmaceutical industry are examples of this.[19] Paradoxically, the anti-psychiatry movement and its particular focus on schizophrenia during the 1960s and 1970s arguably led to its further reification as a psychiatric category. As its adaptability to different scientific and social contexts attests, the continuity of a term does not imply conceptual continuity nor proof of its referent's validity as a phenomenon. Nor is the current conception of schizophrenia based on a single notion, but on a 'patchwork' of understandings, 'made out of clinical features plucked from different definitions'.[20] Arguably, schizophrenia has been an 'omnibus category' from the early twentieth century onwards.[21]

Varied strands of definition of schizophrenia can be identified both over time and at different localities. American psychiatry is understood to have followed the conceptual frameworks of Eugen Bleuler and Adolf Meyer, while Emil Kraepelin is believed to have been more influential in Europe, especially on the mainland.[22] The current historical reappraisal of Kraepelin's work in Germany, via the US, attests to the importance of the transnational flow of knowledge and the creation of confluences of academic interests at particular times. The earlier term, dementia praecox, used by Benedict Morel from the 1850s, was later reconfigured by Kraepelin within the context of wider conceptual changes in the understanding of dementia. Subsequently, in 1907, Bleuler substituted the term with schizophrenia. But this change did not equate to conceptual continuity in the sense of the old dementia praecox essentially slipping into the new clothes of schizophrenia. Bleuler's concept enunciated attributes and understandings that were quite different from Kraepelin's. The two terms were assembled by Bleuler, Kraepelin and others from selected fragments of the old insanities, given new names, and linked up with more or less diverse conceptual frameworks to anchor them to ongoing medical and psychological theory and changing social contexts.[23]

Is it possible to identify to which of the varied concepts Dhunjibhoy subscribed the patchworks of dementia praecox and schizophrenia? To once again use the transportation metaphor, next to whom did Dhunjibhoy sit on the terminological and conceptual omnibuses en route from dementia praecox to schizophrenia? As we know,

Dhunjibhoy travelled widely and kept up to date with the latest publications in his field. We can therefore assume that he was well aware of the prevalent definitional disparities and the exciting and often heated debates about them. It is likely that his conceptual mind-map changed over time.

Judging from the data we have concerning admission policies and patients' socio-demographic background, it is unlikely that there occurred any substantial change in the psychological makeup of the hospital population itself. Therefore, the increase in the figures for dementia praecox from 1925 to 1927 (from 15 to 19 per cent), before apparently stabilising around 20 per cent during subsequent years, is likely to be due to a conceptual shift. However, given that Dhunjibhoy took his patients (and the diagnoses attributed to them) from three different institutions and medical superintendents, the shift would have involved the different diagnostic styles of his predecessors. His peers at Patna, Berhampore and Dacca seem to have been less inclined to assign dementia praecox to patients than Dhunjibhoy. This highlights that institutional statistics may tell us more about the mind-sets of medical doctors than about the psychological condition of their patients.

If Dhunjibhoy was indeed more inclined to make use of dementia praecox as a diagnostic label than his predecessors, what diagnoses would patients have been given before his time? The one category that shows a significant decrease during the relevant period and is likely to have been the prime candidate is mania.

Identifying mania

Mania, too, was a vague category. However, it had been around for many centuries. In Greek antiquity and for centuries afterwards it was conceived of in terms of humoral theory, being characterised by a host of leading complaints in the absence of fever. These ranged from fits of fury and general delusions to confusion, jolliness and excitation to aggression. Siegel noted that mania was then coterminous with madness stating that, 'The word was derived from the same root as the term *mainomai*, to be mad, deranged. In Latin it was called *insania*. The Greek concept of mania comprised a great variety of mental abnormalities. But even in the 18th century Cullen still spoke of mania as *insania universalis*.'[24] Crucially, he points out that the 'ancient usage was not as restricted as the modern meaning of mania'. For Britain, the change towards the modern meaning has been dated to the nineteenth century, when the 'old monolithic view of madness started to break up' and the process of defining mania alongside melancholia as a disorder of the 'emotions' began.[25] Increasingly the term 'psychosis' was used to 'refer to the refurbished insanities'.[26] However, relics of the earlier semantics still resonated alongside and within the plethora of classification guidelines that characterised psychiatric theories and practices during the early twentieth century. The terms 'insanity', 'mania' and 'melancholia' continued to be used in British and British colonial institutions until at least 1940.

Given the coexistence of a multitude of different nosologies, unspecific symptom lists and imprecise definitions that were entangled with earlier and broader understandings, the recategorisation by Dhunjibhoy of a number of maniacs as cases of dementia praecox and, as we shall see, others of circular insanity (the later manic depressive insanity) may not be all that surprising. Mania, dementia praecox and circular insanity shared some characteristics. It has been noted that Kraepelin's conceptualisation of mania had contained a 'confusing multitude of symptoms'.[27] Nevertheless, the 'decline of Kraepelinean mania' in mainland Europe and the concomitant rise of Bleuler's concept of schizophrenia in 1911 led to an increasingly broad definition for schizophrenia and the narrowing down of the definition of mania.[28] In Germany, this process culminated after the Second World War in the 'relegation of mania to the status of a clinical rarity'.[29] Koehler and Sass contend that 'many or even most of the psychoses diagnosed in Germany between 1900 and 1920 would nowadays be considered as schizophrenias' in the Schneiderian sense.[30]

Although Schneider's work was of course not available to Dhunjibhoy in 1927, his more restricted use of mania was in line with what was happening in psychiatric institutions in European countries and the US. There, mania more or less disappeared as a specified main category and dementia praecox/schizophrenia tended to top the list of reported disorders. Dhunjibhoy noted in 1931: 'The high incidence of D. P. is now noticed in almost all the civilised nations of the world. It is high in England, Germany, France, Italy, and highest in America.'[31] He provided statistics from the state mental hospitals in the US, procured during his visits in 1930, which showed dementia praecox as the single most frequently assigned diagnosis (27 per cent), followed by manic-depressive psychosis (16 per cent).[32] Despite mania being increasingly rarely used by psychiatrists across the globe, it was retained in the official report forms in British India and used more widely also in the UK.

The date of Dhunjibhoy's reclassification of patients from mania to dementia praecox in 1927 is significant for a number of reasons. During the first two years of the opening of the new mental hospital, Dhunjibhoy was preoccupied with managerial matters such as dealing with overcrowding, adjusting the diet for patients, developing the fruit and vegetable gardens, identifying suitable nursing staff and responding promptly to outbreaks of cholera and smallpox in the nursing staff quarters and 'sweepers' lines' (cleaning staff's quarters). From 1927 onwards, Dhunjibhoy turned his attention towards the specifics of psychiatric treatment and classification. This was induced not least by his new duties as lecturer for medical students from nearby Patna. The lectures and practical demonstrations of cases were part of the 'intensive training in mental diseases as required by the curriculum of the Patna University for the degree of M.B.B.S.'[33] That same year in December, Dhunjibhoy also delivered a paper at the seventh Congress of the Far Eastern Association of Tropical Medicine, in Calcutta. These activities would have focused his mind on matters of research and any necessary reclassification of patients in terms of the most up-to-date theories.

How did mania figure in the institutional reports at Ranchi during the subsequent period? According to the official nomenclature, up until 1934 it was circumscribed as acute, intermittent or chronic and could be further specified as associated with pregnancy, parturition and lactation (puerperal), epilepsy or old age. There was also a fifth category, 'other forms', which was the most frequently used option. Under the new classification scheme, mania was retained without any subdivisions. The earlier manias related to the female reproductive cycle and old age were subsumed under this umbrella term. Mania sat alongside 10 other main categories (see Table 4.2).

Table 4.2. Form of mental disorder (main categories used from 1934)*

1. Mental Deficiency
2. Manic Depressive Insanity
3. Mania
4. Melancholia
5. Schizophrenia, including Dementia Praecox
6. Secondary Dementia
7. Paranoia and Paranoid States
8. Epilepsy and Epileptic Insanity
9. Toxic Psychosis
10. Organic Psychosis
11. Neurosis and Psycho-Neurosis
12. No Appreciable Disease
13. Not Yet Diagnosed

* Excludes here, for ease of presentation the five subcategories each of Toxic Psychosis and Organic Psychosis.[34]

Dhunjibhoy retained stability in his use of the mania category on occasion of the change of nomenclature in 1933 and 1934. However, figures decreased steadily in the later period, particularly from 1936 onwards. Dhunjibhoy had been on another visit to Europe and the US during the previous year and it is likely that the new ideas he picked up there led him to change his diagnostic practice, using the mania category more sparingly for those patients whom he had been able to observe for a longer period.[35]

Framing melancholia and circular/manic depressive insanity

During Dhunjibhoy's reclassification of mania cases in 1927 not all of the patients were allocated the dementia praecox label. A nearly equal number was subsumed under circular insanity. The long-term incidence trajectory of this category developed in tandem with that of mania – with decreases in the latter being echoed by increases in the former. This requires further scrutiny and needs to be discussed also in relation to melancholia.

Like dementia praecox, circular insanity is a relatively recent category. It was first described in the 1850s as a combined state, showing symptoms alternating between those of mania and of melancholia.[36] Observation over time was crucial in order to differentiate it from mania, melancholia and the exalted state of GPI. The issue of differential diagnosis plagued psychiatrists for many decades. During the late nineteenth and early twentieth centuries, the main characteristics of pure mania were considered to be disorders of thought and delusions, while the mania presented in the combined state of circular insanity was characterised by hyperactivity and elation.[37] The characteristics and boundaries of pure melancholia and of the melancholia as part of the combined state were less clearly established.[38]

In contrast to circular insanity, both mania and melancholia have been used as medical terms in Europe since antiquity.[39] Contrary to the apparent bifurcation inherent in the terms 'alternating' and 'manic depressive insanity' and their modern meanings, these conditions were not understood as polar opposites in earlier periods. Melancholia was referred to as a kind of mania or madness that presented itself in reduced behavioural inclinations. No idea of gloom or dejection was then conveyed by it. It simply meant to be mad. Therefore, 'the ancient diagnosis of melancholy has no correct analogue in modern psychiatric practice'.[40] The meaning of melancholia remained opaque, being used in plural ways over the centuries in relation to spiritual, social, political and cultural contexts, as well as within the humoral medical system. Within the humoral nexus, which dominated in Europe until the modern period, melancholia tended to be linked with bodily fluids.[41]

During the Renaissance in Europe, ancient associations of melancholy with genius found in Aristotle's work made it for a while 'a fashionable sign of nobility of mind in Florentine tradition/aristocratic pretensions',[42] leading historians to consider this period as 'the golden age of melancholy'.[43] A century later, its association with hypochondria led many to consider the period from the late seventeenth to the early eighteenth century as yet another 'age of melancholia'. The meaning of the term remained opaque. When Burton compiled an exhaustive list of melancholic symptoms culled from ancient and modern medical sources for his famous *Anatomy of Melancholie*, he concluded: 'the Tower of *Babel* never yielded such confusion of tongues, as this Chaos of Melancholy doth variety of symptoms'.[44] In the same work Burton attempted to delimit the meaning, giving it the connotation with which current understanding of depression can correspond more easily: 'a kind of dotage without fever, having for his ordinary companions fear and sadness, without any apparent occasion'. Nevertheless, in the early nineteenth century Esquirol was still led to echo Burton's earlier woes, contending that, 'the word melancholia, consecrated in popular language to describe the habitual state of sadness affecting some individuals should be left to poets and moralists whose loose expression is not subject to the strictures of medical terminology'.[45] The term itself had accumulated too much cultural baggage to be considered helpful by him in medical diagnostics.

Despite Esquirol's suggestion to avoid the term melancholia altogether,[46] it remained central to psychiatric nomenclature, with its meaning focusing ever more on affective (emotional) symptoms. Esquirol's attempt to define and delimit melancholia (or lypemania, as he called it) from other conditions, encapsulated some of the main dimensions that were to characterise later efforts to frame the disorder more specifically:

> A disease of the brain characterised by delusions which are chronic and fixed on specific topics, absence of fever and sadness which is often debilitating and overwhelming. It must not be confused with mania which exhibits generalised delusions and excited emotions and intellect nor with monomania that exhibits specific delusions and expansive and gay emotions, nor with dementia characterised by incoherence and confusion of ideas resulting from weakening.[47]

Melancholia was now seen as a disorder to be differentiated from mania and characterised by 'partial delusions'.[48] By the end of the nineteenth century, depression had become a central symptom. It is only with the benefit of hindsight that privileges particular traits post hoc, that we are able to discern a straight-line development from melancholia as one of the allegedly 'monolithic' insanities characterised by lack of motility to depression as an emotional disorder. In fact, it took some time for more precise definitions to be worked out. As Healy has pointed out, well into the nineteenth century 'any state that could lead to under activity or inactivity, for one reason or the other, was diagnosed as melancholia'.[49] What is more, a multitude of different definitions and classification systems were put forward. The rise of faculty psychology and experimental psychology resulted in different strands of thought developing in European countries towards the late nineteenth century, with varied ways of framing melancholia within the national classification systems employed in institutional settings from the early twentieth century onwards.

What is more, just 40 years ago, Kendell pointed out the legacy of the clash between 'the philosophies of the Meyerian and Kraepelinian schools' that could still be felt in the 1970s when he wrote his seminal paper on the classification of depressions, subtitled 'A Review of Contemporary Confusion'.[50] For a while, Kraepelin's understanding of melancholia came to predominate in Germany. In Britain his schema were not reflected in the official nomenclatures, published in 1906 and 1918 but remaining essentially unchanged until after the Second World War. There is evidence to suggest that some British medical doctors admired the German system. Frederick Mott, for example, tried to model Maudsley Hospital on the university psychiatric clinics of Munich, Berlin, Halle and Heidelberg.[51] The authors of an article in the *British Medical Journal* lamented in 1908 that Britain lacked 'so magnificent an instrument for teaching, research and cure as that recently established in Germany under Professor Kraepelin'.[52] However, such sentiments do not appear to have been shared by all colleagues in Britain. For example, Mott was succeeded at the Maudsley in 1923 by Edward Mapother who was hostile to Kraepelin's systematic approach. The nomenclature established in Britain and in British colonies did not follow Kraepelinian classifications.

The disjuncture between Germanic–Kraepelinian and British ways of understanding melancholia, in particular in relation to circular/manic depressive insanity, is an important issue. It helps to locate Dhunjibhoy's diagnostic reference points as he used both approaches.[53] As we will see, he completed institutional records following the prescribed British nomenclature, while availing himself of the Kraepelinean definitions in his overseas lectures and publications. So, how were melancholia and circular/manic-depressive insanity defined during Dhunjibhoy's period at Ranchi?

During the 1920s and early 1930s, melancholia was listed as just one of several subcategories of 'Group II: Disorders of Functions', alongside mania, circular insanity, stupor, and delusional insanity. Delirium, too, was subsumed under functional disorders next to melancholia until 1929, when it was moved to Group III and associated with infective, toxic and other general conditions. Melancholia was described as acute, intermittent or chronic, and subdivided into seven different types.[54] Most of these subcategories did not figure to any great extent during any one year, although they were more frequently applied to newly admitted patients. In 1934, mental stupor and acute delirium were dropped altogether, and melancholia was no longer subdivided. It became one of 11 main disorders in the new institutional record form (see Table 4.2). As in the case of the mania category, the abandoned subcategories were subsumed under the single umbrella term.[55]

Both the pre- and post-1934 nomenclatures used in colonial institutions consistently differentiated melancholia from mania and circular/manic depressive insanity. The Kraepelinean system, in contrast, subsumed a range of conditions under the term manic depressive psychosis. In this category Kraepelin included 'on the one hand the whole domain of so-called periodic and circular insanity, on the other hand simple mania, the greater part of the morbid states termed melancholia and also a not inconsiderable number of cases of amentia'.[56] Kraepelin's scheme was challenged by many of his colleagues in Europe. British and colonial nomenclature kept melancholia in a separate group from mania and circular insanity, referring only to the latter as manic depressive insanity (MDI). The UK's and Kraepelin's systems are not easily mapped on to one another. Dhunjibhoy, so it seems, managed to move between them with great ease although he showed a certain preference for the Kraepelinean classification in his publications.

In a critical exchange in the *Journal of Mental Science* (*JMS*) in 1931 on the prevalence of dementia praecox among different Indian communities, Dhunjibhoy listed the number of cases confined at Ranchi.[57] He referred to the categories of dementia praecox, cannabis insanity and manic depressive psychosis (MDP) – despite the fact that the latter term had yet to be used in the colonial reports (which then still specified circular insanity). Furthermore, he provided a figure of 447 for MDP, while the official records reveal only 87 for circular insanity and 149 for all types of melancholia. Given that the numbers admitted during that year amounted to only nine and four in these two categories respectively, it is clear that Dhunjibhoy had as his blueprint Kraepelin's scheme, subsuming other categories under the heading of MDP. Dementia praecox, too, was used in the Kraepelinian way, as here too the numbers were much higher (419) than those provided in the official end of year report (248). In contrast, the number of cases reported as insanity due to cannabis indica (ganja) exactly equated to the figures indicated in the institutional records. Cannabis insanity was considered a speciality of Indian mental hospitals and hence did not figure in Kraepelin's scheme, making it unnecessary for Dhunjibhoy to recalculate the number of cases.

Dhunjibhoy seems to have reclassified the conditions from the annual report forms, omitting mania and melancholia and referring only to those terms that would have been of interest to learned overseas colleagues such as Kraepelin. Hence, the high number of cases of MDP (447) referred to a selection of cases listed in the Ranchi records under circular insanity (87), mania (215), melancholia (149) and stupor (10).

The fact that Dhunjibhoy employed different nomenclature during professional debate indicates that the terms used in official records do not necessarily reflect psychiatrists' cognitive mind-maps of the diagnoses they consider relevant. Official classifications tend to be based on 'consensus and compromise', as pointed out by Agich in relation to the debates about the Würzburger Schlüssel in Germany.[58] Hospital superintendents may follow the consensus by diligently filling in their forms, yet make use of their own customised nomenclature during scientific debate. It is difficult to reconstruct how exactly Dhunbjibhoy translated the figures in the UK-based scheme into his version of the Kraepelinean nomenclature. The numbers for his MDP do not dovetail exactly with the 1928 figures for mania, melancholia, stupor and circular insanity. How he managed to identify 348 cases of dementia praecox in the official records, but 419 in his *JMS* article is difficult to fathom *post hoc*. It is unlikely that Dhunjibhoy misrepresented the Ranchi statistics in order to prove a particular point about the prevalence of dementia praecox in India. He would have known that manipulation of the figures would have exposed him to attack, if not official censure, especially as he had also recalculated the figures from other institutions (Madras, Bombay, Burma and the Punjab). It therefore seems more likely that he made use of a version of the Kraepelinean scheme in order to substantiate the argument he was putting forward about the high incidence of dementia praecox (and incidentally, of MDP) in India. Recalculating institutional figures on the basis of a nomenclature recognised in Europe and the US moved Dhunjibhoy beyond any possible reproach by colleagues in India. He could always argue that he attempted to make the Indian data comparable to those in other countries.

In another article published in 1930 in the *JMS*, based on a talk he gave at a meeting of the Royal Medico-Psychological Association at the David Lewis Colony at Watford in 1930, Dhunjibhoy provided a concise outline of the classification he preferred to use (see Table 4.3).

Table 4.3. 'Types of insanity commonly met with in India', listed in order of frequency[59]

1. Manic Depressive Psychosis
    a) Mania
    b) Melancholia
    c) Stuporose Phases
2. Dementia Praecox
3. Toxic Psychoses
    a) Indian Hemp Insanity
    b) Alcoholic Psychosis
    c) Confusional States
    d) Psychoses Associated with Infections, Pregnancy or Puerperium
4. Mental Deficiency
5. Further Psychoses
    a) Epileptic Insanity
    b) Paraphrenia and Paranoia
    c) Primary and Secondary Dementia
    d) Senile, Traumatic and Arteriopathic Psychoses
    e) Encephalitis Lethargica
    f) General Paralysis
    g) Psychoneuroses

His lecture was meant to show the high incidence of cannabis insanity in India. This condition was, in order of its recorded frequency at Ranchi, in third place, right behind Kraepelin's dementia praecox (DP) and manic depressive psychosis (MDP) (here, rendered in the singular, in the contemporary Germanic fashion to indicate the psychological meaning in contrast to the use of the plural, 'psychoses', when the individual insanities themselves are implicated).⁶⁰ What concerns us here is the prominence of MDP that subsumed both mania and melancholia along with stuporos phases. Dhunjibhoy's use of a modified version of the Kraepelinean as well as UK-based schemes is similar to what has been observed in regard to German refugees who came to Britain to work at the Maudsley. They too employed two nomenclatures.⁶¹ The German-based schemes accentuated the difference between DP and MDP, privileging these over the old insanities.

Echoing the developments in Germany, Dhunjbhoy came to assign circular insanity/ MDP with increased frequency, even in the official nomenclature, and mania less often (see Figure 4.1).

Figure 4.1. Percentage of patients assigned circular insanity/manic depressive insanity (mainly lower line) and mania (mainly upper line), 1925–1939

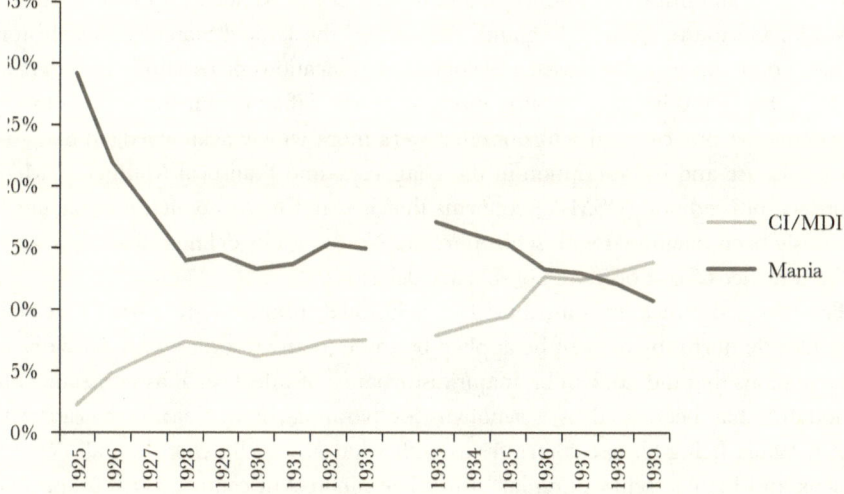

The 50 per cent fall in mania diagnoses between 1925 and 1928 is significant. About 135 mania cases were integrated into the classic twin Kraepelinean categories of DP and MDP (the circular insanity of the UK-based nomenclature used at Ranchi). The trend for both of them, as well as for mania, subsequently remained stable until 1934, when the decline of mania became an inverse image of the growth of what was then officially labelled manic depressive insanity (MDI) – a five per cent decrease for the former and five per cent increase for the latter.⁶² Given that melancholia continued to be attributed relatively consistently after 1934, it is unlikely that melancholic cases were reassigned to the MDI category. The most likely scenario is therefore that the statistical mirror image expresses an actual trend for mania cases to be reassigned to the MDI category. This development would be plausible given that mania and melancholia were used less and less frequently by psychiatrists across the world. The two terms were however retained in the medical registers for England and Wales and in India until after the Second World War.

Over the whole period, mania decreased and MDI increased by a factor of three. It may well be that a similar pattern prevailed during the same period in institutions that were antagonistic to Kraepelinean modes of thinking. Lacking any comparative data, this is difficult to establish. On the basis of the Ranchi data alone, it seems likely that Dhunjibhoy readjusted his diagnostic style in line with mainland European and American practices on two occasions, shortly after each of his extended overseas visits. This highlights the importance of transnational influences and of international scientific networks. 'British colonial psychiatry' would not be an adequate term to grasp the complex circumstances that framed diagnostic processes at Ranchi.

Delusional insanity – paranoia

Delusional insanity was another, relatively recent, category dating from the mid nineteenth century. Both the terms paranoia and delusional insanity have been embedded in different national histories of conceptualisation as Lewis, Kendler and Dowbiggin have shown for Germany, Austria, England, France and the United States.[63] Their histories are also bound up with the varied nosological identifications of psychotic disorders as a whole.[64] Delusional insanity became more narrowly defined from the 1920s onwards, after dementia praecox and schizophrenia were more widely acknowledged diagnoses. It is still in use and its description in the Diagnostic and Statistical Manual of Mental Disorders, fifth edition (DSM-V) confirms that it is not to be applied if a patient has previously been diagnosed with schizophrenia. Nowadays its defining feature is seen to be the presence of one or more non-bizarre delusions.

Previously, the meanings attributed to delusional insanity were varied and before the 1920s the term might even be applied by some to any disorder with delusions and hallucinations that did not exhibit major disturbance of affect (such as in melancholia). Although it has been used as a synonym for paranoia, it was earlier considered as wide ranging, being almost coterminous with what Kraepelin came to call dementia praecox and Bleuler, schizophrenia.[65] In its late nineteenth-century versions, paranoia corresponded most closely with Esquirol's intellectual monomania or partial insanity.[66] Its causation was contested, with Krafft-Ebing, for example, placing paranoia in 1905 among the 'psychic degenerations', accounted for by tainted heredity.[67] In contrast, Kraepelin came to consider it in his later writing as 'a matter of abnormal development which takes place in persons of psychopathic disposition under the influences of the ordinary forces of life'.[68] Dementia praecox, in contrast, remained in his reading a degenerative, neurologically based disorder. In 1907, Kraepelin contrasted the delusions in paranoia clearly with those seen by him to be characteristic of dementia praecox, with the former being 'built out into a coherent system',[69] never 'incoherent' or 'bizarre' and 'without marked mental deterioration, clouding of consciousness or disorder or thought, will or conduct'.[70] However, according to Aubrey Lewis, Kraepelin was 'never comfortable with paranoia' and may have abandoned it as a separate category had he lived longer.[71]

As we have seen, Dhunjibhoy's diagnostic practice was grounded in Kraepelin's classification. This was not necessarily so in the case of other superintendents in India.

For example, in the discussion of delusional insanity in one of the standard reference works, *Lunacy in India* by A. W. Overbeck-Wright, the author reveals the diverse understandings of diagnostic categories of that time, despite the impression of uniformity and standardisation that historians may glean from the official institutional reports. Overbeck-Wright pointed out that 'no one universal classification prevails', noting that he preferred the nomenclature developed by L. C. Bruce because he had worked 'on its lines since 1908' and found it 'the simplest and best for general work and comprehension of the subject'.[72] Bruce had qualified at Edinburgh in 1894 and, failing to obtain a position in the Royal Army Medical Corps or the Indian Medical Service, became medical superintendent at Perth District Mental Hospital at Murthly.[73] Being described as 'a little old-fashioned', he 'concentrated on the physical aspect of mental disease'.[74] Bruce was 'an enthusiast of vaccine therapy' and thyroid treatment. His laboratory-based, scientific work failed to receive recognition, partly because it became quickly outmoded and also because he worked in isolation, being known for being 'the reverse of tactful'.[75] Overbeck-Wright was one of the few who followed Bruce's approach of dividing 'affections broadly into those of non-toxic and those of toxic origin' as outlined in Bruce's, *Studies in Clinical Psychiatry* of 1906.[76]

Overbeck-Wright himself was superintendent at Agra Mental Hospital and lectured on mental diseases at King George's Medical College Lucknow and Agra Medical School. He was the author of *Mental Derangements in India. Their Symptoms and Treatment* (1912), published in Calcutta, and of the more widely received *Lunacy in India* (1921), published in London. He was not in favour of Kraepelin's way of describing paranoia as one of the forms of dementia praecox, alongside catatonia and hebephrenia.[77] This was an 'error', he said, 'for paranoia is of totally different origin from either katatonia or hebephrenia'.[78] Kraepelin too treated these disorders as three distinct 'degenerative processes' with a constitutional basis. However, Overbeck-Wright saw them as having 'not a single feature in common', except that they 'all tend to affect largely young adults of marked neurotic heredity', with katatonia and hebephrenia being due to bacterial toxaemias. In fact, he argued, 'dementia praecox, too, is a misleading term to apply to any of these conditions'.[79] He therefore took to 'ignoring the term *dementia praecox*, and grouping these various conditions under the one head of "Delusional Insanity"'.[80] Overbeck-Wright was correct in his contention that catatonia, hebephrenia and dementia praecox were very different from each other in terms of their appearance (*Erscheinung*, that is, markers such as pulse and temperature). However, Kraepelin's emphasis had been on their perceived shared clinical course, namely that they led to enfeeblement and disintegration of the mind.[81] In Kraepelin's system, matters of clinical appearance were subsidiary to the development of a disorder over time. Both Overbeck-Wright's and Kraepelin's ways of framing disorders had advantages and disadvantages; they were also difficult to match on to each other.

Overbeck-Wright's understanding of delusional insanity was clearly wider ranging than Dhunjibhoy's, as the latter was wedded to Kraepelinian classifications. Such clashes were not unusual or unique to India, having characterised the 'paranoia question' that had engaged psychiatrists' attention during the 1890s.[82] Aubrey Lewis summarised the situation, noting that the 'apparent frequency of the condition consequently varied greatly', and in some hospital reports 'paranoiacs constituted 50% of all admissions, while at the other extreme [Wilhelm] Weygandt, for instance, said that he had diagnosed paranoia on only three occasions, out of 3,000 patients he had seen'.[83] By the late 1920s, the paranoia about paranoia had subsided and, as Berrios has pointed out, the mental affliction became more narrowly circumscribed concomitant on the wider recognition of dementia praecox and schizophrenia. But views such as Overbeck-Wright's clearly lingered for some time. This makes comparisons between institutions problematic, despite the apparent standardisation of classification systems in India.

To make things even more complex, Dhunjibhoy distinguished between dementia praecox and paraphrenia and paranoia. Paraphrenia was meant to designate paranoid disorders that develop later than in dementia praecox, and were milder.[84] This was in keeping with Kraepelin's suggestion of 1912 that:

> If a group of patients with chronic delusions were to be followed up – and if problems such as alcohol [and presumably cannabis for India; WE] and syphilis were to be excluded, about 40% will eventually develop dementia praecox; a larger group will have paraphrenias, and the rest paranoias.[85]

In his publication of 1930, Dhunjibhoy avoided the term delusional insanity, referring instead to paraphrenia and paranoia as 'psychoses' separate from dementia praecox. He noted that paraphrenia and paranoia were 'practically the same as found in the West', brushing over the issue that at the time no consensus prevailed 'in the West' regarding these categories.[86] He highlighted differences in regard to the observed content of patients' delusions, namely that 'among paranoiacs, exalted, querulant or persecutory cases were more common than the amorous, religious or hypochondriacal'. However, his classification boundaries were not clear. He also referred to 'the paranoid and the katatonic types' of dementia praecox, which he reported to have been 'more common in educated and the simple and the hebephrenic in uneducated persons'.[87] Given that Kraepelin changed his views on classifications several times, it is perhaps not surprising that Dhunjibhoy used a variety of terms and overlapping or even mutually exclusive concepts. The real test for any concept's validity is how its meaning relates to other categories within a particular classificatory system.[88] It is difficult to do this post hoc, as we lack a commentated grid of criteria for the full range of categories used by Dhunjibhoy.

Formally, the term delusional insanity (acute or chronic paranoia) was used at Ranchi until 1933, when it was superseded by paranoia and paranoid states. As with most of the previously discussed disorders, from about 1928 onwards its reported incidence remained stable. The aggregate rate for women and men fluctuated around six per cent of the overall patient population.

Dementia, delirium and confusion

The impact on diagnostic practice of conceptual developments in different European countries and the USA can also be pinpointed in regard to other categories. Dementia and confusional insanity were relatively prominent in the Ranchi statistics, albeit less than in the conditions previously discussed. Delirium, on the other hand, was rarely used and was dropped in the new nomenclature of 1934. Focusing on it is however warranted as the historical trajectory of dementia, delirium and confusion are intertwined and best considered together.[89] Furthermore, the problems of placing delirium into the appropriate group in the pre-1934 classification reflect contemporary confusion about this term, raising issues of broader interest to historians of psychiatry.

Dementia, delirium and confusion are now considered as manifestations of related neuropathology or as resulting from physical disorders. Because of their organic aetiology, we might expect them to be more easily identified and delimited from one another than the functional disorders or psychoses. However, this does not appear to be the case – either in regard to current practices or in earlier periods. Even in current historiographic analysis there is a clear contradiction here. On the one hand, dementia and delirium were 'characterised by a surprising phenomenological stability', with robust descriptions despite a multitude of different terms being used since antiquity. On the other hand, the 'kaleidoscopic aspects' connected with them make it 'hard to define and difficult to study' them.[90] The twin problems of retrospective assessment of diagnoses and the widely acknowledged protean manifestations of them are implicated here. Lindesay et al. have noted that current nomenclature about delirium is 'confusing because of the different names used to define and describe it'.[91] The situation is no less perplexing if an attempt is made to dovetail the current term with the 16 or so different words used by Hippocrates for states that we might nowadays consider as delirium.[92] The same applies to the varied terms used for what became dementia the way we understand it today, as a condition clearly delimited from schizophrenia.

There also is and has been much ambiguity surrounding confusional insanity, despite this term only being coined in the middle of the nineteenth century. The fact that it has since been used widely in all countries as a synonym for delirium does not help to clarify the situation.[93] The conceptual overlap between delirium and confusion can be traced to reference to the latter in its nineteenth-century French version, as a syndrome wider than and including delirium, with an emphasis on chaotic thinking and cognitive failure.[94] The narrower understanding of delirium encompassed 'a cluster of mental and behavioural symptoms occurring in the wake of physical disease'.[95] Here the focus was on transient and intermittent features. By the early twentieth century there seems to have been a degree of consensus, whereby the outcome of delirium was either death or full recovery. Its cause was linked to organic factors, while confusion could be due to non-organic causes.[96] The perceived gravity of delirium and its poor prognosis differentiated it from dementia as chronic cognitive impairment involving judgement and memory.[97]

We may then expect this wider historical context of overlaps and entanglement of terminology and conceptual uncertainty to be mirrored in ambivalent institutional nomenclature and unstable statistical trends. However, the Ranchi records reveal formal classification problems only in regard to delirium. The situation for confusional insanity is more difficult to interpret. But even here, diagnostic practice may have been stable, as numerical variation can be explained by plausible external factors. Let us first consider dementia.

Dementia

In his journal article of 1930, Dhunjibhoy had relegated primary and secondary dementia to the last grouping in his house style. Nominally, this category was however substantial. In 1930, for example, the figures were higher than those for cannabis insanity (116 for the former and 102 for the latter). Yet, in his lecture and published article, Dhunjibhoy chose to highlight the Indian 'peculiarity' rather than a humdrum category that had been the bane of psychiatrists all over the world. Many institutions were clogged up with dementia and hence 'chronic' patients. Dhunjibhoy acknowledged this fact, pointing out that primary and secondary dementia 'are also noticed, and the latter contribute[s] largely to the chronic population of the mental hospitals.'[98]

However, the number of patients classified as suffering from secondary dementia at Ranchi steadily decreased. The fall of over 50 per cent during the period is due to the strictures imposed on the admission of chronically ill, yet harmless people. Before and after 1934 only 28 and three new patients respectively were admitted.[99] The decrease in secondary dementia was therefore due to death and discharge. The slight increase in 1934 may have arisen from the abolition of the category dementia with epilepsy and the absorption of these cases at that time and their reclassification a couple of years later, in 1934–35, under the rubric of epilepsy and epileptic insanities.

Under the earlier nomenclature, secondary or terminal dementia was a subcategory of dementia (primary or secondary), listed under Group III (insanity of infective, toxic and other general conditions). In contrast to dementia praecox, which also still belonged to Group III rather than Group II (disorders of function), primary and secondary dementia were subdivided further.[100] In 1934 Groups II and III were disbanded and considerable reassignment occurred in regard to the conditions that had previously been subsumed under Group III. Most noteworthy, dementia praecox was given its own group, as a psychosis, under the label schizophrenia, including dementia praecox. The new phrasing indicates that the two terms were not considered equivalent and that a compromise was negotiated between those preferring schizophrenia and others who favoured the old, more narrowly defined term. Here again, the influence of a variety of different conceptual styles of classification can be discerned. Secondary dementia also came to be its own group, separate from the now segregated groups of toxic psychosis and organic psychosis, under which it had previously been subsumed in Group III. Primary dementia was no longer listed.

Despite Berrios's contention that 'almost identical symptom clusters have been observed throughout the ages', the changes of term (let alone concepts or meanings) appear confusing.[101] It is not clear how these matched up with particular disease entities or even symptomatologies. This may not be entirely unexpected as dementia did not refer to any specific disease but to what we now call a syndrome – a collection of symptoms and signs. Furthermore, in Britain primary and secondary dementia were not differentiated in the *Nomenclature of Diseases*.[102] Dementia continued to refer to both under the umbrella term 'dementia, primary or secondary'. In India, in contrast, the conjoint designation, as well as primary dementia, were abandoned and only secondary dementia was specified in the post-1934 nomenclature. Judging from Dhunjibhoy's figures, there was continuity between the old secondary or terminal dementia[103] and the new secondary dementia. However, it cannot be established what kind of cases were subsumed under these labels.

There is a clear tension between historians' confidence in being able to trace the stability of particular symptom clusters over time post hoc and the recognition that the very conditions these were supposed to denote are even today difficult to delineate and research. A team of psychiatrists have recently observed this, even in relation to the arguably more robust category of delirium.[104] Despite the restricted technological means available to psychiatrists at the time for differentiating the various neurological, psychiatric and medical conditions that could be implicated in secondary dementia, Dhunjibhoy's assessment appears nominally stable. We are left to trust that his patients received the kind of care and attention that helped to ameliorate their experience – regardless of how their condition was classified.

Delirium

During the 1920s and 1930s the term delirium was rarely used. This is partly due to the British *Nomenclature of Diseases* requiring diagnosticians to employ it only when the cause was not known. Episodes of delirium therefore tended to be coded 'under the head of [their] cause'.[105] The other reason for its scarce appearance in the records is connected with the adoption of a more inclusive category. Confusional insanity was framed more broadly, encompassing delirium in its original French definition. The continued use of delirium alongside the confusional insanity category was therefore unnecessary and its eventual abandonment in 1934 was indeed pre-shadowed by its rare use in the preceding years. Only six cases of acute delirium were reported at Ranchi between 1925 and 1933.[106] However, the ways in which the term itself was moved around in the report forms in India prior to eventually being dropped indicates the continued reverberation of a much older conceptual problem.

For a time, delirium had been an epistemological challenge for theories on how physical and mental disease could be differentiated within the Western Cartesian model based on the separation of body and mind. Delirium manifests itself in mental and behavioural symptoms that occur in the wake of physical disease and hence 'created a theoretical conundrum'.[107] Berrios has argued that these conceptual issues had been resolved by the nineteenth century. Delirium was redefined as 'organic in a strong sense' and separate from the functional insanities or psychoses.[108] However, echoes of these earlier uncertainties seem to have resurfaced much later. In the Ranchi records, acute delirium was listed under Group II (disorders of functions) in 1925 and 1926. In 1927, it appeared in its own column, squeezed between Group II and Group III (insanity of infective, toxic and other general conditions), apparently considered as neither one nor the other but perhaps as a bridge between the two. The following year it was moved to Group III, where it remained, rarely used, until 1934.

Lacking detail on the debates surrounding delirium's path towards its destiny as a mental manifestation of organic conditions, we can only speculate that what can be identified in the Ranchi records may be a very belated rehearsal of the debates Berrios dates a century earlier, when it is said to have been aetiologically and phenomenologically redefined. If this interpretation is valid, it would constitute another example of how an investigation of conceptual developments as expounded in the writings of prominent figures does not necessarily correspond with what was happening on the ground.

Confusional insanity

For confusional insanity the situation on the ground was quite different from the delirium pattern. Being used synonymously with delirium up to the present day, this category was consistently subsumed under Group III, indicating its stable status as an organically based condition. The number of cases so identified at Ranchi in the pre-1934 period was much higher (32) than for delirium (6), but overall remained under four per cent of the total population. In view of the low figures, any interpretation of the numerical trend over time is highly speculative. However, Dhunjibhoy indicated that in India confusional insanity was linked mainly to 'starvation and physical exhaustion'.[109] The rise from two to four per cent during the early 1930s may be a reflection of the impact of the worldwide economic depression.[110] Severe hunger cases made 'a speedy recovery with rest and a good nourishing diet' and 'this psychosis [was] one of the few that help[ed] to improve the annual Indian recovery-rate on direct admissions'.[111] Dhunjibhoy estimated the recovery-rate on direct admissions to have been 33.4 per cent.[112] Figures based on the rate of patients remaining in the institution at the end of each year are therefore bound to underestimate the actual number of cases annually treated for the condition. In fact, the total number of patients treated during the pre-1934 period was 334, which differs by a factor of 10 from the 32 cases counted at the inpatient census date each December. The number of admissions over the same period was 204. Cases of confusional insanity were therefore frequently encountered at Ranchi, but as they tended to recover quickly, the turnover rate was high, resulting in low permanent inpatient rates.

Severe hunger took its toll in an area where starvation was endemic concomitant on unequal distribution of the means of living. The 'madness of hunger' has also been documented for other areas of the world, most controversially perhaps by Nancy Scheper-Hughes in regard to late twentieth-century Brazil.[113] Here people affected by severe and common mental symptoms of starvation and malnutrition were prescribed modern drugs while being left to continue to go hungry. In the absence of the mixed blessings bestowed by the pharmaceutical industry during the late twentieth and early twenty-first centuries, Dhunjibhoy applied the basic treatment of nutritional food and rest. What happened to the patients on their recovery and subsequent discharge is a matter for conjecture.

From idiocy and imbecility to mental deficiency

Admission restrictions affected not only cognitively impaired elderly people and the starving, but also those suffering from various kinds of what is now referred to as intellectual disability. If they displayed mostly harmless behaviour and were easily subdued, they were left to fend for themselves within their communities. Hence their number was low at Ranchi, fluctuating around four to five per cent of the overall hospital population during most of the period. The rate in a sample of 10 institutions in England and Wales in 1934 was estimated at 14 per cent.[114] Before 1934, at Ranchi, they were categorised as idiots and imbeciles and afterwards as mentally deficient.

Issues regarding the legal culpability of this group were a main focus of debate in the nineteenth century, alongside concerns about the state's responsibility for providing appropriate care facilities. The accurate delimitation of the intellectually disabled from the mentally ill was another major issue. The desirability of providing separate institutional provision was increasingly mooted and in Britain led to the Idiots Act of 1886 and the recommendation of care and educational facilities for idiots and imbeciles. However, a great number of them continued to be looked after by families or were admitted to work houses and prisons. With the Mental Deficiency Act of 1913, the link between mental deficiency and poor law and penal institutions began to be chiselled away and dedicated school and work 'colonies' were established. Dhunjibhoy visited one of these on the 4th of February 1930 when he travelled to the David Lewis colony at Warford in Cheshire. This colony, established in 1904, cared mainly for people with epilepsy but gradually broadened its scope, providing care also for the mentally deficient.[115]

The Idiots Act of 1886 had referred only to idiots and the imbecile. By the time of the Royal Commission on the Care and Control of the Feeble-Minded (1904–1908), epileptics, the feeble-minded and defective were explicitly specified. The shifts in terminology during the nineteenth and twentieth centuries have been widely researched.[116] A diverse range of intellectual disabilities and even the deaf and dumb have been subsumed under varied terms over the decades, with different nomenclatures emerging in the UK and the USA. For example, mental handicap, mental subnormality, mental retardation, and mental, learning and developmental disabilities are some of the more recent terms employed.

A grading system of sorts containing idiocy (severest type), imbecility (intermediate), and feeble-mindedness (least severe) emerged during the late nineteenth century. In 1908, the British physician Alfred Tredgold published his *Mental Deficiency (Amentia)*, which was to become the standard textbook on the subject and was influential in the development of eugenic sterilisation initiatives. The Mental Deficiency Act of 1913 defined different categories and spelt out the extent of their impairment in relation to the care and supervision required. Idiots were deemed to be 'deeply defective', imbeciles affected in a 'pronounced' way and 'incapable of managing themselves', the feeble-minded required 'care, supervision and control', and moral imbeciles suffered from 'mental weakness with strong vicious or criminal propensities', with punishment having no effect on them.[117] In Britain these terms were used in the *Nomenclature of Diseases*, supplemented by moral imbecility and sexual perversion during the 1930s.

At Ranchi, the nomenclature before 1934 specified only idiots and the imbecile, apparently still following the terms employed in the Idiots Act of 1886. However, as with other categories, these were no longer the only ones used by practitioners such as Dhunjibhoy. He referred to mental deficiency prior to the official introduction of the new nomenclature, noting that in India 'among the certified the imbeciles preponderate over the idiots and the feeble-minded', although the latter subgroup was not differentiated in the records.[118] Ranchi statistics reveal that at least up to 1934 the most severe cases (idiocy) and hence those requiring most care were outnumbered three to one by the more moderately affected mentally deficient.[119]

It has been suggested that definitional consistency in regard to intellectual disability prevailed across time, despite changes in terminology. Scheerenberger, for example, noted in 1983 that 'the major elements (intellectual deficits, problems coping with the demands of everyday life, and onset during the developmental period)' common to the current definition in the United States, were used by professionals as early as 1900.[120] However, as Hoult has shown, in New Zealand institutions the understanding of mental deficiency differed from the late nineteenth century to the 1920s. For example, 'the opinions of doctors at Porirua or Auckland did not always correspond with those of Tokanui's'.[121] The view that organically based conditions were easier to classify and diagnose than mental disorders may be overly optimistic and based on an ungrounded trust in the universal reliability of disease concepts. How Dhunjibhoy differentiated between the various types of mental deficiency is difficult to ascertain.

The merging in India of the earlier two categories in 1934, as opposed to increased differentiation of terms in Britain, reflects the lack of provision in colonial India for people with intellectual disabilities. Dhunjibhoy fell short of criticising the government when he bemoaned this situation in front of the quarterly meeting of the Royal Medico-Psychological Association at the David Lewis Colony in 1930, stating that: 'thousands of India's uncertified defectives are at large and not under State control. In addition, there exist no special institutions for the treatment of defectives.'[122] The British had introduced prisons and hospitals to India, but made no provision akin to the New Poor Law in England and Wales. The practice in Britain prior to the Mental Deficiency Act of 1913, of sending those who could not be looked after by their relatives to the workhouse and other poor law facilities, was not an option available in the colony. In the twentieth century the establishment of specialist care facilities, similar to the school and work colonies for the mentally defective in Britain, was not considered an option either. It is doubtful whether such institutions would have been welcome by the Indian population. Considering the government's laissez-faire approach during the colonial period towards the fate of India's poor in general, and of the mentally deficient in particular, issues concerning the medical categorisation of the latter group were evidently not a priority.

A culture-specific syndrome: Cannabis insanity

At the turn of the twentieth century, Kraepelin carried out research in Java to ascertain the impact of culture on mental illness.[123] The challenge was to fathom whether Western psychiatric nomenclature was universally applicable, despite the different, culturally specific content of delusions manifest in non-Western patients' psychotic episodes. At around the same time, prominent doctors in India mooted the reconfiguration of Western theories. One of Dhunjibhoy's contemporaries, Girindrasekhar Bose (1887–1953), had in 1922 founded the Indian Psychoanalytic Society in Calcutta and argued that Freudian theory required modification to fit the Hindu psyche.[124]

The work of ethnographers and anthropologists such as H. H. Risley and Bronislaw Malinowsky provided a wider context within which debates on culture-bound syndromes could be anchored. They focused on racial and caste typologies and the perceived behavioural, moral and psychological otherness of so-called primitive civilisations and noble savages. Malinowsky's teacher, the eminent, medically trained C. G. Seligman, who became professor of ethnology at the London School of Economics, attracted much attention from psychiatrists such as D. K. Henderson and R. D. Gillespie, John Macpherson and J. R. Lord, when he read a paper on 'Temperament and Insanity in the Far East', at a meeting of the Royal Medico-Psychological Association in 1930. His primary interest was to identify Asians' 'temperament' and learn if they 'reacted to the stresses of life in the same manner as did Europeans'.[125] Henderson contended that 'from the point of view of race temperaments, different peoples tended to react in rather specialized ways'.[126] Gillespie conceded that Seligman's work signalled 'the beginning of something which would be the means of elucidating many problems which were now puzzling us, especially those concerned with the pathology of the psychoses'. He observed that the question of temperament 'was in the air' and that even 'Jung's notions were not particularly useful'. Macpherson contrasted Seligman's findings with Kraepelin's. A minority view was expressed by August Wimmer of Copenhagen, described by the psychiatric epidemiologist Eric Stromgren as 'the most learned psychiatrist whom I have ever met'.[127] Wimmer cautioned against 'attaching too much importance to symptomatology' as well as 'historical researches on insanity'.[128] The former was 'influenced in so many ways by individuality and the particular surroundings of the person concerned'. In the case of the latter, the 'mentality' of people in earlier periods was so different from later ones that 'one could not draw definite conclusions as to the nature of the mental symptoms or disturbances' found.[129]

Views such as those expressed by Wimmer were relatively rare among psychiatrists at the time. Still, the social and cultural peculiarities attributed to Indians raised contentious questions about the universality of psychological and moral predispositions and about particular communities' social inclinations. At the same time, anti-colonial strife and increased national consciousness and nationalist movements among Indians articulated new ideas about Indian identity and valorised its uniqueness as well as India's right to join the global guild of independent nations.[130] The extent to which Western diagnostic categories and psychological theories were appropriate to the Indian context was therefore widely debated. It still is today, albeit within the post-colonial context of a quite different concept of culture and a widespread assumption that all branches of science have been and need to be subject to successful globalisation. Modern psychiatrists and psychoanalysts have highlighted 'specific culture-bound syndromes seen in India'.[131] Kakar suggested that 'the "hegemonic narrative" of Hindu culture as far as male development is concerned, is neither that of Freud's Oedipus nor of Christianity's Adam …[but] that of Devi the great goddess, especially in her manifold expressions as mother in the inner world of the Hindu son.'[132] How these suggestions apply to different religious communities and social strata of society in South Asia has however not been articulated.

The issue of the postulated 'average Indian's' difference from the 'average Caucasian' is still a matter of discussion among psychiatrists in South Asia, as attested by Avasthi's recent presentation to the Indian Psychiatric Society entitled 'Indianizing Psychiatry'.[133] Are diagnostic criteria derived from clinical observations in Western countries also valid in the Indian context? Is there a need to globalise or conversely to Indianise and, more generally, localise psychiatry? As Avasthi points out, there has been a tendency to the former, with any psychological problems puzzling to Westerners being considered 'ethnic' and 'culture bound'. *Dhat*-syndrome or the fear of semen loss is one such condition. It is included in the current International Classification of Diseases (ICD) as both an 'other specific neurotic disorder' and a culture specific disorder (in the ICD 10 Annexe). It is diagnosed in relation to male patients who attribute their fatigue, weakness and multiple somatic complaints to the loss of semen through nocturnal emission, urination and masturbation, and has until recently been considered specific to South Asia.[134] Given *dhat*'s status as a neurosis, patients suffering from it were unlikely to be admitted to institutions dedicated to the reception of the dangerous and violent. No such case was mentioned by Dhunjibhoy.

Cannabis insanity was another condition considered to be a 'culture bound' phenomenon, namely, as Dhunjibhoy put it, a 'special form of mental disease' that was 'commonly met with' and peculiar to India.[135] At Ranchi, its statistical mode was a stable 10 per cent, in line with the reported incidence in some other institutions.[136] Dhunjibhoy published on this phenomenon in the 1920s.[137] By doing so, he established himself as an expert on a mental disease allegedly unique to India, ensuring a lasting legacy by continuing reference to his article.[138] Dhunjibhoy's publication was also timely as it reverberated with a number of wider social and academic debates. For example, it fits in with Western psychiatrists' concerns about how the toxic psychoses should be recategorised in light of new insights derived from chemical analyses and developments in pathology. Moreover, the first chair of pharmacology was established at the Calcutta School of Tropical Medicine in 1921, and its incumbent, Cambridge-educated R. N. Chopra, surveyed 'toxic insanity cases' in Indian mental hospitals from 1928 onwards. From 1930 to 1931, Chopra was to head the high-profile Drugs Enquiry Committee, which led to the Drugs Act of 1940.[139] Dhunjibhoy would have been aware of these developments in his area of expertise. Chopra was to cite his Ranchi-based colleague's observations in his and his co-author's article for the World Health Organization in 1957.[140]

Western eyes, too, turned to the potential dangers and the exploitation of the Indian pharmacopoeia as new drugs were sought, while in India access to cheaper indigenous medicines during a period of economic austerity was seen to require adequate knowledge about the composition, purity and efficacy of ingredients. The professionalisation along Western lines of Indian medical approaches such as Ayurveda, Unani and Siddha went hand in hand with further examination and control of the drugs used by them.[141] There clearly existed a wider policy and scientific context for the reassessment of cannabis both as a drug used in indigenous medicine and as potentially implicated in mental disease. Dhunjibhoy was therefore bound to make an impact on discussions in the fields of psychiatry and pharmacology as well as on policy debates about the control of drug addiction and the role of narcotic drugs in indigenous medical systems. Overseas interest was further heightened by him framing his insights in an idiom imbued with eugenic connotations and references to 'defective stock', while providing alluring exotic details of Oriental customs and practices. For example, in regard to the connection of hemp drugs with crime he surmised:

> Excessive or prolonged use of hemp drugs degrades the mind and character of the consumer and predisposes him to commit crime. Thus hemp is one of the most effectual means of increasing the criminal classes in India. It is also largely consumed by bad characters to fortify themselves for crime. Bhang is a very useful weapon in the hands of criminals for looting ornaments [i.e., jewellery] from women of easy virtue, and the sweetmeat majum for looting ornaments from children. It is also a known fact that some persons fortify themselves with an excessive dose of ganja, generally mixed with dhatura [*Datura*] seeds (stramonium), for premeditated murders, whether for gain, grudge or revenge. Similarly, sudden or prolonged use of large doses of hemp mixed with dhatura seeds are responsible to some extent for such serious crimes as unpremeditated murder, running amok, grievous hurt, rape, etc., which occur daily in a country like India.[142]

These views corresponded with contemporary eugenic concerns and Orientalist preconceptions across the world.[143] In other passages Dhunjibhoy used the preferred psychiatric terminology of the time, referring to the condition as 'hemp drug psychosis', rather than 'insanity', and its diagnosis, prognosis, post-mortem examinations and treatment. Large parts of his narrative however relied heavily on earlier publications, going back to the mid-nineteenth century.[144] Although some of the formulations and arguments advanced are nearly identical, the wider context of the previous debates, and hence the meanings attributed to particular assessments, were quite different. During the earlier period, medical and public debates on the politics and morals of the Opium Wars of 1839–42 and 1856–60, as well as fears about the degeneration of racial stock and the reported connection of particular drugs with 'criminal tribes'[145] and so-called criminal castes provided the background against which reports of cannabis-related insanity were read. The fact that alcohol consumption among European troops in India constituted a severe problem for military discipline and soldiers' health, with cases of *delirium tremens* and alcohol-related mental derangement reported increasingly by asylum staff, led to attention also being paid to Indians' preferred drug habits. While the Europeans' vice was alcohol, the Indians' was hemp. Both became subjects of medicalisation.

There were of course continuities and overlaps in medical, political and public discourse on these various aspects during the late nineteenth and early twentieth centuries. However, the ways in which the term cannabis insanity has been discussed has generally been notably ignorant of the specific contexts that drove different conceptualisations under the same or similar terms. Furthermore, earlier highly selective and anecdotal evidence has been reproduced uncritically, up to the present day reflecting various political interests and legal, moral and medical concerns around the prohibition or legalisation of cannabis use. Let us first consider the evidence Dhunjibhoy used in his article.

Dhunjibhoy's observations were principally based on his clinical experience at Ranchi, from 1925 to 1928, and at Berhampore some years earlier. At Ranchi alone he would have treated 126 to 136 patients diagnosed with 'insanity due to cannabis indica or its preparations or derivates'. His criteria for the diagnosis were based on the patients' behavioural histories, the absence of hereditary factors, and clinical observation of symptoms and physical signs:

> A patient admitted to an Indian mental hospital with intense excitement, grandiose ideas, tendency to wilful violence and destruction, the peculiar eye condition [conjunctival congestion in the horizontal vessels of both eyes] [...], total amnesia of all events, with an attack of short duration followed by complete recovery, with a history of the drug habit and without a psychopathic or neuropathic heredity is a typical case of 'hemp insanity'.[146]

Dhunjibhoy suggested that hemp drugs 'produce a special form of mental disorder, which is characterised by a definite train of symptoms which is fairly uniform in character'.[147]

In terms of symptomatology, Dhunjibhoy and current psychiatrists would certainly agree on the main features exhibited by patients apparently suffering from cannabis-related mental disorder. The observed phenomenon has survived to the present day in the shape of the diagnostic category used in India: cannabis-induced psychosis. It is listed as 'substance-induced psychosis' in ICD10 (F12.5). Ajit Avasthi, a leading psychiatrist based in Chandighar, describes it in the following way. Typically, it is a florid presentation, with multiple delusions and hallucinations, often in several modalities (auditory and visual) and with content laden with religious-spiritual themes and the context in which cannabis is used (for example, 'seeing' and 'hearing' Lord Shiva and believing that the person is endowed with special spiritual powers). The duration of such psychotic illness is typically brief (days to a few weeks at the most) provided further cannabis use is halted. According to Avasthi's experience, some go on to continue with a full-fledged independent psychotic condition like schizophrenia even in the absence of further cannabis use. These cases are then no longer diagnosed as cannabis-induced psychosis but re-classified as schizophrenia or other psychotic disorders. Most cases, however, recover completely and do not show any relapse unless heavy cannabis use is resumed.[148] Other researchers back up the notion of a discrete set of symptomatic behaviours characteristic of cannabis psychosis. Research from 1976 on cannabis psychosis and paranoid schizophrenia in India suggested that a group of 25 cases of the former 'substantially differed in terms of behavioural manifestations' from the latter. Patients tended to be violent, panicky and show bizarre behaviour, with rapid ideation and flight of ideas, but possessed some insight into the nature of their illness. The 25 cases of paranoid schizophrenia showed these characteristics less frequently, mostly presenting the 'characteristic thought disorder'.[149] Similarly, in 1999 research by Basu et al. indicated that cannabis psychosis showed distinctive features that justified 'its separate nosological status vis-à-vis that of acute schizophrenia', cautioning against over-diagnosing the latter condition.[150]

On account of the varied clinical picture which may include symptoms seen in manic psychosis (namely inappropriate and excessive cheerfulness, euphoria, increased talking and movements, and grandiose content of thought), some researchers believe, as Dhunjibhoy did, that the condition ought to be framed as cannabis-induced mania. Others, like Basu and Avasthi argue that the broader term, cannabis psychosis, is preferable on account of the presence of other features that are not characteristic of mania.[151] However, whether the predominant clinical features of a potential case of cannabis psychosis are closer to mania or schizophrenia was not yet an issue during the 1920s and 1930s. During this period, the question of how the functional psychoses ought to be delimited was only beginning to be settled.

Dhunjibhoy conceptualised hemp insanity by reference to the classificatory frameworks at the time as cannabis-induced mania rather than cannabis-induced psychosis. He differentiated three different 'types' of Indian hemp insanity: acute mania, chronic mania and dementia. However, in his view, the difference between them was only a matter of degree. The first type was the 'result of prolonged and excessive use of the drug in any form', with symptoms 'resembling those of ordinary acute mania', but with important differences. The first typical symptoms consisted of mostly visual and auditory hallucinations, which related 'as a rule, to beautiful women who are supposed to talk and copulate with the patients'. Another involved a 'characteristic dare-devil demeanour with an irresistible impulse to wilful damage'.[152] Unlike in mania, Dhunjibhoy observed that the duration of the attack was shorter and relapses were less frequent if the drug was stopped at once, with recovery then being the rule. While chronic mania and the acute type of hemp insanity shared similar symptoms, in the latter condition they were less severe and 'the patients are generally cheerful and boastful, with a sense of well-being'. Occasional complete, if temporary, loss of speech was reported. Only a 'very small number of chronic cases' gradually lapsed into secondary dementia.[153]

Cannabis-induced psychosis and mania both remain in use as distinct and unique entities in South Asia and other non-Western countries. India-based researchers such as Basu and Avasthi contend that there is a subgroup of patients in whom cannabis is both a necessary and the sufficient cause of the psychosis, which would not have appeared without cannabis and subsides when cannabis is stopped, but recurs with repeated use.[154] Western researchers, in contrast, now tend to believe that any such cases are better framed as schizophrenia which is simply precipitated or 'unmasked' by cannabis use or, in other words, that any such patients would have manifested schizophrenia anyway, with or without cannabis.

In Dhunjibhoy's time, little had been written by psychiatrists about the condition. I. C. and R. N. Chopra, in their *Use of the Cannabis Drugs in India* of 1957, provide a very short reading list indeed, with just seven other authors who had published on the topic between 1870 and the 1950s (excluding themselves, Dhunjibhoy, and United Nations and government reports).[154] Although the Chopras' bibliography is not comprehensive, missing some vital material that they may, nevertheless, have consulted, it indicates that research in the field was limited during the early part of the twentieth century. In fact, a large portion of the Chopras' as well as Dhunjibhoy's work used evidence from the same, rather obsolete sources such as N. Chevers' *Manual of Medical Jurisprudence* (1856) and L. A. Waddell's *Lyon's Medical Jurisprudence for India* ([1888] 1921). Waddell revised his handbooks to fit in with the latest nomenclature in medicine and law, but continued to draw heavily on Chevers' cases and his highly circumstantial evidence derived from selected asylum reports, travellers' observations and hearsay of colleagues of over half a century earlier. This is the kind of material that served to supplement Dhunjibhoy's and the Chopras' clinical and legal observations.

Dhunjibhoy had also followed the example of eminent contemporary researchers, engaging in 'self-experimentation' in order to judge 'the peculiar and important property' of 'temporary amnesia' that had been so important in some legal cases.[156] In regard to one of these, the infamous Bhawal case, documented by Partha Chatterjee in his *A Princely Impostor*, Dhunjibhoy had even been called as an expert witness, together with Berkeley-Hill.[157] The experiment involved him, 'in company with friends', drinking a moderate dose of bhang and smoking a pipe of ganja. Apart from inducing amusement in his friends about his antics whilst drugged, he experienced first hand the 'amnesic property of the drugs, and in future', he noted, 'I shall not hesitate to believe anyone who commits acts of violence under the influence of drugs and pleads complete amnesia of the crime on recovery'.[158] During the trial of the alleged impostor of the Kumar of Bhawal he testified against the plaintiff, finding his alleged 'amnesia' inauthentic.[159] This would have made him unpopular as the wider public strongly supported the pretender's case, with Berkeley-Hill providing favourable evidence during cross-examination.[160]

While cannabis-induced psychosis and mania remain well-established and apparently valid categories in South Asia, some of the historical phenomena and conjectural findings reported by Dhunjibhoy and his contemporaries are more dubious. Examining them does however reveal preconceptions about particular Indian communities and the highly selective and contradictory assessment of evidence produced in relation to cannabis. For example, Dhunjibhoy omitted to state that Chevers, one of his and Waddell's, and to a certain extent also the Chopras', main sources, had actually questioned the link between cannabis and 'true' insanity. Chevers made the following statement in the introduction to his chapter on insanity:

> Late in their miserable career, the gunjah-smoker and the opium-eater become utterly shattered, alike in mind and body; but I have not met with or heard of any case in which true Insanity has been caused by these practices; the opiumeater sinks into the condition of a hopeless driveller, the gunjah smoker and bang-drinker often remain chronically inebriated, and are sometimes excited to acts of frantic violence, but these states may be readily distinguished from true Insanity.[161]

Chevers' views by no means clashed with those of all of his colleagues', as the civil surgeons' annual reports of the lunatic asylums in Bengal and the northwestern provinces reveal.[162] There was no consensus among European doctors on the validity of a separate diagnosis for cannabis insanity during the second half of the nineteenth century. Many held that, given the widespread use of cannabis in India, it was only to be expected that a proportion of the insane would happen to have a history of drug use, which may be incidental to their mental illness. Others, like Chevers, argued that,

'In some rare cases, these pernicious habits, doubtless, hasten the advent of Insanity in individuals otherwise predisposed.' Drug use was, in contemporary understanding, an 'exciting factor', rather than the cause. He added: 'This would certainly much embarrass diagnosis'.[163] Dhunjibhoy clearly did not follow Chevers' line of argument in this respect. The Indian Hemp Drugs Commission of 1893–94 reiterated some of Chevers' observations, but stressed the effects of moderate in contrast to heavy drug use:

> In the case of specially marked neurotic diathesis, even the moderate use may produce mental injury. For the slightest mental stimulation or excitement may have that effect in such cases. But putting aside these quite exceptional cases, the moderate use of these drugs produces no mental injury. It is otherwise with the excessive use. Excessive use indicates and intensifies mental instability. It tends to weaken the mind. It may even lead to insanity. [...] It appears that the excessive use of hemp drugs may, especially in cases where there is any weakness or hereditary predisposition, induce insanity. It has been shown that the effect of hemp drugs in this respect has hitherto been greatly exaggerated, but that they do sometimes produce insanity seems beyond question.[164]

The Commission's report consisted of eight volumes and was based on the evidence of over 1,000 witnesses from a wide range of people: doctors, yogis, fakirs, hemp cultivators and dealers, tax gatherers, army officers, and priests. However, some prominent medical professionals from the turn of the century onwards did not accept the Commission's findings. Waddell, whose line of argument Dhunjibhoy followed, along with that of G. F. W. Ewens (1904) and A. W. Overbeck-Wright (1921), suggested that the Commission's conclusion had 'distinctly underestimated' the effect of hemp drugs in the causation of insanity in India, while 'popularly speaking' it was 'overrated'.[165] No evidence was provided by Waddell to substantiate this contention. The incidence figures for cannabis insanity he provided varied considerably, from a little over 10 per cent (for 1907) to 20 per cent as suggested by Ewens in 1904. Like Chevers' evidence, most of Waddell's was speculation. The discussion was highly contentious and prior strong views trumped reliable data. This was partly due to the fact that one of the main motives for the investigation of 1893–94 had been to identify the social and economic effects of drug taking. The Commission referred to these concerns in its report as well as the difficulties of procuring hard evidence to substantiate existing fears of social decay and economic stagnation concomitant on drug use.

> The injury done by the excessive use is [...] confined almost exclusively to the consumer himself; the effect on society is rarely appreciable. It has been the most striking feature in this inquiry to find how little the effects of hemp drugs have obtruded themselves on observation. The large number of witnesses of all classes who professed never to have seen these effects, the vague statements made by many who professed to have observed them, the very few witnesses who could so recall a case as to give any definite account of it, and the manner in which a large proportion of these cases broke down on the first attempt to examine them, are facts which combine to show most clearly how little injury society has hitherto sustained from hemp drugs.[166]

Being narrowly concerned with clinical matters of diagnosis and treatment, Dhunjibhoy's assessment, like that of his medical peers, provided an insufficiently contextualised and highly selective appraisal of the debates on cannabis insanity. His account of the history of the phenomenon was similarly skewed, despite the fact that simply reading Chevers' volume more thoroughly, for example, would at least have helped him to compare some of his own conjectures against the assumptions of other authors. Chevers had suggested that both opium and hemp were popular among Hindus as well as Muslims and that 'from very early periods, these two poisons have been made to supply the place of fermented liquors, by some of those who pretend to be the strictest abstainers among both Hindus and Mahomedans'.[167] His case studies included hemp users from Hindu, Muslim and Sikh backgrounds. Dhunjibhoy noted that the narcotic properties of hemp were mentioned in the *Atharva Veda* – an important Hindu text currently dated to 2000 BCE. However, he attributed the first description of mental derangement by use of hemp to Iban Beitar (Ibn al-Baitar al-Malaqi, 1197–1248 CE), a Muslim physician, acclaimed for his pharmacopeia and encyclopaedia of treatments for a great variety of specific diseases. He also referred to the work of Makrizi (al-Maqrizi, 1364–1442 CE), a Sunni preacher and lecturer from Cairo, who had published various compilations of historical narratives. Al-Maqrizi had reported that severe ordinances were passed in Egypt against the use of hemp drugs in the year 78 AH (657/8 CE), with extraction of teeth having been the punishment for non-compliance, and that 700 years later, by 799 AH (1378/9 CE), hemp use had 're-established itself with more than the original vigour'.[168]

However, contrary to his own historical account and Chevers' evidence, in his journal article Dhunjibhoy seemed to suggest that hemp use was a problem mainly among Hindus and Sikhs, being linked, as he pointed out, to these communities' religious and social customs. He contended that it was 'in no way connected with the social or religious customs of Mohammedans, as the Mohammedan religion condemns such practices'.[169] Nevertheless, as Chevers and even Dhunjibhoy's own quote from al-Maqrizi reveals, Muslims used hemp drugs at particular periods despite harsh sanctions. Dhunjibhoy chose to trace knowledge of the medicinal properties of hemp to the Hindu classics and the first observation of insanity from cannabis to the period around the end of the Islamic Golden Age, suggesting that cannabis consumption came to be identified as disorder or even crime during Muslim rule. Muslim governance in Egypt and the colonial state in India shared concerns about drug consumption, though for different reasons. Dhunjibhoy's uncovering of an Islamic history of social and religious concern about the perceived dangers of cannabis use as well as the Hindu embracement of the drug sat happily alongside ethnological commentaries on the widespread contemporary permissiveness and perceived depravity of Hindu traditions on the one hand, and the medical profession's identification of the health issues seen to be connected with such socio-religiously sanctioned practices on the other.

To conclude, the category of cannabis insanity had emerged within Western medical discourse during the nineteenth century when concerns about the disciplinary, social and economic effects of alcohol and narcotic drug consumption became acute. It established itself as a permanent feature of psychiatric nomenclature in the course of the increased medicalisation of drug use more generally. Despite similar descriptions of its symptoms, course and prognosis at different periods, it is important to consider the varied socio-political contexts within which cannabis insanity flourished. It would be problematic to base current debates on the dangers and benefits of hemp drugs on the evidence produced by Dhunjibhoy and his contemporaries without critical and rigorous historical awareness of the contexts within which it was produced.

General paralysis of the insane (GPI): A Western culture-bound condition

Within the wider contexts of colonialism, Westernisation and globalisation, anthropologists and psychiatrists have come to think of culture-bound syndromes as characteristic only of non-Western cultures. Conditions such as cannabis psychosis and *amok* have been linked with particular Asian cultures. GPI, in contrast, was considered rare among Indians. For a while, the condition came close to being discussed as a culture-bound syndrome specific to Western contexts. Dhunjibhoy, like many of his peers in India, subscribed to the continued myth that the East was different from the West and that, consequently, the bodily and mental constitutions of Indians were also different from those of Westerners.[170] This contention was supported by ideas on the impact of warm climates on the body and mind and beliefs in racial difference. These notions reflected Europeans' experiences in India as well as military statistics that revealed high incidence of syphilis among European troops and low numbers among Indian soldiers. Ewens pointed out in 1908 that GPI (dementia paralytica, paretic dementia) was, 'like Tabes Dorsalis, unknown among natives of India'. He provided only 'a very brief summary of the disease' in his psychiatric textbook, stressing that 'the majority of practitioners out here will never probably have an opportunity of seeing an instance of the affection'.[171] Some doctors in India held on to this position for a couple more decades.

Overbeck-Wright's views were quite different. In 1921 he pointed out that, at the very same time when an article in the *Indian Medical Gazette* of January 1912 commented on how 'very rare among Indians' GPI was, he happened to be in charge of 'twelve typical cases among Indians in the second and third stages of the disease' at the Agra Asylum – a few more were 'taken out on security by relatives, while one had died in the asylum'.[172] He concluded: 'I am of the opinion that if properly looked for and diagnosed it would be found to be much more prevalent among Indians than it is at present generally believed to be'. Overbeck-Wright's was however a minority view – GPI continued to be diagnosed only rarely by his colleagues for at least one more decade. Although his textbook was widely referred to by his contemporaries, some of his suggestions do not appear to have had an impact on clinical practice.

Overbeck-Wright summarised his favoured scientific perspective on the matter: GPI was a 'progressive degeneration of the central nervous system' and it was 'only very rarely that cases uncomplicated by mental disease are met with'.[173] Referring to Bruce, he contended that 'many alienists have jumped at a wrong conclusion and described as one entity what is really two separate conditions, classing G.P.I. among mental diseases, when [...] they are really dealing with two diseases – a purely nervous one, G.P.I., complicated by an intercurrent attack of some form of insanity'.[174] Overbeck-Wright was aware that views were changing slowly and remarked polemically:

> For many years practitioners in India had it drilled into them that G.P.I. was unknown among Indians who had never left their mother-country. During the last few years prior to 1913 this had been modified to 'extremely rare', but the result was the same, and many medical men in India would never dream that a case could possibly be G.P.I., even though all the cardinal symptoms were obviously present, and would pooh-pooh the very suggestion of such possibility as absurd. [The returns of asylums in India for 1913 and the census reports of 1901 and 1911] show that some, at least, of the Presidencies and Provinces are unbiased in their diagnosis, while others seem to be waking to a broader view of the matter.[175]

He insisted that 'syphilis is as rife in India as anywhere' and argued that even if they thought that GPI was rare, practitioners should 'not be afraid to diagnose it' and should use available diagnostic aids such as the Wassermann reaction (the test for globulin and a lymphocytic count) in doubtful cases.[176] He considered the smaller reported incidence in contrast to England to be due to 'a species of partial immunity which exists among Indians and Persians to syphilis'.[177] Dhunjibhoy's views could not have been more different. He steadfastly maintained as late as 1930 that, 'This psychosis [GPI] is extremely rare in India though syphilis is very common.'[178] He claimed that he had 'not yet seen a case of general paralysis in an Indian who has not been abroad'. The only two 'undoubted cases' he had observed were 'in Indians who had been to Europe, and had a history of exposure to infection'.[179] In fact, no cases were reported by him and his predecessors at Dacca, Berhampore and Patna.

During his lecture at the meeting of the Royal Medico-Psychological Association in England in February 1930, Dhunjibhoy referred to the lack of consensus among practitioners on the issue of syphilis and GPI, conceding that, 'Some observers in India claim that they have seen and treated cases of general paralysis among Indians who have never left their country.'[180] His own view was that although various theories 'have been propounded', he found 'none so far [...] convincing'. His audience was intrigued by this position. E. J. Fitzgerald, who had gained his medical qualifications at the National University of Ireland and was involved in research on syphilis and on a range of new diagnostic techniques, challenged Dhunjibhoy's views.[181] He argued, 'There was a popular opinion that G.P.I. was rare in Ireland (except perhaps in Dublin and Belfast), and that the native Celts who had not mixed with foreigners did not develop syphilis or G.P.I'.[182] In contrast, Fitzgerald believed that 'the alleged comparative absence of venereal disease in Ireland would not bear laboratory investigation'. In fact, he pressed Dhunjibhoy to let the audience know the 'result of the Wassermann and the gold-sol reactions in the cerebro-spinal fluid of admissions to native Indian hospitals'. Fitzgerald also rejected the assumption that exposure to malaria was a safeguard against syphilis, claiming that he had 'under his care at present Europeans who had both syphilis and malaria in India' who were 'among the worst cases of G.P.I.'.[183]

Still, Dhunjibhoy continued to insist as he had done earlier that syphilis was 'very common in the ordinary population', while general paralysis was not. Besides, he noted,

'India was not as backwards as one might imagine'. 'They had', he pointed out, 'fully equipped laboratories and good routine, and some research work was done'.[184] In fact, Kraepelin had been expected to visit Ranchi together with his pupil and assistant, Johannes Lange, to carry out research and in particular Wassermann testing on Indian patients in early 1927.[185] Dhunjibhoy and his German-educated wife, Silla, had assured the two famous psychiatrists from Munich in three letters, written in German, that they would make them feel *gemütlich* (comfortable) at their house in Ranchi. Lange was due to publish his highly influential book *Crime and Destiny* (1930). As the German title *Verbrechen als Schicksal* (crime as destiny) presages, Lange was, as Shorter put it, 'rightwing'.[186] He argued that a person's personality was determined almost exclusively by hereditary factors. Lange was involved with the Nazi sterilisation programme and was listed posthumously as one of the editors of the fifth edition of the Nazi tome *Grundriß der menschlichen Erblichkeitslehre und Rassenhygiene* (Outline of the laws of human heredity and of racial hygiene). A visit to an institution where 44 per cent of patients were certified criminals would have been a boon for Lange's research as well as contributing to debates about the aetiology of GPI. Alas, Kraepelin died in 1926 and the research plans had to be cancelled. As Dhunjibhoy was right to point out a couple of years later to his audience in London, the need for further investigation into GPI in India remained.

Dhunjibhoy's views were shared by some of his colleagues at Ranchi. For example, P. C. Das, who filled in for Djunjibhoy while he was oversees, also held that GPI was not prevalent in India.[187] The hospital statistics reflected this, as diseases considered to be sexually transmitted were not mentioned in relation to deaths (where tuberculosis features highly), nor in relation to illnesses (where malaria appears to have been a main problem). Although Wassermann testing had shown positive results in 1928 and 1929, Dhunjibhoy merely reported that most of the affected patients (96 out of the 105) benefited from a 'full course of anti-syphilitic treatment' and that its effect had been restricted to physical improvements only, with no alleviation of patients' mental condition.[188] It took many years of debate among psychiatrists to agree that syphilis was the cause of GPI, following Noguchi and Moore's identification in 1913 of spirochetes in the brains of paretics, and for the link to become more widely accepted. It is surprising therefore that a practitioner like Dhunjibhoy, well attuned to the latest professional debates, would not have explored the situation further. The tables he and Das collated for types of insanity and for aetiological factors and associated conditions showed for the former zero figures for syphilitic insanity (which referred to GPI and dementia from local cerebral syphilis) and until 1930 only one case of syphilis for the latter (as an 'exciting' rather than 'predisposing' factor).[189]

On his return from Europe, the first patient, a woman, was assigned the diagnosis dementia from local cerebral syphilis in 1931. The number of those whose mental state was attributed to syphilis increased from zero in 1930, two in 1931, five in 1933 to ten in 1934.[190] In 1933, Dhunjibhoy noted, 'one patient taken away from "Mania – other forms" and shown under head "General Paralysis of the Insanes" as he has subsequently been diagnosed as such'.[191] GPI had clearly begun to feature more for Dhunjibhoy than it had during the 1920s. However, the number of patients given the diagnosis of cerebral syphilis remained extremely low, at two patients only – until 1939 when six new admissions were assigned this label. The change was a little more pronounced in regard to the aetiological factors and associated conditions. Invariably, the number of those cases listed under 'Toxic. Syphilis Acquired' and 'Toxic. Syphilis Congenital' (until 1933) and 'Infections. Incidence of Syphilis' (from 1934 onwards) was higher than the figures for those diagnosed with GPI and dementia from local cerebral syphilis (until 1933) and cerebral syphilis (from 1934). In most cases syphilis was given as the exciting as opposed to the predisposing cause.

Dhunjibhoy did not explain what had caused him to employ GPI/syphilis as a diagnosis and assumed cause from the early 1930s – albeit only rarely. The challenging debate on occasion of his talk in London in 1930 may have been one factor. There had also been changes in the mental hospital for Europeans just 'next door'. Owen Berkeley-Hill had, in 1930, done away with segregation on sexual lines and let his patients freely intermingle, causing much debate, outrage and interest.[192] Berkeley-Hill was most vocal about his views on sexuality, which were informed by ideas on sexual development as put forward by Freud and other psychoanalysts at the time, as well as by his own escapades, which are documented in his autobiography, *All too Human*. What is more, in an article published in the *Indian Medical Gazette* in 1921 he had noted that nearly 40 per cent of patients in the European Mental Hospital (73 out of 186) were infected with syphilis, arguing that this high figure can only be accounted for by the widespread infection of Indians with it. Placing the blame of Europeans' condition on the Indians, he estimated an incidence rate of 75 for them.[193]

Another influencing factor may have been the appearance of a new clinician in a high-profile position on the local scene. Pacheco had been appointed at the European Mental Hospital as the temporary replacement for Berkeley-Hill who retired in December 1933. Pacheco was then in the process of completing the manuscript for his book *Modern Methods in Psychiatry*, which was to be published in 1935. He lived and worked just a short walk from the Indian Mental Hospital and may have caused Dhunjibhoy to reconsider his stance on GPI. Pacheco did not subscribe to the idea that GPI was rare among Indians. Attention to GPI at Ranchi increased even more when Pacheco was made the locum for Dhunjibhoy during most of 1935.[194] It was then that the issue of neurosyphilis was dealt with fully for the first time. Pacheco provided clear information on the results of the Wassermann tests (for blood and cerebrospinal fluid). Out of a total of 653 blood samples tested over a three-year period, 529 (or 81 per cent) were positive. The figures for the 122 cerebro-spinal fluid (CSF) samples were 94 (or 77 per cent). Pacheco rightly pointed out that the CSF testing provided more accurate results 'in the diagnosis of neurosyphilitic conditions, especially general paralysis of the insane'.[195] He was clearly well informed about the latest diagnostic and treatment methods in relation to GPI. He did not criticise Dhunjibhoy directly, but he pinpointed what he considered to be misperceptions still prevalent in India at the time:

> The general belief in medical circles, that general paralysis of the insane is a comparatively rare disease in Indians, still holds, with the result that the diagnosis […] is often overlooked. This disease is, I am of opinion, by no means rare, and if the cerebro-spinal fluid is examined as a routine measure, the more frequent will a proper diagnosis of general paralysis of the insane be evident.[196]

On his return from leave on 17 February 1936, Dhunjibhoy was faced with Pacheco's triennial report that had brought neurosyphilis into the limelight. He began to cover in more depth this topic in his own subsequent reports, albeit still in a cursory way, with little detail on what exactly his position was. During this period, the professional literature was full of investigations into the alleged phenomenon that the incidence of neurosyphilis was low in areas where malaria was endemic and the observation that patients who had contracted a febrile disease during the early years of their syphilitic infection almost never developed neurosyphilis.[197] It is puzzling that Dhunjibhoy did not refer to the observation of extremely inconclusive results concerning the veracity of Wassermann testing in areas where malaria was present, as this would have lent support to the assumption that syphilis was rare and that the positive Wassermann tests at Ranchi might have been linked with the high incidence of malaria rather than indicating a high syphilis rate. False positives for Wassermann tests were after all reported in 10 out of 11 publications worldwide after 1930.[198]

GPI was clearly not one of Dhunjibhoy's favourite research topics. The debates surrounding GPI highlight the impact of social as well as epidemiological and medical factors on the frequency with which particular diagnoses are assigned. Amongst these were the deep-seated social preconceptions about Europeans' and Indians' different physical and mental constitutions; the flawed extrapolation to the wider population and to mental hospital patients from select military statistics that showed high incidence of syphilis among European troops yet low numbers among Indians; and the conjecture that exposure to malaria provided a certain level of immunity against syphilis developing into GPI, which seemed to be verified further by the positive effects of malaria therapy in Europeans affected by GPI. Fitzgerald, who had challenged Dhunjibhoy's views during his talk in England, alluded to yet another reason for the tendency of practitioners to avoid reference to syphilis. Contending that syphilis seemed to be under represented – while tuberculosis and cancer were over represented – in mortality statistics, he concluded: 'Cancer and tuberculosis freely appear on the death certificate; they are respectable diseases.'[199]

Male and Female Maladies?

Gender is relevant to a number of the diagnostic categories used by Dhunjibhoy at Ranchi. The records show the preponderance of women among some and of men among others. Cannabis insanity, melancholia and delusional insanity, for example, were more frequently applied to men, while mania, dementia praecox/schizophrenia, circular insanity/manic-depressive psychosis and confusional insanity were more frequently diagnosed in women. How can we account for these differences? Are they indicative of culturally specific male and female maladies or are they artefacts of the diagnostic process and shifting conceptualisations of particular categories? Did the trajectory of gender differences in the allocation of diagnostic labels change over time? And are there any differences between Ranchi and other institutions in terms of gendered patterns of diagnosis?

As with any analysis of incidence rates of particular conditions, it is important to evaluate trends in any one diagnosis within the wider spectrum of categories during a specific period as well as over time. The higher male rates for melancholia, for example, require discussion of the frequency with which alternative diagnoses were attributed to women. Just as gender needs to be conceptualised as a relational category, so do diagnostic labels and the phenomena they encapsulate. Furthermore, a combination of factors, some of them not strictly medical, will have had an impact on the rate with which a specific diagnosis was assigned to men and women. Lacking access to detailed case records enables us only to advance general speculative explanations. The higher female incidence rate for confusional insanity is arguably the easiest to fathom in these terms.

Confusional insanity and female reproduction-related disorders

The female rates for confusional insanity (3–5 per cent) were consistently about double those for men (0–3 per cent). They peaked immediately after the opening of the institution and again during the early 1930s. The earlier trend can partly be explained by the lack of accommodation constraints and necessary admission restrictions in the female compound during the 1920s in contrast to the male section. The second peak affected both men and women and may, as argued above, have been due to the worldwide economic depression. There was a perceived link between confusional insanity and economic hardship. Ideas such as those of Conally Norman, who practised in Dublin during the 1890s, resonated with Indian practitioners' observations in a country periodically scarred by famine, paralleling the situation in Ireland during British rule. Norman had noted that confusional insanity was not recognised as much in England as in Ireland. Yet in his view it generally was the most common of all forms of insanity. Given the high levels of poverty in Ireland and the high incidence of confusional insanity among prisoners reported by Krafft-Ebing, locale-specific factors were likely to have influenced Norman's views on and use of this category. Like others, he also linked the condition with puerperal insanity and prolonged lactation.[200]

In light of the widespread preference given to male offspring in India, and discrimination against women in terms of health-preserving measures, their chance of suffering from food-related deprivation was increased. This phenomenon has been widely documented to the present day.[201] Bearing in mind these issues, it may not be surprising to find that women were reported to show severe symptoms of confusion proportionately more frequently than men, arguably as a consequence of starvation. Dhunjibhoy explicitly linked confusional psychosis with starvation and physical exhaustion.[202] Overbeck-Wright, too, had pointed out this connection. The disorder continued to be referred to as exhaustion insanity. In 1913, for example, Ewens used the terms exhaustion psychosis, acute hallucinatory insanity, acute confusional insanity and Meynert's amentia interchangeably to refer to 'a very definite condition supervening in extreme bodily exhaustion'.[203] Ewens did not explicitly connect any of these terms with a particular gender.[204]

Overbeck-Wright, in contrast, did spell out gender-specific aetiologies for exhaustion insanity. His focus was on its link to women's reproductive cycle, noting that the condition was 'occurring as a sequel to exhausting diseases and typically seen as the result of prolonged lactation'.[205] While it was observed in men almost exclusively during the 'late adult or senile periods of life, when the natural reparative powers of the body begin to fail', it presented in women at 'much earlier age periods' and particularly 'owing to prolonged lactation'. He explained that prolonged lactation was implicated 'specially' in India, 'where the habit prevails, certainly among the lower classes, of suckling the children for two or even three years'.[206] In Western countries, in contrast, authors like Kraepelin had referred to lactation psychosis, which was reported to occur three to five months postpartum. It is intriguing to note that despite Overbeck-Wright's criticism of some of Kraepelin's nosological practice, he was close to Kraepelin's assessment of the link between lactation and exhaustion psychosis. He also concurred with Kraepelin's insistence that a separate nosological entity for postpartum psychoses was not justified. As Overbeck-Wright put it in 1921, in the context of his discussion of insanities of toxic origin:

> 'Puerperal insanity' is a term better left unused. Any type of insanity may follow on the puerperal condition, and none are peculiar to it. It is but small wonder that cases do occur as its sequelae, when one considers the exhaustion and pain of parturition, the loss of blood, and the liability to septic infection which occur in this condition.[207]

Dhunjibhoy did not follow this suggestion – at least not until the change in the official nomenclature occurred in 1934. Until then he used the categories of puerperal mania and puerperal melancholia alongside confusional insanity. There was a correlation between the percentage decrease in puerperal mania and the increase in confusional insanity rates for women between 1926 and 1931. This might indicate that Dhunjibhoy began to follow the contemporary practice of subsuming cases of puerperal mania under the heading of confusional or exhaustion insanity. However, the numbers were too small for the former and fluctuated too much for the latter to verify this. Kraepelin had held that disorders of the lactation period were present in about five per cent of women treated in mental hospitals.[208] At Ranchi, the figures for puerperal mania dipped from a high of three per cent reported in 1925 to one per cent between 1927 and 1931, stabilising subsequently at around two per cent. From 1934 onwards reproduction-related disorders were no longer diagnosed at Ranchi. However, in contrast to puerperal mania, Dhunjibhoy did use puerperal melancholia with increasing frequency prior to 1934. Here too the numbers were small, ranging from one per cent in 1925 to three per cent in 1933. On balance, it seems that only a small proportion of confusional insanity cases may have been attributed to conditions related to women's reproductive cycle. The predominance of women in confusional insanity throughout the period is likely to have been due to general starvation and exhaustion. If so, the raised gender-specific rates for confusional insanity would have mirrored gender discrimination in society at large. In spite of the focus on admission of dangerous cases, fewer accommodation constraints on the female wards may have facilitated the confinement of women patients who did not constitute a danger to the public but did suffer from severe hunger.

Cannabis and alcohol insanity

In India, cannabis insanity was applied almost exclusively to men. Alcohol-related insanity, in contrast, figured much less prominently and was assigned marginally more often to women. Male predominance among those being treated at Ranchi for the former condition can be explained by the well-documented connection between cannabis and crime[209] and its reported customary use within groups of men gathering in public places in a village or city.[210] Ewens was even slightly bemused about men's joint meetings, as 'curiously enough, all the smokers are mixed and not necessarily of one caste'.[211] Overbeck-Wright, too, believed that it was 'seldom that any native, except perhaps a faquir, indulges in any form of the drug by himself'.[212] Given the social restrictions on women among many Indian communities in regard to their presence in public places, these observations may indeed explain the reported almost exclusively male face of cannabis insanity.

Most authors, including Varma, one of Dhunjibhoy's successors at Ranchi, made a point of emphasising that no women were admitted to a mental hospital for cannabis psychosis.[213] Ewens suggested that 'this was a habit practically unknown among women and they therefore escape the disease'.[214] He reported that he had 'never heard of a woman addicted to this habit'.[215] Dhunjibhoy's data, too, confirm that for most of the period, cannabis insanity was found exclusively among men. However, towards the late 1930s a few women began to appear in Dhunjibhoy's statistics and some cases were also reported at the institutions in Madras province. How can this change be accounted for? We can only speculate that earlier observations such as those of Ewens may have previously nurtured a disinclination among superintendents to explore women's history as diligently as men's. They may not have been alert to what were considered the tell-tale signs of cannabis use, particularly in those cases where the symptoms women presented could be classified by means of categories considered to be characteristic of female insanity, such as mania and dementia praecox. Epidemiological and cultural factors together with the replication in diagnostic practice of wider social perceptions about gender differences regarding the use of drugs may account for the overwhelming male predominance in diagnosis of cannabis psychosis.

The situation is more opaque in regard to alcohol. The historical dimension of alcohol consumption in India has barely been investigated. Current research seems to suggest that considerably more men than women overindulge in alcohol, although severe prohibition laws in some Indian states and the practice of home-brewing make it difficult to ascertain valid figures. Against this background the Ranchi pattern of a – albeit minor – prevalence of women among those diagnosed with alcohol-related psychosis is intriguing. Of course, we cannot conclude from this that female alcohol consumption was equally widespread among women in the wider population. The frequency with which particular psychiatric categories are assigned to patients in mental hospitals is not necessarily indicative of incidence rates of mental illness among non-hospitalised populations. Nor do hospital figures reveal consumption behaviours prevalent among the general population. Mental hospital-based data are limited to a very specific group of people.

In contrast to Ranchi, women in the two mental hospitals at Calicut and Waltair in Madras province were not diagnosed more frequently than men with alcohol-related insanity. The number of women in that category was in fact extremely low. This may point at the implication of socio-cultural factors, such as alcohol overconsumption having possibly been more frequent in the northeast provinces than in southern regions, although evidence for this is not available. It is equally plausible to assume that the diagnosis of alcoholic psychosis, as Dhunjibhoy referred to it in 1930, was not applied consistently across Indian institutions. What is more, early twentieth-century authors as well as their nineteenth-century predecessors tended to construe alcohol-related madness as a predominantly European condition, despite the fact that alcohol-related disorders were well known in indigenous Indian medicine. This may have skewed some doctors' diagnostic judgement, resulting in the low incidence rates for the disorder even at Ranchi (only about two per cent for both genders combined during the 1930s).

On the basis of his experience at Agra Mental Hospital, Overbeck-Wright suggested in 1921 that:

> Alcohol is not so frequent a cause of mental and nervous disorders in India as in countries where European races constitute the bulk of the population, mainly because of caste and religious customs, which prevent the Indian on the whole from indulging in it. [216]

Dhunjibhoy, basing his observations on northeastern regions merely noted that alcohol 'is largely consumed in those parts of India where the hemp drug is difficult to obtain or is unknown'.[217] His own data suggested that alcohol-induced psychosis was present in Bengal, Bihar and Orissa, but it figured prominently neither at Ranchi nor at Waltair or Calicut. In regard to the 'types of alcoholic psychosis' seen at Ranchi, Dhunjibhoy's view again differed from Overbeck-Wright's. He suggested that they were 'the same as one sees in the West'.[218] Overbeck-Wright insisted on influential racial differences stating that, 'The effects of alcohol vary greatly, not only between individuals, but between races.'[219] Given the colonial context it is perhaps not surprising that a man of European heritage should put emphasis on race while Dhunjibhoy, the Parsi from India, stressed commonality in disease presentation. Neither commented on issues of gender. The history of alcohol and gendered consumption patterns in Indian communities as well as the varied frequency with which alcohol-induced psychosis was observed in different mental hospitals requires further research.[220]

Epilepsy

Today the term epilepsy encompasses a wide range of chronic neurological conditions characterised by seizures and highly diverse symptoms. Conditions that manifested themselves with seizures have a long history in both Western and non-Western societies, often linked to the sacred or the demonic.[221] Since the late nineteenth century epilepsy has straddled the disciplines of psychiatry and neurology; for neurologists its psychiatric manifestations are 'complications'.[222] Attempts to pinpoint the meanings of the concept at different periods have been hampered by the possibility that the clinical presentation of some mental symptoms may have changed over time.[223] In South Asia epilepsy was recognised within the main medical traditions, as *mirgi* ('small death')[224] in Unani Graeco Arabic medicine, and in the Ayurvedic tradition as *apasmara* ('loss of recollection/consciousness').[225] As with any medical corpus, significant changes over time occurred in

Indian medical systems.[226] Nevertheless, in Ayurveda the general trend was for *apasmara* to be differentiated from *unmada* (insanity), the former being conceptualised primarily in relation to the humours and in organic/bodily terms. Metaphysical or spiritual aspects – possession by the *Grahas* – were merely acknowledged by some (as in the various versions of *Carakasamhita* and *Susrutasamhita*, for example), and emphasised by others (Vagbhata's *Astangasamgraha*, for example).[227] To identify which definition patients and their practitioners had in mind when they referred to 'epilepsy', *apasmara* and *mirgi*, would require in-depth study of specific cases in context.

In line with European debates on the 'combined psychoses', in 1908 Ewens suggested that epilepsy presented frequently in conjunction with 'various forms of Insanity'.[228] In India, he argued, this led 'more frequently' than in Europe to sufferers' detention on account of the 'dangerous and troublesome nature' of such cases.[229] He pointed out the great danger to a patient's own life, as 'the fits occur suddenly without warning, and the patient having no means of protecting himself may fall and drown in 6 inches of water, or may burn himself to death'.[230] But his observations focused particularly on the threat that these fits posed to others. 'After a fit', he held, 'instead of the stupor and mental confusion which is a typical ending, the patient may suddenly pass into a condition of fury, of wild maniacal rage in which they will tear, rend, murder and mutilate'.[231] Ewens warned: 'Such patients are, without exception, the most dangerous of all insanes, and it is in view of the possible occurrence of such events that all epileptics are to be regarded with suspicion.'[232] This fear of and wariness towards epileptics has a long history and was prominent in Western medical and public attitudes towards such patients during Ewens' time.

Overbeck-Wright, in 1921, too, noted some epileptics' potential for violence, considering such episodes as symptoms of post-epileptic psychoses. 'These are of various kinds', he argued, 'and are of the utmost importance to the medical jurist on account of the frequency with which acts of homicide have been committed by persons suffering from this condition'.[233] His response to any such 'violent attack of mania' that replaced the more usual coma in some cases was more matter of fact than Ewens'. Acknowledging that 'while in this condition the patient is in a state of frenzy, shouting, kicking, biting, scratching, and committing even homicidal assaults on any and every one', he concluded soberly: 'As a rule this condition is quite transitory, lasting for a few hours only.'[234] Given the admission restrictions at Indian mental hospitals, it is likely that the majority of patients classified as epileptic belonged to those who had shown threatening behaviour and committed a violent crime.

The diagnostic labels used in the annual reports up to 1934 were 'mania associated with epilepsy' and 'dementia from epilepsy'. The latter was rarely applied to patients at Ranchi (about one per cent only). The former figured a little more prominently, amounting to between three and four per cent for both sexes combined over the period. This is a higher rate than that reported by Overbeck-Wright for the Agra Mental Hospital, where epileptic mania and epileptic dementia combined accounted for only 1.5 per cent of the cases treated during the year and for 4.13 per cent among admissions. Overbeck-Wright explained the discrepancy between the rates for patients treated and admitted. In his view it was due to 'many cases of idiocy originating from or being complicated by this disease'.[235] This statement is an indication of how blurred the lines between epilepsy and idiocy, as well as other categories, were. As Ewens had contended a little over a decade before him, 'insanity with epilepsy may simulate almost any form of mental disease'. His diagnostic preference had been to identify epilepsy in combination with a particular mental condition rather than the other way round, as suggested by the nomenclature then in place in India. Ewens argued:

> Cases apparently of katatonia or other forms of stupor or of Dementia Praecox, melancholia and mania have been admitted and diagnosed as such until after a short observation [...] an epileptic convulsion has shown the error, and longer residence has clearly shown that the case was essentially one of epilepsy.[236]

Confirming the observed initial confusion created by what Overbeck-Wright considered as a 'toxic'[237] disorder exhibiting a range of mental symptoms, he speculated that 'the real proportion of epileptics in Indian asylums is considerably over the percentage shown among admissions'.[238] Psychiatrists became increasingly aware of this problem during the 1920s and 1930s and epilepsy ceased to be a 'psychiatric' disease.[239] Patients were reclassified, as Ewens had suggested. This is borne out by the Ranchi statistics, which show an increased use from the later period onwards of the epilepsy and epileptic insanity diagnosis.

From 1934 onwards, when mania associated with epilepsy was replaced with epilepsy and epileptic insanity, dementia from epilepsy was no longer specified and the small number of such cases seem to have been absorbed by secondary dementia. Classification practices (but not official nomenclature) changed further in 1935, when a higher number of patients were reclassified under the new diagnostic label by Pacheco. Which diagnoses these patients had previously been assigned is difficult to ascertain, as Pacheco did not comment on this issue. Incidence of mania, secondary dementia and confusional insanity show a decrease at that time. Epileptics classified under the label secondary dementia are the most likely to have been reassigned to the epilepsy and epileptic insanity category.

Although the increased rates for epilepsy and epileptic insanity from 1935 onwards are minor in statistical terms (only one percentage point), the timing of the change of terminology was significant, as it paralleled the rapid changes that occurred during the 1930s in regard to how conditions under this label ought to be understood, identified and treated. The reconstitution of the International League against Epilepsy (ILAE) in 1935 in connection with a meeting of the International Neurological Congress in London marked a new era of research into epilepsy. Dhunjibhoy attended the Congress. He was also one of 32 doctors from 14 countries who decided to revive the ILAE, which had been founded in 1909 at the International Congress of Medicine in Budapest, but had lost its momentum following the First World War. At Ranchi, epileptics were treated in separate wards in the mental hospital and, given the debates in Europe on the desirability of special 'colonies' for this group, keeping all of them together, regardless of their particular mental manifestations, may have been considered more in line with contemporary thinking.[240]

What concerns us here is the slight but stable preponderance of men (ranging from two to four per cent) categorised with mania associated with epilepsy/epilepsy and epileptic insanity from 1925 to 1939. The pattern for dementia from epilepsy in the pre-1934 period also showed male predominance, but the difference was much smaller (a fraction of one per cent). The numbers involved may have been low, but the case of epilepsy may indicate that gender predominance is not always necessarily and exclusively due to gender-based social discrimination or gender-biased diagnostics. Current research on both the incidence and prevalence of epilepsy among populations across the globe reveal, with few exceptions, higher rates for males than females.[241] While the gender-specific differences are not statistically significant, their consistency across different studies in varied localities suggests, in current risk-factor-focused language, that 'males are at higher risk than females for unprovoked seizures and epilepsy'.[242] Whether these findings would also apply to early twentieth-century trends among communities in northeast India is difficult to ascertain retrospectively. Nor can community-based trends be taken to reveal institution-based patterns of diagnosis. What can be said is that current research indicates a similar pattern to that presented in the Ranchi records of a marginally lower likelihood for women to be diagnosed with epilepsy than males.

Dhunjibhoy differentiated epilepsy patients in terms of three main categories: *grand mal, petit mal* and *status epilepticus*. He pointed out in February 1930, during his visit to one of the then few specialist 'epilepsy colonies' in England, the David Lewis Colony at Warford, Cheshire, that:

> The majority of the epileptic population of the hospitals suffer from *grand mal; petit mal* seems to be more prone to attack the children and turn them into epileptic idiots. Patients often suffer from *status epilepticus*, and many a homicidal act in India reminds one of the existence of epileptic equivalents.[243]

It would be vain to attempt to map these broad categories on to current diagnostic concepts and the gendered epidemiologies connected with them today. In fact, although there seems to be 'broad agreement between studies that females have a marginally lower incidence of epilepsy and unprovoked seizures than males', particular kinds of epilepsy are more common among females (for example, idiopathic generalised epilepsies), while others predominate among males (*status epilepticus*).[244] Some researchers explain the slightly higher overall rates for males among Indian communities by presumed 'local types' of epilepsy (such as 'hot-water' epilepsy in Karnataka), and the varying prevalence in particular localities, and the varied impact, of infectious diseases on the sexes.[245] Assumed social factors relevant in regard to current health-seeking behaviours relate to the 'Denial of epilepsy in women, especially those in younger age groups who may fear social stigma'[246] and, in the peculiarly judgmental words of Baviskar et al., to women's tendency to 'follow false beliefs than sound practices', namely to be more likely to consult Indian traditional practitioners.[247]

Judging from the current state of research on epilepsy and the marginal predominance of men among those subject to the varied conditions subsumed under this term, 'epilepsy is still a puzzle', as is suggested even on the website of the International League Against Epilepsy.[248] It would have seemed so also to Ewens, Overbeck-Wright and Dhunjibhoy, despite the rapid developments in the field especially during the 1930s. How to account for the predominance of men, however marginal, in epilepsy, while women seemed to figure slightly more (by one to three per cent) in regard to mental deficiency, also requires explanation. We may be tempted to suggest that in relation to the former category a tendency prevailed to conceal girls' and women's epilepsy and prevent their hospitalisation in order to enable them to be married off. In regard to the latter, we could suggest that girls and women were valued less than men by their relatives and hence families sought to unburden themselves from them through institutionalisation. Taken separately, both of these explanations may sound plausible, fitting in with cultural perceptions and clichés about Indian gender discrimination. We might even have evidence to corroborate them. However, how they fit together is more difficult to fathom, particularly in retrospect. It is equally hard to say whether the male predominance was linked to gendered admission patterns, influenced by wider social preconceptions; doctors' gendered views of a particular condition; or due to biological predisposition and socio-biologically grounded variance in how epileptic states presented during the 1920s and 1930s. Given the complexities of the matter, it is vital to consider all of these aspects.

Male melancholia – female mania and schizophrenia

Apart from cannabis insanity, the gendered patterns of the conditions discussed above are not numerically significant. In contrast, the trends for the five categories to be focused on in the following discussion are represented by high numbers. They are also highly relevant to current debates about gender and mental illness. We will consider three predominantly female and two male diagnoses, namely mania, schizophrenia, and manic depressive psychosis (MDP) for the former, and melancholia and paranoia for the latter. The high male incidence rate for melancholia may strike us as the most intriguing as this condition is usually equated with today's depression, which has in Western countries been seen as the archetypical female disorder – particularly since American feminist psychologist Phillis Chesler published her *Women and Madness* in 1972. However, in Western countries, too, cultural representations of melancholia varied with time and place. As Schiesari and Radden have shown, women did not figure in European Renaissance discourse on melancholia, as this condition was then associated with artistic genius and intellectual depth.[249] It was only when melancholy became increasingly medicalised during the nineteenth century that its association with women became more widespread, illustrating the dynamics between medical conceptualisations and cultural norms of gender. Within this context, psychiatric debates on melancholia contributed, as Hock argues, to 'the naturalization of gender difference by assigning cultural meaning to clinical observations' or, in other words, 'nineteenth-century psychiatrists were caught between the scientific demand for objective clinical observation and the gender norms of the culture to which they belonged'.[250]

Leaving aside for the time being feminist assessments of the social construction of diagnostic processes, it is also vital to reiterate that patterns in mental hospital-based data are quite different from those relating to primary care settings and wider population trends. Prevalence data for mental illness in the wider population may vary considerably from those influenced by admission restrictions, service access and utilisation factors. While Chesler's 1960s, 1970s and present-day America and Europe have been arguably characterised by parity of access to institutional healthcare for both sexes, the situation was and is different in India. Davar has noted that in the West, 'Comparisons of community survey rates of mental illness and hospital rates do not grossly differ' in regard to gender.[251] However, the social hierarchy in Indian families tends to mean that women's mental health needs are neglected. Decision-making about women's health rarely rests with them but is undertaken by their parents or their husbands' families.[252] Therefore, conclusions about the gendered prevalence of mental disorders based on hospital samples are not only methodologically flawed but also politically misleading.

Davar's argument is particularly pertinent to hospital-based research from the 1970s, which recorded male predominance in depression. This conflicted with trends reported in the West, where women were more likely to be diagnosed with severe depressive disorders. Whether the case Davar is making is relevant also for the Ranchi data, which relates to the 1920s and 1930s, remains to be assessed. It is clear however that if we are inclined to see treatment in a mental hospital as a positive thing, the strongest argument about social discrimination against women is their low representation among the hospital population overall. Only one of five patients at Ranchi was female. If we see confinement in a mental institution as an imposition and manifestation of social control, we would consider the disadvantage to have rested with men. Either way, the question is how to explain that a higher percentage of hospitalised men than women were diagnosed by Dhunjibhoy as suffering from melancholia.

At Ranchi, the male incidence of melancholia was consistently higher than that for females. The difference amounted to approximately three per cent. Dhunjibhoy had pointed out that while the 'types of melancholia' were the same, 'the number of the agitated cases is certainly far less compared to those seen in English hospitals'.[253] So, what kind of patients did he have to deal with? Assuming that the mental, behavioural and physical symptoms presented by patients in Indian institutions did not change between 1908 and the 1920s and 1930s, we could rely on Ewens' rich description of what he considered 'as a rule, one of the easiest forms of insanity to assure oneself of'.[254] Ewens noted that whatever the names of the various varieties, 'in all cases there is intense mental pain, the patient feels miserable – looks so'.[255] There were other symptoms that would have been observed not only by the psychiatrist but also by the family prior to a patient's confinement in the mental hospital:

> Either the patient is slow, self-absorbed, sitting down alone and rarely moving, or he is constantly full of gestures of intense grief; he has always the eyes full of tears or is actually weeping; he wrings his hands, clasps them, sighs, groans or bows his head back and forward for an indefinite number of times, or sits clasping it with his hands or roams ceaselessly about, huddled in a blanket, moaning and complaining, breaking out into fresh complaints at the sight of a visitor, frequently, instead of complaining, emitting one monotonous ejaculation of God if a European, Ari Bap if a native, slowly and without variation.[256]

If we remember Davar's suggestion that 'social hierarchy in Indian families would ensure that women's mental health needs are neglected', the display of symptoms like those described by Ewens may not have led to favourable responses if displayed by female relatives.[257] Melancholic patients required constant vigilance and doting care. Ewens noted:

> All the symptoms are aggravated at night, especially towards the early hours of the morning at about two or 3, at which time in those predisposed to suicide, there is the greatest danger. Many, indeed a majority of melancholics, have a tendency to suicide, and if fully determined to do so, nothing will prevent them short of unceasing surveillance. The danger must never be forgotten, and if it is desired to prevent it once the suspicion is aroused, such a patient must never for one instant or second, night or day, sleeping or waking, be left alone.[258]

Within the context of discriminatory social structures, this kind of round-the-clock vigilance may have been less commonly employed by families in female cases of melancholia. Melancholic women may have had more opportunity to take their lives, while men may have had a greater chance of being presented for admission to a mental hospital once the pressure on family to keep them safe became too much. Force-feeding was common in such cases and on admission to Ranchi many patients were reported to have suffered from 'some defect of nutrition'.[259] Would women within extended families have been fed as adequately as men? As Ewens pointed out, some 'ordinary chronic melancholics' were 'difficult to tend and need constantly being supervised, to see that they are fed and clothed'. Often, he noted, they were 'carried off by intercurrent diseases, phthisis or chronic dysentery'.[260] It is likely, we might argue, that women melancholics may have been more likely to die before they had a chance to be admitted to a mental hospital.

Another factor may have been implicated. Two in five patients at Ranchi were classified as criminal lunatics; men predominated in this group. A number of these may have been classified as melancholics. Ewens contended that 'a certain blunting of the moral sense' was a 'frequent' attribute of melancholics and that such patients were 'seen among the criminal insanes of this country'.[261] Although no data were provided, Ewens suggested that they formed 'a large proportion of the criminal lunatics (guilty of homicide) seen in India'. He contended that 'no man of this character ought to be allowed out of the asylum' as they had:

> no delusions, will speak perfectly sensibly, keep themselves clean and tidy, but seem to have always an idea of personal injury; they are always lowering, morose, difficult to please, and above all liable to fits of uncontrollable diabolical rage from trivial occurrences which it is difficult to foresee and impossible to prevent.[262]

It is not clear if Dhunjibhoy, too, would have diagnosed this kind of patient with melancholia. If so, this might be a factor in the male predominance in the melancholia category. But, there may also have been personal factors that influenced diagnostic practice. For example, was Dhunjibhoy more likely than his colleagues to assign melancholia disproportionately to men? How do the statistics for other Indian institutions compare to Ranchi's?

Figure 4.2. Percentage of men and women (of total number treated) assigned the diagnosis 'melancholia, other forms', 1933

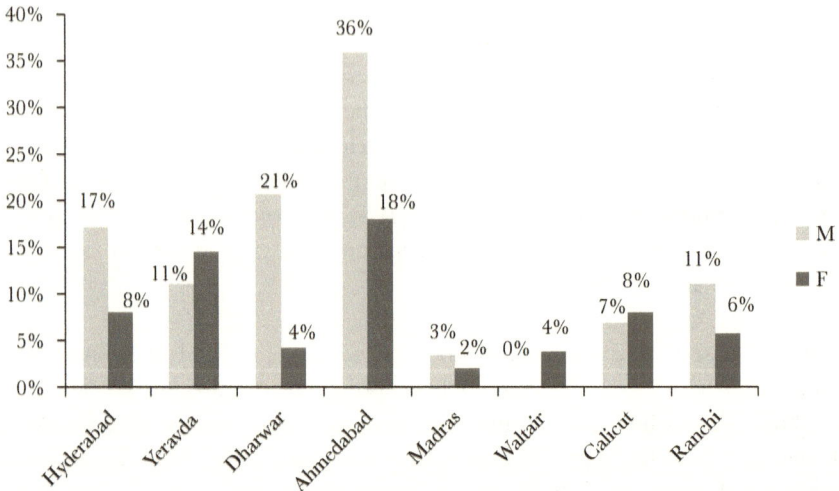

If we put aside issues concerning the comparability of the individual data sets for the different institutions, three major points are evident in Figure 4.2.[263] Firstly, there was considerable variation across institutions in the frequency with which melancholia was assigned. Second, the overall number of patients attributed this label in the eight institutions amounted to 419 men and 109 women; men were given it nearly four times as often. Third, at three hospitals the incidence of melancholia was seen to be higher amongst females. In two of these, overall patient numbers were however much smaller than at Ranchi (namely one melancholic woman out of 27 at Waltair and eight out of 100 at Calicut).

The institution most comparable to Ranchi in terms of reputation for clinical excellence, standard of institutional provision and number of inmates was Yeravda. Dhunjibhoy had been sent there in 1928 to make himself familiar with the latest developments in modern hospital management.[264] Yeravda was however special in the sense that it provided for both Europeans and Indians. The percentage of men diagnosed with melancholia was almost exactly equal in Yeravda and Ranchi. However, the female rate was considerably higher at the former institution. Could it have been the case that the presence of European patients resulted in the emergence of a pattern that was allegedly characteristic of institutional trends in Western countries? In numerical terms this is unlikely, as only 16 per cent of the hospital population at Yeravda were Europeans, of which 40 per cent were women. Of the Indian patients, 35 per cent were women. More importantly, suggestions regarding female preponderance in depression in Western countries have so far been substantiated only for the decades immediately before critical feminist scholarship emerged. The higher female Indian rate at Yeravda in contrast to Ranchi therefore remains an open issue. What we can say is that Yeravda seems to have been an anomaly with Ranchi being more in line with diagnostic practices in other Indian institutions.

Alternatively it could be suggested that the different gender rates are not so much a product of classification, as they are of the variably gendered prevalence of melancholia among highly diverse communities in northeast, northwest and southern India, and in urban in contrast to rural areas. Yeravda served an arguably more Westernised conurbation than, say, Ahmedabad, or even Ranchi. Hence a pattern akin to that postulated (yet not substantiated) by historians for Western countries could be expected, albeit only if the patient population at Yeravda was Westernised in ways that had a bearing on the manifestations of mental illness. Clearly, there are far too many factors involved to allow for a straightforward interpretation of the gendered data.

How do the patterns of the melancholia data compare to those of equally or even more distinctly gendered trends for other conditions? In the case of dementia praecox/schizophrenia, for example, the gender differential in favour of females was, during the 1930s, a stable six per cent.[265] For mania it varied, with a steadily falling trend, between an earlier fifteen per cent and later two per cent. Delusional insanity/paranoia and circular insanity/MDP showed more complex patterns, with male predominance in the case of the former. All of these conditions had to be differentiated by doctors from melancholia during the diagnostic process. In some cases this posed difficulties, as reported by Ewens, who pointed out, for example, that in relation to delusional insanity it was 'extremely difficult to class some of the varieties of insanity' in which 'a delusion forms almost the only symptom':[266]

> In India where of all countries of the world it is most rare to get any reliable family history or clear account of the origin of a disease, it is not always easy to distinguish from these cases those of a maniac or melancholic who has lost all his acute symptoms.[267]

Given Ewens' awareness of the problem, we might infer that he took particular care not to mistake cases of delusional insanity for other conditions and that therefore a significant proportion of patients would have been diagnosed by him with delusional insanity. The reality was far from this. In fact, Ewens contended that in India they were fewer than in Europe,[268] 'only forming about 2 to 4 per cent of those in European Asylums and infinitely less in Indian ones'.[269] What is more, he held that the condition was 'more common in men than women'.[270] While male predominance fitted in with the trend at Ranchi, the figures did not. Under Dhunjibhoy, the male ratio fluctuated steadily between seven and eight per cent, with the female ratio some three per cent below this.[271] In contrast, Overbeck-Wright held that the condition 'affects the sexes equally', referring to an aggregate figure of about five per cent.[272] How can we account for these three different observations and figures?

Ewens' observations drew on his experiences during the last decade of the nineteenth century and the first decade of the twentieth, whilst Overbeck-Wright's were based on figures mainly from the 1910s, and Dhunjibhoy's on those from the 1920s and 1930s. These differences would have been crucial, as there were considerable changes in nomenclature and the conceptualisation of mental illness during these periods. The difficulties of differential diagnosis commented on by Ewens, which were exacerbated by rapid developments in the field, may have been another factor, leading to gendered or un-gendered trends respectively and to prevalence figures dependent on doctors' diagnostic mind-sets at particular times.

We know already, for example, that Overbeck-Wright chose to 'ignore' dementia praecox as he grouped the 'various conditions' (paranoia, katatonia and hebephrenia) that he thought were assigned this label by others 'under the one head of "delusional insanity"'.[273] In contrast, Ewens and Dhunjibhoy employed both dementia praecox and delusional insanity. At Ranchi, women outnumbered men for dementia praecox by at least four per cent most of the period. It may well be that Overbeck-Wright's integration of dementia praecox cases into delusional insanity effected an equalling out of the gender ratio. This would indicate that un-gendered or gendered patterns for specific conditions – in this case delusional insanity and dementia praecox – were due to superintendents' preferences for particular categories rather than reflecting actual gender differences for any one disorder (that would in any case have been subject to shifting and different conceptualisations). A similar suggestion could be made in regard to circular insanity/MDP, which was assigned more frequently to women at Ranchi, significantly so from 1935.[274]

At Ranchi the average gender differential for this condition varied between zero and seven per cent. As in regard to the rising aggregate numbers discussed previously, the widening of the gender gap in 1936 may have been due to changing preferences in the allocation of particular categories over time and the changing ways in which they were conceptualised. The rise of MDP is mirrored by the decline of mania, particularly so in the case of women, with the gender difference narrowing towards the end of the period for mania and widening for MDP. At Ranchi the gender differential was by 1939 comparable only to that of cannabis-induced psychosis (which had been consistently an almost exclusively male category) and dementia praecox (which showed a stable female prevalence throughout the period).

The rise of circular insanity in India from its earlier French conceptualisation as *folie circulaire* to its later, Kraepelin-influenced incarnation as MDP, can be mapped in Ewens', Overbeck-Wright's and Dhunjibhoy's writings. During the 1910s Ewens was aware that circular insanity or *folie circulaire* was 'believed by some to be a distinct disease', but he remained sceptical:

> Whether the condition is a special disease or no[t], the alteration of the two forms, mania and melancholia, has been often described, and such cases possibly form the basis for the new entity, manic-depressive Insanity, instituted on the Continent.[275]

He speculated that 'in India such a regular alternation must be of extreme rarity, and has certainly never come under my own notice'.[276] Reframing this statement in less opaque terms, he referred to his own clinical experience:

> Mania in all its varieties is peculiarly frequent in this country and in this province, but among all the many instances of it that have been treated here, no single one has exhibited such an alternation of symptoms as to warrant its being considered as corresponding to the type of disease under consideration.[277]

Like Ewens, Overbeck-Wright kept his observations about the condition that he preferred to frame as *folie circulaire* crisp and brief, despite both circular insanity and

MDP being used more frequently during the 1920s. He classed it under insanities of toxic origin (namely 'Insanities in which there is evidence of Bacterial Toxaemia') together with katatonia and hebephrenia.[278] He was consistent in his rejection of Kraepelin's juxtaposition of MDP with dementia praecox (which subsumed, at the time, paranoia, katatonia and hebephrenia).[279] Yet, unlike Ewens, he clearly acknowledged *folie circulaire* as a discrete entity, providing a succinct description of its different stages. Dhunjibhoy, as we already know, was familiar with continental diagnostic debates and he increasingly employed Kraepelinean categories from the 1930s onwards. It is clear that the ways in which particular categories were conceptualised and matched up with patients' symptomatic behaviours by Ewens, Overbeck-Wright and Dhunjibhoy varied greatly. The statistics produced by superintendents on the official report forms suggest standardisation of some kind – but it was simply standardisation of the mechanics of record keeping.

The figures recorded in the institutional report do not by themselves reflect diagnostic practices nor the meaning attributed to particular terms by those who filled in the forms. The standardisation of nomenclature hides variation. Individual superintendents employed variously conceptualised categories as mooted in Britain, Germany and France as and when they filled in their end-of-year report forms. This can be illustrated to a certain extent by a comparison of the prevalence rates reported at different institutions in 1933 and 1939 respectively for the two main types of what we might today consider as depressive disorders: melancholia and MDP.

Institutions compared: Longitudinal trends in gendered diagnoses

Statistics are available for 1933 and 1939 for a number of institutions in British India, including the provinces of Bombay and Madras. Let us assess the longitudinal data for two mental hospitals dedicated to Indians in Bombay province (Dharwar and Ahmedabad) and Madras (Waltair and Calicut) as well as those that treated Europeans, Eurasians and Indians (Yeravda in Bombay, and Madras). We can then compare these with Ranchi (covering Bengal, Bihar and Orissa) and the Parsi-funded Sir Cowasji Jehangir Mental Hospital, located at Hyderabad (Sind), in today's Pakistan. The latter provided for a majority of Hindus and Muslims as well as a small number of Indian Christians and Parsis.

If we contrast Figure 4.2 for 1933 with Figure 4.3 for 1939, the following trends can be discerned in relation to the frequency with which melancholia was assigned to men and women at the different institutions.

The average male and female ratios for all hospitals except Ranchi reveal that melancholia remained a predominantly male disorder, with gender differentials of six and five per cent for 1933 and 1939 respectively. At Ranchi, too, melancholia continued to be assigned more frequently to men, albeit less so in 1939. While the Ranchi rate remained at a stable eleven per cent for men, it increased for females from six to nine per cent between 1933 and 1939. The institutions that admitted both Europeans and Indians showed very different patterns. Madras rarely made use of melancholia and reported no gender difference. Yeravda, too, assigned the diagnosis less frequently overall, but

Figure 4.3. Percentage of men and women (of total number treated) assigned the diagnosis melancholia, 1939

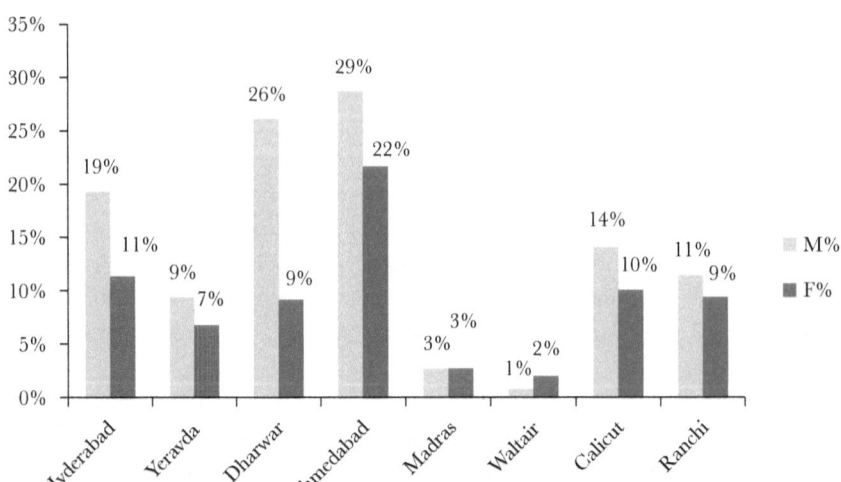

reversed the female preponderance reported in 1933 to male predominance in 1939. Hyderabad showed a completely different pattern, with increased use of melancholia and stable male preponderance. The pattern for the exclusively Indian institutions was no less diverse. Like Madras, Waltair assigned melancholia extremely rarely, while Calicut further increased its use of the category and even reversed its gender trend towards male predominance. As at Calicut the assignment of melancholia at Dharwar in Bombay showed an upward trend, but maintained the highest level of male predominance of all institutions. The other institution administered by Bombay, Ahmedabad, showed a very different pattern, with melancholia being diagnosed less frequently for both male and female patients, with male predominance narrowing.

Diversity is no less apparent in the case of MDP, despite the trend for most institutions (Madras and Calicut being the exceptions) towards an increase in the use of this diagnosis (see Figure 4.4 for 1933 and Figure 4.5 for 1939). In fact, Ahmadabad's and Waltair's figures shot up from one per cent for males and zero per cent for females to 17 and 20 per cent and 16 and 29 per cent respectively. In the other institutions the increased use made of this diagnosis was not quite as pronounced, but still considerable.

In regard to gender predominance, striking variety prevailed. At Ranchi MDP became a more markedly female disorder, with its gender ratio in 1939 being well above the combined average of the other institutions (it had been close to the average in 1933). Madras on the other hand continued to use the diagnosis so rarely (a fraction of one per cent) that no significant gender difference could be ascertained in 1939. Hyderabad and Calicut exhibit nearly equal gender ratios, but while the former increased its use of the diagnosis, the latter reported a decrease. Two institutions (Ahmedabad and Dharwar) showed male predominance and two others (Waltair and Yeravda) female preponderance. The gender differential at Waltair was particularly pronounced, with 17 and 29 per cent for men and women respectively.

Figure 4.4. Percentage of men and women (of total number treated) assigned the diagnosis manic depressive insanity/psychosis, 1933

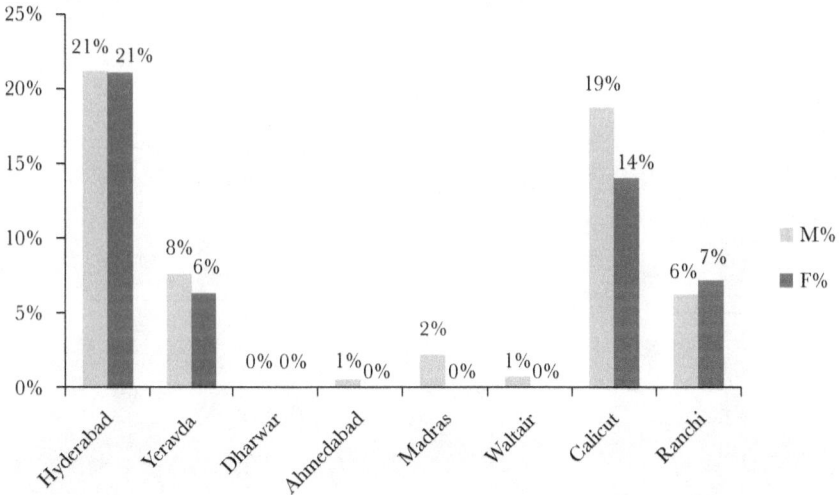

Figure 4.5. Percentage of men and women (of total number treated) assigned the diagnosis manic depressive psychosis, 1939

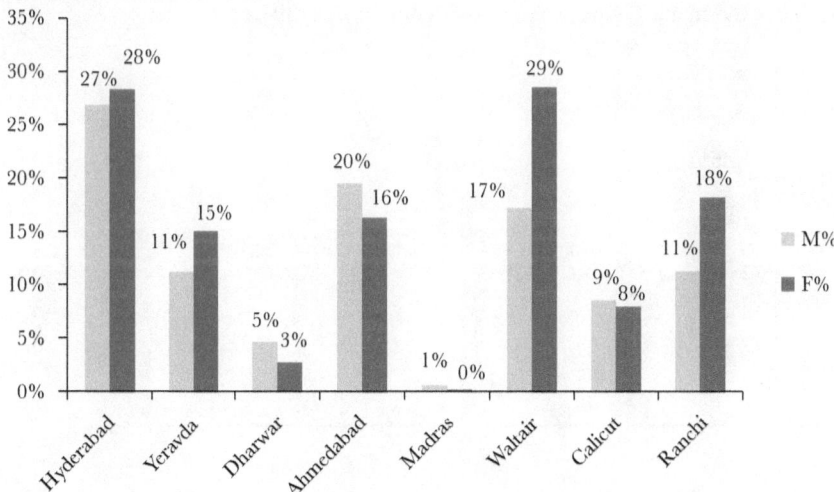

These complex trends become no less puzzling if we consider the aggregate figures for both diagnoses (see Figures 4.6 and 4.7, for 1933 and 1939 respectively). Such combination of datasets for individual conditions is often done to enable researchers to identify trends for a particular group, such as those classed as mood disorders.

The most conspicuous feature revealed in the figures below is the overall rise in the diagnosis of the two depressive disorders: from 21 per cent for males and 14 per cent for females in 1933, to 27 and 23 per cent respectively in 1939. This upward trend is mirrored

Figure 4.6. Percentage of men and women (of total number treated) assigned the diagnoses melancholia (other), and circular insanity/melancholia and manic depressive psychosis, combined, 1933

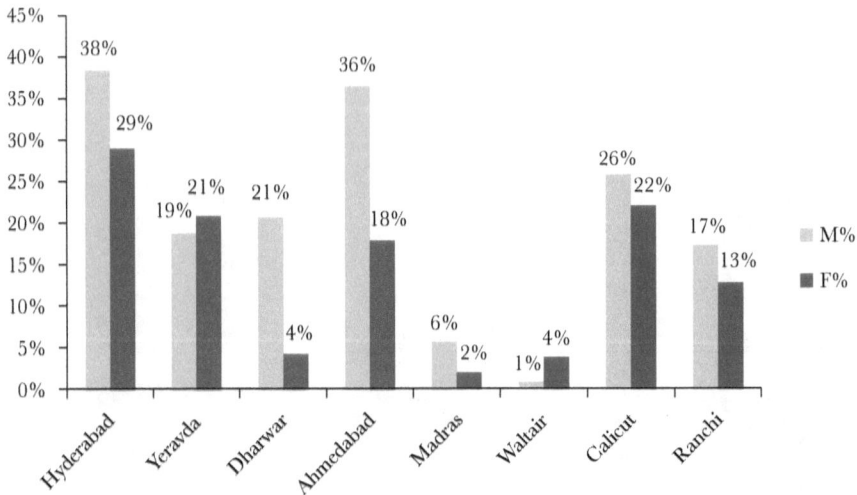

Figure 4.7. Percentage of men and women (of total number treated) assigned the diagnoses melancholia and manic depressive psychosis, combined, 1939

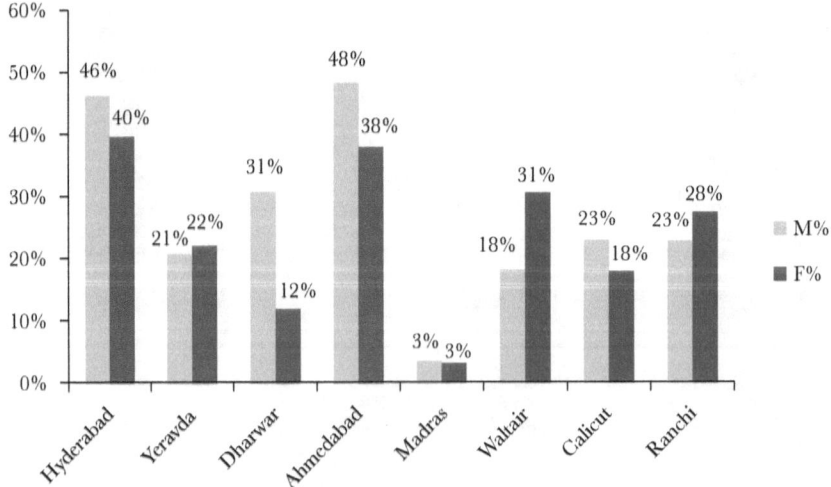

at Ranchi.[280] However, overall the gender differential narrows from seven per cent in 1933 to four per cent in 1939, effecting a decrease in male preponderance. Only Madras retains a consistently low use of the depressive disorder categories – this is evidently out of step with what is happening at the other places. Despite these general trends, a high degree of variation between and within institutions is still discernible for the aggregated diagnoses. In contrast to the prevailing trend, at Ranchi and Waltair (and to a very minor extent, Yeravda), the depressive disorders combined assumed a female face by 1939. The inversion of the earlier male gender predominance at Ranchi occurred in 1936. Yeravda's aggregate trend suggests continuity of gendered diagnostic practice, but hides the reversal of gender predominance in melancholia and MDP that occurred between 1933 and 1939.

So, what are we to make of the general trend towards the increased application of the two depressive disorder categories commonly used during the 1930s and the apparent narrowing of male predominance? It may be tempting to explain the former as an early indication of a trajectory leading to the current high rates of depression reported worldwide. The narrowing and eventual reversal of gender predominance poses more difficulties. Given the heterogeneity of the institutional patterns, any selective equation of one particular institutional trend with popular representations, such as the gendered face of depression in literature, would be misleading. In fact, the high level of intra- and inter-institutional heterogeneity of diagnostic practices allows us to postulate almost any gendered pattern that fits our preferred analytical perspective, conveniently enabling us to apparently substantiate such hypotheses by means of carefully selected evidence from a particular mental hospital.

The cases of melancholia and MDP have shown that the analysis of one institution, even in depth and over time, does not legitimate any generalisations about, for example, depression in Indian mental hospitals or depression in India as a male malady. Such statements would rest on misconceptions regarding the representativeness of the currently available evidence. Nor would a focus on the aggregate or average trend in a range of institutions over time be more illuminating as these figures hide highly diverse and contradictory patterns. Only an in-depth assessment and comparison of the whole spectrum of diagnoses and the changing meanings of the terms over time at a wide range of individual institutions enables us to arrive at appropriately nuanced and hence, perhaps less clear-cut propositions regarding the connections between wider cultural perceptions of gender and mental illness, diagnostic practices, and the institutional prevalence rates for particular conditions.

Aetiology – 'the outstanding problem of psychiatry'

'The question of causation is the outstanding problem of psychiatry', noted Dhunjibhoy in his report of 1937.[281] He went on to suggest, 'There are so many causes which may contribute to a mental break-down that in most cases one cannot specify any one in particular.' He listed 'Toxic agents, epilepsy, various bodily illnesses and life's stresses of various kinds' as the main ones, but affirmed that 'the cause of mental disorders does not lie in any one of the above stated aetiological factors alone, but is the resultant of many such factors'. The large number of potential causes that were listed on the institutional report form confirms Dhunjibhoy's observation. By the 1930s these had been reduced to 22 from the earlier 48. Although on average only 18 of these had actually been used under the old report template (15 from 1933 onwards), the number and variety of potential causes were still considerable while the aetiology of mental illness remained a contested enigma. Dhunjbhoy concluded: 'The patient must be considered as a biological problem.'

The reference to biology is grounded in a strand of contemporary thinking that identified heredity and physical factors as the decisive causes of mental disorder. Dhunjibhoy himself considered 'inherited taints' as main causes, likening their 'heredity' to that assumed to be the case in tuberculosis. 'The child does not inherit the disease itself but certainly inherits a predisposition to contract the disease under suitable conditions.'[282] Contemporary psychiatric theory postulated that, as Ewens had put it in 1908, 'predisposing and exciting causes are both necessary', with the 'predisposing (physical) one in the patient's constitutional tendency' being 'derived from hereditary influence'.[283] Although some causal elements could be both predisposing and exciting (syphilis and alcohol, for example), the latter were 'frequently moral ones'.[284] By the 1930s the terminology and the meanings attributed to 'moral' had changed, with 'psychic' causes, 'mental stress' and 'environmental' factors becoming more prominent phrases in scientific debate. Dhunjbhoy explained:

> Next in importance to 'Heredity' are 'Environmental factors'. Some Psychiatrists attach great[er] importance to 'Environmental factors' than 'Heredity'. But I for one feel convinced that 'Heredity' does play an important role in the causation in [the] majority of the cases combined with the anxieties and increased stresses of modern every-day life.[285]

Dhunjibhoy's insistence on the priority of hereditary factors (predisposing causes), whilst acknowledging the relevance of mental stress or, as he put it in 1932, the link between 'modern civilisation and mental strain', was in line with contemporary thinking.[286] As his own publications and hospital reports suggest, he was familiar with the latest developments in psychiatry through consultation of the relevant British and North American journals and textbooks. His German family connections and visits to his in-laws in Berlin nurtured a strong appreciation of Kraepelinean ideas, and travels to Vienna and Zürich kindled a certain appreciation of Freudian and Jungian thinking. Dhunjibhoy had also read, and at times used near verbatim quotes from, prominent textbooks and other work published in India, such as that of Macpherson, Ewens and Overbeck-Wright. Given that the aetiological schemes promulgated by these theories were very different and even at odds with each other, Dhunjibhoy's phrase that the causation of mental illness was an 'outstanding problem' reflected his own situation as much as that of psychiatry more generally. Above all, he had to reconcile his own thinking with the headings used in the prescribed forms, which, as has been shown in relation to diagnoses, lagged behind established wisdom in India and Britain. There was agreement of sorts on the assumed existence of both predisposing and exciting factors, but if and how these could be differentiated and what their relative role was, remained highly contested and subject to shifting definitions.

Ewens had drawn on C. A. Mercier's classification of causes, which differentiated heredity and stress.[287] The latter included diseases, fevers, Indian hemp, alcohol, as well as worry, over-education, syphilis, sexual excess and masturbation. Like many others at the time and later, Mercier's scheme did not map in any straightforward way on to the juxtapositions of 'physical' and 'moral' or of 'predisposing' and 'exciting', which were also widely used. 'Heredity' included not only 'the presence of Insanity, nervous disease, etc., in the parents', but also 'alcoholism or syphilis' and 'Tubercle' in the parents[288]. Dhunjibhoy's likening of the hereditary transmission of mental illness to that identified for TB was imbued with Ewens' and Mercier's earlier understandings of causation.

Another reference text for Dhunjibhoy was Overbeck-Wright's *Lunacy in India*, which in turn drew on L. C. Bruce's understanding of mental illness. Bruce's 'toxic theory' was not generally adopted fully in Britain, but Overbeck-Wright subscribed to it to the letter.[289] In late nineteenth-century India, J. Macpherson most prominently mooted the 'toxic basis of all forms of insanity', although he conceded that it was 'a presumption for which there is fairly good foundation but no proof'.[290] Macpherson's division of types of toxaemia had consisted of three principal groups. These were; a) autointoxication (as result of physiological instability, defective metabolism, defective gland secretion, autointoxication from alimentary tract, liver and kidneys); b) intoxication from microorganisms; and c) voluntary intoxication by alcohol and drugs.[291] As in most schemes, these causes were often seen to be prevalent in combination. In both the pre- and post-1934 official report forms, toxic causes were listed alongside others, but in the former period they included only alcohol, drugs, fever, TB, syphilis, plague and other toxins, whilst in the latter they subsumed a bewildering assortment of toxins, alongside the former ones, namely physical, bodily illness, pregnancy, childbirth, climacteric, epilepsy, and head injuries. From 1934 onwards, the 'toxic' categories were differentiated from mental stress and infections. The causes listed under infections are no less intriguing for modern observers, ranging from *encephalitis lethargica*, influenza, syphilis, and 'other infections of old age', to hereditary predisposition. The meanings attributed to particular medical terms at different periods are evidently highly context specific.

Elements of the lists of aetiological factors of both Ewens' (based on Mercier) and Overbeck-Wright's (based on Bruce) were prevalent in Dhunjibhoy's and other psychiatrists' classifications, as were ideas on degeneracy and heredity, which enjoyed a heyday during the early twentieth century. In contemporary understanding predisposing factors, heredity and degeneration were invariably linked. Ewens did not even discuss the 'constitutional tendency derived from hereditary influence' but simply referred the reader 'in this particular [...] to the Chapter on "Degeneration"' in his book.[292] The main authority cited by him was the American physician Eugene Talbot and his *Degeneracy: Its Causes, Signs, and Results*, which had been edited in 1898 by the sexologist Havelock Ellis. Talbot's work, as Seitler puts it, 'provides an example of the extraordinary inclusiveness with which medical discourse forged links among diverse social, racial, gendered, and sexual subjects'.[293] Like many of his contemporaries, Talbot used degeneracy as an umbrella term to describe a host of regressive 'disorders', ranging from alcoholism to hermaphroditism, prostitution, pauperism and moral insanity, to giantism and negro degeneracy. From today's perspective, this reads of course like an incoherent medley of physical, social and behavioural factors and ideological categories.

Overbeck-Wright's understanding of hereditary predisposition was similarly wide ranging. It included not only 'those born of insane parents' but also offspring of syphilitic, gouty, rheumatic, phthisical parents, as well as 'defects' such as 'extreme nervousness, eccentricity, alcoholism, hysteria, epilepsy, vagabondage, and any want of balance in the mental development – *e.g.*, extreme brilliancy in one direction combined with deficiency in others'.[294] 'Whatever the exciting cause of insanity may be', he contended, 'undoubtedly the *chief predisposing cause* is an unstable mental heredity'.[295] Dhunjibhoy drew heavily on Overbeck-Wright's thoughts and on his formulations regarding heredity in his extended triennial report for 1930 to 1932. He listed a sample of 'exciting causes' that could, in his view, be found in the annual report 'of any institution for the insane':

> Business and domestic worries, loss of property, disappointment in love, domestic troubles, excessive study, loss of near relatives, political excitement, sexual frigidity or starvation, tyranny by mother-in-laws, cruelty and neglect by husbands, excessive religious tendency, etc.[296]

He went on to ask the rhetorical question:

> How many of us must have suffered at sometime or other from some or perhaps all of these so-called above stated exciting causes of insanity and yet despite this fact we find that sanity is the rule – insanity the exception.

This, he claimed, 'therefore proves beyond doubt that whatever the exciting cause of insanity may be, undoubtedly the chief predisposing cause is *unstable mental heredity*'.[297] Using Overbeck-Wright's phrasing, he explained that, 'the term "hereditary predisposition" here has a wider application than to those born of insane parents only.' His list of 'such defects' was slightly different, but equally colourful, including:

> Extreme nervousness, eccentricity, alcoholism, epilepsy, vagrancy, child marriage, faulty upbringings, lack of moral training and any want of balance in mental development. In addition to this, the offspring of syphilitic, gouty, rheumatic and phthisical parents are infinitely more liable to suffer from mental disorders than those sprung from healthy stocks.[298]

As was characteristic of the degeneration and mental hygiene school of thought during this period, social problems and the consequences of inequality and discriminatory political structures were being medicalised and represented as problems of tainted biology. However, unlike Overbeck-Wright, who disliked any ideas that were not based on Bruce, and in particular Freudian and Jungian ones, Dhunjibhoy embraced the latter, alongside those mooted on the hereditary causation of mental illness. He noted:

> A great deal of what heretofore has been regarded as hereditary predisposition is now regarded by the psycho-analysts as 'quite possibly individual' and due to causes which almost are preventable. In a certain sense a large number, if not all of the psychoses, can be considered as life reactions. That is, a defect of adjustment only develops upon the basis of some weak point in the personality make up and that weak point can be traced to its developmental beginnings in the early life. The presence of unconscious complexes cause reactions such as anxiety and obsessional neurosis, hysteria, etc., which seem to be constitutional only because the real causes are buried from sight.[299]

Dhunjibhoy's reflections highlight two important aspects. Firstly, the plurality of approaches to mental illness that flourished alongside each other during the 1920s and 1930s. Secondly, the opportunities this offered to eclectically draw on several strands of thought simultaneously, or as appropriate within different contexts. The Brucean purist, Overbeck-Wright in contrast had derided 'the theories promulgated by the Austrian schools of Freud and Jung', arguing in 1921 that 'now psychologists are practically unanimous in affirming that their theories are unsound'.[300] He even found it 'needless to cumber such a book as [his] aims to be with an exposition of their theories and doctrines', given 'the probability [...] that in another twenty years their teaching will be forgotten or only stored as curiosities in scientific libraries'.[301] Overbeck-Wright's judgement seems to have been refuted by history also in regard to another 'prevalent view held at present', namely the theory that 'disease originates *de novo* in the deranged cells and fibres of the cortex of the brain, and that the physical symptoms concurrent with such disease are directly the result of the pathological changes in the cerebral cortex'.[302] He suggested, 'on a little consideration', that this theory was 'rather too sweeping a statement'. After all, this theory

> palpably assumes that the brain is immune from the results of disease affecting the body as a whole, takes no note of the physical symptoms which in the majority of cases precede insanity, and ignores altogether the fact that, in practically all cases, physical improvement precedes any change for the better in the mental condition.[303]

In contrast, he proclaimed, 'with the theory of the toxic origin of insanity no such fault can be found' – after all, Bruce postulated that 'a physical cause in all cases must precede mental symptoms, and, therefore, that a physical improvement must take place before any hope of improvement in the mental condition can be held'.[304] Overbeck-Wright was very adamant, not to say obstinate, about his allegiance to one particular theory of causation, more so perhaps than Ewens and Macpherson had been before him. Unlike his prominent European colleagues in India, Dhunjibhoy's mind-set was more accommodating, arguably on account of a lack of exclusive identification with British-bred theories or, to put it in the language of transnational networks, his cosmopolitan connectedness with varied strands of thought in different localities around the globe. As one of few Indians in senior positions within the colonial service still frequently subject to censure by his European superiors, he may also have had to learn to be more diplomatic and conciliatory than some of his more dogmatic colleagues by integrating varied approaches into his own thinking and practice.

This is not to say that practitioners in Europe and North America were not also similarly eclectic in regard to psychiatric theory and practice, nor that the potential tension between hereditary and environmental theories was irreconcilable. Dhunjibhoy constituted a good example for the latter, when he included reflections on 'modern civilisation and mental strain' in one of his reports, in 1932.[305] The trope of social and economic progress leading to mental breakdown and unhappiness has had a long and chequered history. In Western literature and science it was refuelled during the early twentieth century by ideas of racial and social hygiene as well as anthropological research that postulated the adverse effect of modern civilisation on people from different racial or cultural backgrounds.[306] This process established common ground between models of degeneration on account of tainted heredity and those that highlighted the role of mental stress due to rapid socio-economic progress. 'Tainted' or 'unstable' mental heredity included, as Dhunjibhoy had observed, a number of social, psychological or 'moral' factors and sat comfortably alongside theories of social decline on account of mental strain caused by modern life.[307] Dhunjibhoy noted:

> We live in an age dominated by machinery and this has increased the speed at which we work and play and carry on many other activities to a rate which is far in excess of our capacity for biological adaptation. This accelerated tempo of living is productive of enormous mental tension and fatigue.[308]

Such considerations followed on seamlessly from his reflections on the predominance of tainted heredity in the causation of mental disorder. His wider aim during the 1930s was to argue the case for 'a well organized programme of mental hygiene', contending that 'the Indian corporations, municipalities and district boards must help to make it a success'. In a nutshell, he argued:

> It may well be stated that the increasing prevalence of mental diseases comes from the very nature of modern civilization and as India is fast adopting all the methods of modern Western civilization in order to be on equal footing with the civilized nations of the world, it might as well also provide ample facilities for the treatment of its mental and nervous breakdowns.[309]

The official response by Dhunjibhoy's senior, Colonel L. Cook, indicates that despite the apparent internal logic of his conception of the link between civilisation and mental stress, the argument failed to entirely convince this gatekeeper of colonial administration and finances. The opening statement of Cook's riposte was of a simply pragmatic, yet ultimately irrefutable, nature. It read as follows: 'Whether this epoch is advancing slowly or rapidly, the effective repercussions of the administration to meet such a situation will, as at present, depend on financial considerations.'[310] More importantly in this context, Cook did what Dhunjibhoy had failed to do on this occasion, namely provide evidence. He used the most recent census data, freshly released in 1931, to investigate whether Dhunjibhoy's conjectures could be substantiated by statistical evidence. Almost inevitably he noticed that the figures 'would appear to indicate that insanity is less prevalent in India than in the West.'[311] However, being aware of the problems of the census enumeration process in India, revealed by those in charge of data collection, he conceded that 'it is not improbable that the figures given in the Indian Census return do not include all the half-witted or feeble-minded that would be included in the census for England and Wales'. Cook's decisive argument concerned the tension between hereditary and social causes:

> One might infer from these comparative figures that the majority of the population is not yet subjected to the strain of living which is extant in the West, and that if a large number of feeble-minded have not been included in the Census figures, that these

feeble-minded are perhaps the result of hereditary defects rather than any acceleration in the tempo of living.[312]

However easily Dhunjibhoy was able to reconcile a number of different aetiological models in his mind, Cook made use of their potentially contradictory nature to great effect against his subaltern's proposal.

Given the power structures of the medical service, Dhunjibhoy perhaps wisely chose not to respond to Cook's incisive, if simplistically binary, analysis of heredity versus environment. It was not until five years later, in 1937, that Dhunjibhoy raised the issue again. A new inspector-general of civil hospitals had replaced Cook, and Dhunjibhoy restated the case for mental hygiene, outlining a number of measures to be taken, including 'eugenic sterilization of all known adult defectives of both sexes'.[313] On this occasion, some flaws in the evidence provided by Dhunjibhoy became apparent. He provided figures and vague estimates that were meant to substantiate the 'preponderance of inherited taints in major Psychosis and defects'.[314] Yet the figure for 'inherited abnormalities' in one set of disorders – schizophrenia and dementia praecox – was just 50 per cent.[315] The figure given for manic depressive psychosis ('the greatest inherited taint') was only an estimate, as was that for mental deficiency ('a very high percentage of forebears of mental defectives are alcoholics or the subjects of nervous disease'). Only in the case of epilepsy was the figure provided a conclusive 80 per cent, with transmission being thought by Dhunjibhoy to be 'frequently direct'. What was the statistical evidence for the preponderance of inherited factors at Ranchi?

As there is no data on causation for particular disorders, we must therefore rely on an analysis of the 'probable causes of insanity' tabulated for the annual reports. In these there is a clear and consistent trend over the period for hereditary causes to be recorded less frequently than those relating to mental stress. However, while the former were considered to be predisposing, the latter could be either predisposing or exciting. Heredity tended to trump mental stress as a predisposing factor. This was the case, despite the fact that the nomenclature prescribed in the report forms changed in 1934. During the earlier period, heredity had to be differentiated into separate categories (insane, epileptic, neurotic, marked eccentricity, alcoholism), while from 1934 there was only a single category, namely hereditary predisposition. Conversely mental stress became disaggregated and more clearly circumscribed. The earlier two rubrics of acute and chronic for mental stress gave way to moral, business worry, and domestic worry. (The fourth subdivision, 'stress of military service', was not applied at Ranchi, but its inclusion in the forms signalled official acknowledgement of the impact of war trauma on soldiers' mental health). It is likely that the aggregated categories referred to the same range of causes as did the subdivided ones. The figures provided under the relevant headings in 1933 and 1934 suggest this, as they were of a similar order. However, this cannot be confirmed.

We can only glean the frequency with which particular causes were assigned, whatever their meaning at particular periods. In 1925, heredity was given as the cause of mental illness of only eight per cent of the patients admitted to Ranchi from their previous institutions (with 95 patients being reported to have been the offspring of an insane and four of a neurotic parent). This was only the fifth most frequently reported category overall, if we consider both predisposing and exciting causes. This was similar in subsequent years, when heredity was on average in fourth position. Mental stress came third in 1925 (14 per cent), with a sharp increase to 48 per cent in 1933, when heredity equalled 19 per cent. However, if we look at the cause most frequently considered as predisposing – rather than both predisposing and exciting combined – then hereditary emerges as the clear main category. Still, the gap narrowed as by 1939 hereditary predisposition was reported in 15 per cent of cases, whilst the three main divisions of mental stress were implicated as predisposing factors in 13 per cent of cases of mental illness.

The statistical pattern for mental stress is more complicated than that for hereditary predisposition. The latter was, by definition, always a predisposing and never an exciting cause. Mental stress, on the other hand, was reported as both a predisposing and exciting cause to varied degrees over the period. During earlier years, when only 'sudden' and 'prolonged' mental stress were differentiated from one another, it was reported as an almost exclusively exciting cause in 1925, 1930 and 1931. It was listed as mainly predisposing in 1926, and mainly exciting in 1928, 1929, 1932 and 1933. In some of these years, it trumped heredity as the most frequent predisposing cause. Under the new nomenclature the pattern became more nuanced. Stress due to business or domestic worry was generally listed only or principally as an exciting cause. Moral stress, in contrast, changed from zero attribution in 1934 to a still rare and exclusively exciting cause in the following two years (2 per cent in 1935 and 4 in 1936). It became a frequently assigned category in 1937 (20 per cent), which could be both predisposing and exciting, and finally a mainly predisposing cause (10 and 21 per cent) in the last two years of Dhunjibhoy's superintendence at Ranchi. In 1940, when his deputy, Das, was in charge of the institution, mental stress reverted to being listed only as an exciting cause.

How do we explain the rise of the category of mental stress generally, from 1932 and, more specifically, as a predisposing cause, from 1937 onwards? Different reasons may account for these two trends. Dhunjibhoy attributed this cause with significantly increased frequency among female patients from the very year when he raised the issue of mental hygiene in India for the first time – 1932. The female rate jumped from nine per cent in 1931 to 49 in 1932 and 71 in 1933 (while the male rate remained around a stable 24 to 25 per cent). The elevated trend prevailed also under the new nomenclature, with continued high rates for women and considerably raised ones for men. The male rate jumped to 63 per cent in 1934, fluctuating subsequently between a low of 31 (when Pacheco was in charge) and a high of 73 per cent in 1939. In the last year of Dhunjibhoy's time at Ranchi, domestic worry was assigned as a cause (mainly exciting) to 86 per cent of the women admitted to the institution. In contrast, heredity figured, as a predisposing cause, in only 15 per cent of patients at that point.

The second shift in the frequency with which mental stress was attributed occurred in 1937, the year when Dhunjibhoy formulated his second epistle on 'Mental Defectives of India', advocating the adoption of eugenic sterilisation as 'a means of ridding the race of its defective germ plasm'.[316] Arguably, Dhunjibhoy's tracts in 1932 and 1937 on issues of mental hygiene had an impact on the kinds of cause that were attributed to the patients admitted during those years. The rate for business worry among men increased from 24 per cent in 1936 to 43 per cent in 1943 and from zero to three per cent for women. This was higher than that reported for moral causes, which amounted to only 22 per cent in the case of women and 18 per cent for men. However, business worry was only an exciting cause, while the majority of moral cases were reported as predisposing factors.

Another question arises from the fact that moral, business and domestic worry were identified separately under the term mental stress from 1934 onwards. Were moral causes assigned also under the pre-1934 nomenclature? The category used during the earlier period that came closest was moral deficiency, which was one of the causes listed under mental instability alongside congenital mental defect, eccentricity and previous attack. All of these were considered as predisposing causes. Alas, moral deficiency was used only in one year, in 1926, when it was applied to two men. How is it that moral causes, which figured so prominently in the wider psychiatric, literary and public discourse during this period, were not prevalent in Ranchi's statistics until the late 1930s? One explanation may be that, as Ewens pointed out, 'moral causes are said to be more effectual (they are certainly more frequent) in the more "civilised" countries'.[317] Once psychiatrists in India began to frame the epidemiology of mental illness in relation to a perceived progress towards the kind of civilisation alluded to by Ewens, identification of the adverse effects of modern life could begin to be identified in India. Why then did Dhunjibhoy not use moral deficiency as a potential cause from 1932 onwards, when he had mused so eloquently on the impact of civilisation and mental stress? We can only speculate on this. It could be argued that the category of moral deficiency, the only one that accommodated moral causes until 1934, was not considered suitable, as these were then still seen, as in Ewens' time, as mainly exciting rather than predisposing factors such as those listed under mental instability. This requires further research.

Dhunjibhoy's contention of 1932 that hereditary predisposition was wider ranging than simply its application to 'those born of insane parents only', raises similar questions as he did not comment on why the statistics failed to substantiate the theories he argued for so strongly.[318] During that particular year, being born to insane parents was in fact the most frequently assigned cause (in 21 out of 23 cases) under the label heredity. Some of the other defects he claimed to be part of his broader definition were in contrast sparsely represented: 'extreme nervousness' (1), 'eccentricity' (0), 'alcoholism' (0) and 'epilepsy' (1). There was no category for vagrancy or child marriage, but they could, in line with one strand of contemporary thinking, have been subsumed under moral deficiency, together with 'faulty upbringings, lack of moral training and any want of balance in mental development'.[319] Alas, that year not a single patient was assigned this cause and only two patients were reported under congenital mental defect.

There are other important issues that warn against over-interpretation of the available statistical and circumstantial evidence. These relate to the high level of unknowns in the hospital data. Causes could not be ascertained by the superintendent for between 14 and 65 per cent of cases from 1926 to 1938. The extent to which background information on patients' conditions was missing varied significantly over the period. The figures for unknowns were at their highest in 1931 and 1932 during the trade recession (63 and

65 per cent respectively). They decreased sharply when the new nomenclature was introduced in 1934 (from 36 per cent in 1933 to 19 per cent in 1934) and slowly declined thereafter (to 12 per cent in 1938). Whether the economic situation during the early 1930s and the change of nomenclature in 1934 were indeed linked to the rising and falling pattern cannot be substantiated, not least because it is not clear what exactly was meant by the term 'not ascertained'. During the pre-1934 period, superintendents were able to identify two different reasons for lack of data, these were: 'no causes assignable' and 'no cause ascertained – history'. This made it possible for them, in principle, to clarify whether causes could not be provided because information on the patients' circumstances was missing or, alternatively, because the medical officer was unable to assign any causes despite such information being available. The latter was not really an option for a trained professional as it would have reflected poorly on his expertise. The 'no cause assignable' category was therefore used only in 1925, when the patients were transferred from their previous institution, and in 1927, when the two columns for 'not assignable' and 'not ascertained' appear to have been reversed accidentally. The decision in 1934 to drop the former category therefore made sense.

Any assessment of the aetiological factors that superintendents did manage to identify needs to take into account that during some years the unknowns far outweighed the number of ascertained cases. Crucially, during most of the period the figures for 'not ascertained' were higher or just equal to those for heredity/hereditary predisposition. The situation was similar though not quite as pronounced for mental stress during the pre-1934 period. After 1933, domestic worry was pinpointed in between 37 and 75 per cent of cases, whilst even the lowest rate for unknowns from 1934 to 1938 was a still significant 12 per cent. However, the acknowledgment of moral causes from 1934 and the reported rise in all subdivisions of mental stress during the later period may have led to the fall in 'unascertained' cases.

Missing data on Indian patients' background had been a well-documented phenomenon throughout the nineteenth century. By the turn of the century, Ewens confirmed that even then it was 'peculiarly difficult especially in this country to obtain any history at all […] or a true one'.[320] Overbeck-Wright, too, complained about lack of details, stating that 'Asylum statistics in India on [heredity] are most vague, owing to the meagre information as a rule received with each patient, fully 50 per cent. coming to the asylum without any family history whatever.'[321] Efforts to obtain more background details during a patient's presentation for admission were no less inconclusive. For example, in the case of 'C.D, a rifleman in the –th Gurkha Rifles', Overbeck-Wright reported that, 'On asking about him [he] received the usual statement in such cases, "*pagal hua*" [gone mad].'[322]

Given the circumstances described by Overbeck-Wright, it appears that much depended on the superintendent's skill during the anamnestic process as well as his tenacity in tracing more information by interrogating the person who accompanied the patient. The fact that patients were often taken to the hospital by a *peon* did not facilitate the process. A *peon* could be anybody, from a watchman, office orderly, policeman and soldier to an odd-job person. These people were supposed to ensure the patient's comfort and the safety of those around him and would not usually have been familiar with medical let alone psychiatric considerations. Language problems and the need for the medical officer to rely on an interpreter during the admission process constituted a further challenge. The patients admitted to Ranchi came from three large provinces and belonged to a number of different cultural and linguistic communities. In 1925, when Dhunjibhoy reported the reception of 1,274 patients, he had sufficient information on predisposing and exciting causes for only 176 men and 32 women.[323] In 1931, when the rate of 'causes not ascertained' amounted to a hitherto unmatched 63 per cent of those admitted during the year, Dhunjibhoy felt compelled to explain that, 'In [the] majority of cases no causes could be assigned due to practically no information being supplied by the police in the descriptive roll of the patients.'[324]

Despite the uncertainties regarding medically relevant background information, superintendents like Ewens and Overbeck-Wright did not hesitate to ponder on the possible causes of mental illness among Indians. They contrasted these with the aetiology seen to be typical of Europeans and presented their reflections as if they were valid assessments rather than conjectures based on selective personal and professional experience and hearsay. The question is of course to what extent this kind of evidence tells us more about individual doctors' Eurocentric perceptions of the causes of mental illness in India than about the factors actually implicated in patients' mental breakdown.

Overbeck-Wright held particularly strong views about the different causes affecting people in Europe and in India. He also highlighted the ideas that he considered most prevalent particularly among 'the laity'.[325] Europeans, he claimed, considered the cause of insanity to be 'due to an unstable brain readily thrown into disorder by physical causes, nervous shock, or mental strain, and that this instability is transmitted from one generation to another'. He provided two examples for this position. When a 'parturient woman becomes mentally deranged', factors such as 'physical cataclysm, the pains of labour, the excitement, mental and bodily, the exhaustion, the loss of blood, septicaemia, the sudden diversion of the stream of vital energy from the uterus to the mammae, the reflex disturbances on an unstable brain from the reproductive organs' are seen to be responsible. In cases such as 'when a man who has suffered monetary losses, or a mother who has lost her child, becomes insane, the condition is at once believed to be directly due to the mental effect of such losses'.[326]

According to Overbeck-Wright a different view of causation was prevalent among Indians. He described it as follows:

> The causes most commonly – in fact, almost universally – given, are demoniac possession, a curse for slighting some faquir or sadhu, a visitation for the defiling of some grave, or a punishment for neglecting to sacrifice to some of their numerous deities, or desecrating some tree, tank, or shrine dedicated to them. Next in frequency, but a very poor second, indeed, comes disappointment in love, the patient in such cases generally having squandered, not only his own, but much of his employer's money on some well-known prostitute, who in the end has discarded him for some richer lover.[327]

Overbeck-Wright's representation of European and Indian ideas about mental illness was highly flawed. He cited in regard to the former one particular strand of thinking that was not so much based on the laity's views, as on contemporary, but increasingly out-dated, scientific rationales (such as Thomas Clouston's, who had revised his highly influential *Clinical Lectures on Mental Diseases* of 1883 for a wider public during the first decade of the twentieth century). For the Indian view he provided a list of common beliefs. He thus contrasted European rationales anchored in what could then still be counted as science with Indian ones grounded in what the British considered to be superstitions. The reference points for his comparison were therefore not equivalent, but based on different constituencies. To achieve a degree of parity he would have needed to either contrast European with Indian non-science based rationales or European popularised science with its contemporary Indian equivalents (such as popular thinking drawing on Ayurveda, Unani or even Daktari medicine[328]).

Leaving aside these issues of culturally skewed medical perceptions among Europeans, Overbeck-Wright did not consider the popular science-based British perspective, nor the alleged Indian lay position to be appropriately grounded, and instead favoured Bruce's aetiological model. Like other practitioners, then and now, he did not rely on his patients' and their relatives' causal attributions and instead drew on the aetiological theories and classifications promulgated within the medical profession. In regard to the relative frequency of particular causes among Indians and their culturally specific manifestations, doctors expressed slightly different views. Ewens, for example, held that

> In Europe, it is said, that domestic worry frequently causes it in the female, and commercial, pecuniary in the male, but in this country one sees that the most frequent cause in both is worry connected with family – the loss of several members of it (as by plague, etc.), with the male the publicity of wifely infidelity.[329]

He concluded that 'it is very clear indeed, that worry and constant anxiety are pre-eminently the indirect causes of insanity'.[330] Overbeck-Wright, in contrast, contended that among 'male admissions into asylums in India undoubtedly the most common exciting cause of insanity is the abuse of Indian hemp (*Cannabis indica*) in some one or other form'.[331] He claimed that in 1913 nine per cent of the male admissions were 'due to this cause alone'. The Ranchi statistics reveal a pattern that differed from both Ewens' and Overbeck-Wright's observations. Here, mental stress was attributed significantly more frequently to women than men from 1932 onwards (double and nearly three times as often in 1932 and 1933 respectively). Under the new nomenclature, there prevailed a highly significant male predominance for business worry among men and a trend towards female preponderance for domestic worry. This was closer to what Ewens considered to be typical of the European situation, for which the separation of the public and private spheres was seen to be a characteristic feature. In regard to Indian hemp, the Ranchi rates for men fluctuated between four and 28 per cent (on average 15 per cent) from 1925 to 1933, and between five and 21 per cent (on average six per cent) in the post-1933 period. While the average figures compared reasonably well with Overbeck-Wright's nine per cent, they were considerably lower than those for many other causes and hence did not substantiate the contention that cannabis insanity was the 'most common exciting cause' among men.[332]

There were further perceptual discrepancies in the observed frequency of particular causes of mental illness. Overbeck-Wright had pointed out that 'practically no females' were admitted owing to the abuse of Indian hemp, while the 'most common causes' among women were 'fever, lactation and childbirth, and mental stress'.[333] At Ranchi too cannabis consumption was rarely assigned to women as a cause, but neither were causes related to childbearing (pregnancy, puerperal, lactation), from 1925 to 1933, or toxins (pregnancy, childbirth), from 1934 to 1939. However, mental stress, as illustrated previously, figured highly at Ranchi – whatever the varying definitions of this category at different periods. In his first report as the new superintendent at Ranchi, following Dhunjibhoy's assumption of military duties in Karachi, Das commented on the 'principal predisposing and exciting causes amongst the new admissions during the year'. He referred first of all to mental stress explicitly including 'privation and malnutrition'.[334] This highlights again how categories, such as mental stress, were defined in various ways by individual superintendents. Privation and malnutrition did not appear in the post-1934 nomenclature. This was in contrast to earlier practice when privation and starvation had been listed alongside malnutrition (in early life), over-exertion (physical), and sexual excess under the heading of physiological defects and errors.

Madness that was seen to have been caused by hunger was a significant factor between 1925 and 1933, and was assigned with higher frequency to women between 1927 and 1929, and 1932 to 1933. This led to the emergence of the female face of confusional insanity during these years, as discussed previously. The issue that remains to be explained is what happened when hunger could no longer be identified in the records as a cause of mental illness from 1934 onwards. Das seems to have included such cases under mental stress, presumably under business, or domestic worry. Had Dhunjibhoy done so, too? It is difficult to say. Judging from his commentaries on the statistics provided in the annual reports, Dhunjibhoy seems to have been more interested in the relationships between civilisation, mental stress, heredity and degeneration. Hunger did not figure in these reflections in any pronounced way, despite the fact that he mentioned, in other contexts, the relative ease with which patients admitted in a severely compromised physical condition would recover quickly if fed properly for some time. We find occasional remarks that may hint at the matter, such as in 1931, when Dhunjibhoy referred to 'prolonged mental and physical stress' and, more expressly, in 1932, when he listed starvation among many other causes such as tyranny by mothers-in-law and sexual frigidity that he considered as merely exciting and therefore secondary to an underlying predisposing 'unstable mental heredity'.[335] This is perhaps particularly puzzling to modern audiences, given that his preferred wider definition of hereditary predisposition that he shared with Overbeck-Wright included factors such as vagrancy, child marriage and faulty upbringings. Listing them under 'chief predisposing causes', Overbeck-Wright commented on the effect of child marriages:

> *Child marriages*, which are so common, especially among Hindu communities, are undoubtedly a factor to be reckoned with in the aetiology of mental diseases in India. In such cases the parties to the union are liable to suffer from the evil effects of premature sexual congress, the offspring suffer at first from the immaturity of the parents, and later

from the vitality of the parents, lowered, as it must be, by such premature sexual indulgence. The lives of the widows of such marriages, often bereft of their husbands while yet even children, is wretched in the extreme, and well calculated to produce melancholic and delusional conditions as a result of the prolonged misery and mental strain.[336]

His thinking was more opaque in regard to the role of 'consanguineous marriages and the greater stress of modern civilised life in the production of mental disease'.[337] He contended that these were 'at times brought forward as predisposing factors'. He further differentiated their respective roles. While the former, he argued, 'can only influence [mental disease] as tending to inte[n]sify a bad heredity', the latter, stress, was 'a very questionable item, at least in countries where civilization and learning have progressed slowly through the centuries and allowed an equivalent development of the mental faculties'. Here he referred to Europe. He then went on to argue in relation to places such as India:

> Where [...] the nation has vegetated for some centuries, and then, waking suddenly to its position, strives to attain at one bound the acme of civilisation and learning attained by other countries after years of laborious struggle, the result must be very different. In such cases there is not time for the necessary increase in mental development, early associations, customs, and beliefs are rudely torn away, and the minds are incapable of grasping adequately and complying with the new conditions. Such a country, therefore, must be prepared to pay a heavy bill in mental and nervous breakdowns in the course of the pursuit of its ambitions.[338]

In India, therefore, the 'greater stress of modern civilised life' acted as a predisposing cause, as it '*impairs the general vitality* [and] weakens resistance to bacterial invasion'.[339] A similar rationale held true for '*Faulty upbringing and a lack of moral training*', as these 'common and potent factors' also caused 'a deficiency in the development of volition and self-control, as well as the formation of undesirable dispositions and associations, which exert an undesirable influence upon the whole of the after life'.[340]

Dhunjibhoy had followed the same line of argument in his epistle on 'Modern Civilization and Mental Strain' – with one important difference.[341] He tended to stress the commonalities between Western and Eastern propensities rather than accentuating the differences between Europe and India. Dhunjibhoy referred, in a generalising way, to the increased 'speed at which we work and play', suggesting that this was 'productive of enormous mental tension and fatigue'. His understanding of the impact of stress was universal and inclusive, as when he pronounced that 'we' live in an age dominated by machinery.[342] Dhunjibhoy's resistance against reiterating the contemporary East and West dichotomy in regard to the role of the main factors implicated in the aetiology of mental illness constituted a break with his European colleagues' perspective as well as contemporary anthropological research. His point of reference had become the kind of universalist agenda mooted by organisations such as the American Foundation for Mental Hygiene and the League of Nations. In contrast, Ewens' and Overbeck-Wright's commentaries on aetiological factors were imbued with colonial attitudes and racial premises. These were increasingly challenged by Indian doctors such as Dhunjibhoy.

Chapter 5

TREATMENTS

'The treatment received by the patients in this hospital is up to the level of the latest modern methods employed in all the modern mental hospitals.'

—J. E. Dhunjibhoy, 1927

Ranchi was, Dhunjibhoy liked to claim, a 'modern mental hospital' that benefited from the introduction of 'all the latest approved Western methods of treatment'.[1] The evidence provided in his regular reports and publications fully substantiates this claim. When he was not travelling to 'keep abreast with the rapid advancement of the science', Dhunjibhoy read profusely.[2] His library books and journals at the Ranchi Indian Mental Hospital have been well preserved and are testimony to his profound and wide-ranging knowledge of hospital management and therapeutics. There are books that he might have acquired well before the institution's inauguration and which would have helped him to set up the institution from scratch, and complete sets of some of the most authoritative journals, considered vital reading by Western-trained psychiatrists around the world. These included, *American Journal of Psychiatry* (from 1923), *British Medical Journal* (from 1927), *Journal of Mental Science* (from 1921), the *Lancet* (from 1927), the *Practitioner* (from c. 1929), *Psychoanalytic Review* (1921–42), *Psychological Bulletin* (1927), *Psychiatry – Journal of the Biology and the Pathology of Interpersonal Relations* (1938, 1939), *International Journal of Psychoanalysis* (1920), *Brain. A Journal of Neurology* (from 1927) and *The Journal of Abnormal and Social Psychology* (from 1928).[3]

The number and variety of journals is impressive, representing diverse schools and approaches, ranging from biologically to psycho-dynamically orientated perspectives. In 1934 Dhunjibhoy noted,

> As usual strict watch was kept over the latest mental and medical journals for anything likely to influence in a direct or indirect way the course of the malady, and neither expense nor trouble is ever allowed to stand in the way of the employment of the latest discoveries if thereby the patient can in any way be benefited.[4]

While the former was clearly the case, the latter was a gross overstatement as severe financial constraints put limitations on the treatments available at Ranchi. Indeed, the attempts to identify indigenous drugs that were efficacious, provided new treatment options cheaper than European medication.

Indigenous Herbs

Two medicinal drugs, commonly used in Ayurveda, Unani and Siddha and by folk practitioners in India, were under trial at Ranchi: *Ocimum basilicum* (sweet basil) and *Rauvolfia serpentina* (Indian snakeroot). The former came from a small shrub indigenous to Persia and Sindh and was widely cultivated in South Asia. Dhunjibhoy knew about the plant's prevalence in indigenous modes of healing and referred to its Latin (*Basilicum citratum*) and its Sanskrit names (*Bisva Tulasi*) as well as Sindhi versions (*Sabji, Subji,* or *Sabajhi*). He also explained in his report of 1936 that the juice derived from it was 'largely used as a cure for insanity' by, as he put it, 'the Fakirs and Sadhus in India'.[5] His reference to *fakirs* and *sadhus* (wandering ascetics) instead of *hakims* and *vaidyas* (medical practitioners of Unani and Ayurveda) is intriguing. The former, although known to have administered drugs, were not primarily engaged in medicine, while the latter were experts in highly sophisticated learned medical systems. Was Dhunjibhoy indifferent to the finer points relating to indigenous medical knowledge and treatment practices? Or did he feel more comfortable aligning indigenous drugs with folk practices rather than learned Indian medicine? The timing of his assessment may be crucial to answer these questions.

Three years earlier, when Dhunjibhoy had observed 'encouraging results' following the application of sweet basil, he had explained the herb's geographical provenance but not its common use by both learned and folk practitioners.[6] He had even started growing the shrub in his own garden 'for the purpose of further experiment'. Specifying how it was applied at Ranchi, he stated that 'the leaves contain a yellowish green essential oil and if 5 or 6 drops of this oil are poured into each nostril of a highly excited patient, it allays the excitement and serves as a powerful hypnotic.'[7] Following his positive evaluation in the annual report, Dhunjibhoy received a number of enquiries about his trial, from India as well as England. However, three years later, on his return from his latest visit to what he then wittily described as the 'famous Psychiatric shrines of England, Europe and America', he declared that he had 'widened' his 'knowledge and experience'.[8] Following experiments 'on a larger scale' he contended that the indigenous drug worked as a powerful hypnotic only 'at times' and that 'the results were rather disappointing'.[9] The drug showed an effect 'in two cases only', while 'the majority remained unaffected by it'.[10] For the time being, this disappointing result would have settled Dhunjibhoy's enquirers on the question of the efficacy of this indigenous drug within the context of modern institutional treatment of the mentally ill. At Ranchi its use appears to have been discontinued.

Dhunjibhoy was also sceptical about a number of recently synthesised modern drugs. His rejection of an indigenous herb could therefore be considered as another experiment that resulted in a negative outcome. On the other hand, given that he had earlier omitted any allusion to the use of basil in Indian medicine, explicitly referring to it only after his tour of modern institutions abroad, he may have reconsidered his position on the use of indigenous drugs in a hospital that saw itself located at the cutting edge of modern, science-based psychiatry. His British colleagues' attitudes towards practitioners of indigenous medicine were at the time divided, with some supporting legislation aimed at institutionalising traditional medical systems such as Ayurveda, Unani and Siddha along Western lines by making them subject to scientific scrutiny. Others objected to any recognition being given to what they saw as un-improvable, outmoded and unscientific practices. Dhunjibhoy's seemingly casual remark on *sadhus* and *fakirs* may therefore be indicative of an attempt to distance himself from traditional practices and Indian drugs as part of the pharmaceutical arsenal of modern medicine. He did however contend that there still was a place for the herb, in locations not yet touched by modern development. He argued that 'the drug is well worth a trial in Indian villages or places in India where hypnotic drugs or injections are not available at a moment's notice, because this shrub is abundantly found in the remotest corner of India'.[11] The message was that indigenous drugs had a role to play in the plural field of healing, but not within one of India's reputedly most successful and modern mental hospitals.

There may also have been a problem of mistaken identity. There existed another basil variety, known as holy basil (*Ocimum sanctum, tulasi*), with which *sadhus* and *fakirs* were particularly closely linked. Ayurvedic, Unani and Siddha practitioners as well as ascetics made use of this herb, known as Krishna *tulasi* and Vishnu *priya*. As the name suggests, it was not only a medicinal plant, but also an important element in religious ritual. It was revered and seen as a potent way of preparing body and mind for spiritual practices. It is evident from the records that Dhunjibhoy trialled sweet basil rather than the sacred basil or *tulasi*. However, he may have linked up folk and ritual practices involved with *tulasi* with those relating to the use of sweet basil. (Incidentally, the classification of the basil/Ocimum genus has only recently been resolved satisfactorily.[12])

As to the second indigenous drug trialled at Ranchi, similar issues regarding Dhunjibhoy's stance on the use of folk medicine arise. His assessment of *Rauvolfia serpentina* (Indian snakeroot) was even more perfunctory and brusque. Alongside the second set of experiments with basil, he trialled snakeroot in 1936, immediately on his return from overseas leave. Dhunjibhoy provided much evidence in that year's report of being full of fresh ideas about modern psychiatry. He contrasted Ranchi favourably with the old institutions: 'The care and treatment of insane to-day in a modern mental hospital can only be fully appreciated by a comparison with conditions which existed in the one-time old asylums of India.'[13] He went on to argue:

> The armamentarium of medicine in general and of Psychiatry in particular has enormously increased and it has become one of the functions of the Ranchi Indian Mental Hospital to bring all these various diagnostic and therapeutic agencies which have been developed through the years to the service of its patients.

Most importantly in the current context, he contended the following: 'Modern mental hospital[s] offer outstanding opportunities for medical research.' Alas, as we shall discover, he missed one such opportunity in his examination of Indian snakeroot.

The experiments in 1936 were a retrial, as a first run had been done the year before. In 1935, during Dhunjibhoy's fourth extended visit to Europe, the Calcutta School of Tropical Medicine had sent an alcoholic extract of the drug to Ranchi with the request to 'try this medicine as it is renowned as a specific for insanity'.[14] Dhunjibhoy's locum, Pacheco, duly administered it 'both orally and by injections' to 26 male and 14 female patients suffering from acute excitement, diagnosed with either mania or catatonia.[15] Pacheco provided a small table in his report to illustrate the results of the trial, which he thought showed that 'as a hypnotic' the drug was 'very efficacious specially in allaying restlessness of excited patients'.[16]

Table 5.1. Results of *Rauvolfia serpentina* trial, 1935

	Male	Female
Cured	6	1
Improved	1	4
Unimproved	19	9
Total	26	14

When Dhunjibhoy returned from Europe in 1936, another batch of the drug had arrived. In contrast to Pacheco's findings and without providing any figures, he reported that, as in the case of sweet basil, 'the results were rather disappointing'.[17] In his view, 'apart from its mild hypnotic effects the drug did not produce any beneficial results and [the] same results could be achieved by any other hypnotic drugs.' The conflicting assessments by Pacheco and Dhunjibhoy require explanation. One issue relates to the substance sent for trial. Pacheco had referred to it under its Latin as well as Hindi name *chota chand*; Dhunjibhoy, on the other hand, used in addition one of its popular Western Indian terms: Hassan Imam's root.[18] Both mentioned that they had been sent an alcoholic extract, but it is of course difficult to evaluate if the alkaloid compounds they received were identical in chemical terms. If they were not, this may have been responsible for the different results reported by Pacheco and Dhunjibhoy.

In 1931, S. and R. H. Siddiqui of the Research Institute at the Unani and Ayurvedic Tibbia College in Delhi had managed to isolate an alkaloid from snakeroot that they named *ajmaline* (after the physician Hakim Azmal Khan, the founder of the Institute). However, another five alkaloids that they tested later on frogs 'did not exhibit any properties of interest', leaving them, presumably, hopping mad.[19] M. M. G. Sen and K. C. Bose of Calcutta, on the other hand, found that the drug known in northern India as *pagal-ki-dawa* (medicine for the mad) did indeed have an impact on mental illness. It was apparently also widely used, in Bihar in particular, to put babies to sleep. Sen was an Ayurvedic practitioner from Bengal also trained in Western medicine and played an important role within the Ayurvedic revival movement during the early twentieth century. His view was that, 'If Ayurveda is not scientific, it is not worth pleading for.'[20] Bose was a director of India's first pharmaceutical company established in 1901, the Bengal Chemicals and Pharmaceutical Works. Together they published an article in 1931 titled 'Rauwolfia Serpentine, a New Indian Drug for Insanity and Blood pressure', explaining that 'doses of 20 to 30 grains of [*Rauvolfia*] powder twice daily produce not only a hypnotic effect but also a reduction of blood pressure and violent symptoms'.[21] In contrast to these success stories, the research team based at the

Chemistry Department at the Calcutta School of Tropical Medicine (CSTM), led by R. N. Chopra, spent more than ten years on *Rauvolfia* and its alkaloids. They published their findings in 1933, confirming that *Rauvolfia*. had the propensity to reduce blood pressure.[22] However, although 'they also demonstrated that crude extracts of the root had powerful sedative properties', they were unable 'to isolate an alkaloid with sedative activity'.[23]

The varied results produced from the samples under trial at Ranchi may well have been due to the CSTM research team's failure to provide a verifiably active chemical compound.[24] On the other hand, Dhunjibhoy may have understated the effects of the material he had been sent. He compared them to other drugs that had just been developed, such as Evipan Sodium, a barbiturate derivative with hypnotic and sedative effects, which was fast-acting and used as an anaesthetic in surgery. Reporting its effects in his report of 1936 Dhunjibhoy noted: 'In some [cases of acute excitement where other drugs failed to quieten the patients and to induce sleep] it worked like a charm and the patients remained quiet from 24 to 48 hours after an injection'. He 'strongly' recommended this powerful drug. The indigenous drug, in contrast, showed only 'mild hypnotic effects'.[25] We do not know whether Dhunjibhoy came to regret his lukewarm assessment of *Rauvolfia* when a colleague gained much fame for his work on the drug only a couple of years later. In 1938–39, Rustom Jal Vakil, another Parsi trained in Western medicine, started research into the effects of *Rauvolfia*. Vakil subsequently published a path-breaking scientific paper and is, as Isharwal and Gupta put it, 'to be credited with introducing Rauwolfia to the Western world, thereby giving it the 1st effective antihypertensive drug and enabling the elucidation of other therapeutic uses of Rauwolfia, such as the treatment of schizophrenia.'[26] Vakil's work from 1949 onwards led to conclusive evidence of the sedative-hypnotic and antipsychotic properties of reserpine and other *Rauvolfia* alkaloids. During the 1950s reserpine was successfully applied in psychoses;[27] it is still in use in some cases of refractory schizophrenia and Huntington's disease.[28]

Might Dhunjibhoy have been the one to gain fame by substantiating *Rauvolfia*'s efficacy in mental illness, had he focused less eagerly on the latest Western developments? It is difficult to say, not least because even Pacheco's trial data were not quite as conclusive as he had suggested. It is tempting though to postulate that Dhunjibhoy, the Parsi from India, may have, in his ambition to emulate modern cutting-edge treatments, been blinkered regarding the potential of drugs commonly used by indigenous practitioners and folk healers. The irony of this is heightened by the fact that his Eurasian colleague, Pacheco, harboured misgivings if not a disparaging attitude towards indigenous practitioners. In his report he had bemoaned the public's tendency to present patients for treatment belatedly, 'after a disappointing trial of Ayurvedic or Kabiraj nostrums'.[29] However, unlike Dhunjibhoy, who appears to have shared Pacheco's reservations about Indian medicine, he had willingly acknowledged the efficacy of the Indian remedy once he had tested it himself. The divide between modern European medicine and indigenous modes of healing did not necessarily or exclusively follow the lines of nationality or ethnicity. As the cases of Dhunjibhoy and Pacheco demonstrate, perceptions of indigenous drugs and of modern medicine were complex – among Indians as well as Eurasians and Europeans.

'Modern' Drugs

Despite Dhunjibhoy's enthusiasm for the latest modern treatments, his evaluation of their effects was not always positive. He experimented on his patients as soon as successful trials were reported in the scientific literature. In 1933, for example, when Dhunjibhoy ran his first experiment with sweet basil, he also tried four sedatives and hypnotics. These were Nembutal, Soneryl, Somnifene and Hypnol. Nembutal and Soneryl were barbiturates, first synthesised in 1930 and 1921 respectively. Nembutal is now administered in doctor-assisted suicide and capital punishment, and is also known as a recreational drug. Of the other two, a modified version, Rohypnol, has come to recent public attention as a date rape drug, while Somnifene gained prominence during the 1920s and 1930s within the context of 'prolonged sleep therapy' as practised at the Burghölzli clinic in Zürich under J. Klaesi.[30] Dhunjibhoy found all of them 'useful', reporting 'encouraging results', but only 'in some cases of excitement and insomnia'.[31] Still, he believed them to be 'worth trying [in cases where] other ordinary drugs fail to allay excitement and bring about sleep in highly refractory cases'.[32] This had been, and continued to be a standard phrase in the annual reports. The 1920s and 1930s lacked specifics in the treatment of mental illness and doctors were keen on finding the quickest and most long-lasting ways of sedating excited patients.

There was a clear shift over the period towards use of the most recently synthesised drugs at Ranchi. In 1928, classic mainstays of the nineteenth-century pharmacopoeias were still listed alongside recently developed drugs. For example, hyoscine hydrobromide was 'extensively given' in cases of Parkinsonian tremors and 'worked wonders', leading to 'speedy improvement'.[33] Bromides, long used as sedatives and in epilepsy, were listed alongside Medinol, a paracetamol compound, and the sedative and muscle relaxant sodium luminol (which had been available since 1912 as Luminal). They were found to be 'very satisfactory'. Dhunjibhoy was less impressed by sulphonol, trionol, veronol and Dial, which he had also trialled in cases of insomnia.[34] Luminal, which has been described as the 'king of the barbiturates', re-emerged at Ranchi after Dhunjibhoy's overseas trip in 1930.[35] He had witnessed in Zürich Hospital Klaesi's 'prolonged sleep therapy'.[36] The results at Ranchi were 'very encouraging but unfortunately the benefit was temporary'.[37] The same was the case in 1932. The short-lived effects of some of the barbiturates trialled were clearly a concern.

Dhunjibhoy also reported mixed results with other drugs that were widely used at the time. In 1930, he applied paraldehyde by means of deep intramuscular injections, 'daily for a fortnight in highly excited cases'.[38] The results were not surprisingly 'very encouraging' but, again, the 'benefit was temporary'. Two years later he noted that it 'worked like a charm in some cases', but 'failed in others'.[39] By 1937, after many sets of experiments with a multitude of sedatives and hypnotics, he finally sang the praises of this drug. Not only was it cheap and relatively safe, with 'no depressing effect on [the] heart', but also 'the most useful sleep producing drug at our disposal'.[40] He employed it for '"prolonged continuous narcosis" in highly intractible [sic] maniacal cases'.[41] Dhunjibhoy was particularly taken by one of his 'highly excited patients, who showed no signs of improvement or abatement of excitement in spite of vigorous treatment by all the known hypnotics and sedatives at our command, showed marked improvement by this method'. He was very pleased, as 'after the first-day treatment the patient remained quiet for three consecutive days and slept at a rate of 14 to 16 hours a day'.[42] The only drawback reported by Dhunjibhoy was that patients 'require to be thoroughly watched' due to 'a risk of respiratory failure'.[43] He noted that in 1938 'we nearly lost one of our patients during this treatment'.[44] The dose administered was consequently cut down.

Correct dosage of drugs was a general problem with sedatives and narcotics, particularly so when 'heroic' amounts were given for extended periods as in the Zürich treatment.[45] No less dangerous were barbiturates like Evipan, which was used for clinical anaesthesia from 1932 onwards, but had also been celebrated as a 'new sleeping remedy'.[46] Its effects were rapid but also short-lived and here too an overdose could be fatal. Still, Evipan was seemingly a godsend for psychiatrists as it worked, as all barbiturates did, 'like a charm'.[47] In the case of Evipan 'the patients remained quiet from 24 to 48 hours after an injection'.[48] Although it has been suggested that deep-sleep treatments were going out of fashion once insulin and Cardiazol shock therapies came on the scene, the evidence from Ranchi suggests otherwise. Apart from sedatives and hypnotics, Dhunjibhoy experimented with a range of other drugs, some of which proved to be ineffective.

For epilepsy, for example, the tried and tested bromides continued to be administered at Ranchi and were found 'very satisfactory' during the early period.[49] The use of mercury iodide pills, as recommended by L. J. J. Muskens of the International League Against Epilepsy in his book *Epilepsy* (1928) was tried by Dhunjibhoy in the same year. He administered the pills in five 'inveterate cases of epilepsy where other treatment had failed' and, in 1929, in 17 'old cases', but could only report that 'unfortunately the results were not encouraging in our series'.[50] The application of 'detoxicated snake venene' from South Africa was tried on two epileptics in 1932, but its effects were 'thoroughly disappointing'.[51] In 1938, following reports of the successful treatment of 'many epileptics' with antirabic vaccine by Dr Nikitin of St Petersburg, Dhunjibhoy procured the vaccine from the Pasteur Institute at Patna and administered it to eight male and two female 'confirmed' epileptics.[52] The results were 'not encouraging'. This was confirmed in a similar trial in the United States that Dhunjibhoy duly cited.[53] During that same year another negative result was reported for a drug that had been used widely in the treatment of epilepsy – atropine. On this occasion, it was given in cases of mania, as suggested by Karl Leonhard, who gained fame for his nosological classification of psychoses.[54] Dhunjibhoy noted: 'Our patients did not get much benefit by this treatment.'[55]

Radium therapy, as trialled at Ranchi by Pacheco in 1935, was not to become a standard treatment either. Perhaps this was due to Pacheco having purchased the necessary 'Radium emanation apparatus' at his own expense, taking it away with him on Dhunjibhoy's return.[56] Given that the treatment involved 'injections of Radio Active Water', as recommended by 'continental workers',[57] discontinuation of the trials may not actually have been to patients' disadvantage. At the time, Pacheco reported that out of 'several cases' two diagnosed with acute mania showed 'considerable improvement' and that a case of 'ringworm' had 'markedly improved after a few injections'. What exactly these improvements consisted of remains subject to conjecture. In regard to epileptic cases the results were however 'disappointing'.[58]

While the treatment of the psychoses by means of barbiturates clearly flourished at Ranchi during the 1930s, fewer drug treatments were reported for melancholic states. In fact it is not until 1936 that the first drug aimed specifically at 'Melancholics and cases of Endogenous depressions' was mentioned. Hoematopophyrin was, as Dhunjibhoy put it, 'now largely used for melancholic conditions and is sold under the trade name Photodyne'.[59] The drug had been known in Europe for a few years but did not attract attention in North America until 1934.[60] It was observed that the substance increased the 'available energy of the individual'.[61] By 1936 a flurry of articles was published, some of which confirmed its efficacy, whilst others did not. Dhunjibhoy's observation, after having given the drug to 'six patients with marked endogenous depressions', as well as using it in his private practice, was 'not encouraging'.[62] Only one of his patients had improved. It is not clear if he continued to use the drug. Benzederine (an amphetamine) was also only briefly commented on in 1937, being referred to as 'very useful in cases of mild depression either of exogenous or endogenous origin'.[63]

It seems that, at least at Ranchi, shock therapies did not supersede the barbiturates (sedatives, hypnotics, anti-epileptics), but both of these treatments were more prominent than what came to be known as anti-depressants. The fact that institutions with a high percentage of violent or excited patients had an interest in pacifying rather than increasing the available energy of the individual would have been an important factor.

Wonder Cures

Glandular or organotherapy was an approach that was widely used in psychiatry and in other fields from the 1890s onwards. It was developed following C. Brown-Sequard's suggestion in 1889 that 'a juice extracted from the testicles of animals' had invigorating effects that led to the rejuvenation of men.[64] The substance was marketed as an extract and became known as 'the elixir of life'.[65] It was still popular during the 1920s, alongside material derived from the thyroid and pituitary glands of pigs, for example, as well as raw liver and brain, which were used almost as cure-alls. An M.D. from Pittsburgh listed the 'most common' indications of organotherapy in an article in the *Journal of the National Medical Association* in 1923: 'vomiting of pregnancy; insufficient breast milk (agalactia); sub-involution of the uterus; dysovarism; hyper-thyroidism and hypo-thyroidism; treatment of backward children; hypertrophy of the prostate; asthenia following infectious diseases; obesity; tuberculosis; high blood pressure, and many others.'[66] Organotherapy, he claimed, 'already unfolds before the astonished view of the seeing eye, a land of promise beside which the discoveries of Lister and Pasteur are destined to pale into honourable insignificance'.[67]

Even Kraepelin had applied 'preparations of every possible organ, of the thyroid, of the testes, of the ovaries and so on' in cases of dementia praecox – 'unfortunately', he noted, 'without any effect'.[68] At Ranchi, too, glandular therapy showed 'disappointing results', even when it was tried 'on a larger scale' in 1928.[69] Raw brain was given in four 'stuporous cases' in 1933 and 1934 but abandoned on account of 'no appreciable improvement' being noted.[70] The treatment was continued despite regular reports that 'with few exceptions' the results remained, as before, 'not encouraging'.[71] Those few exceptions may have kindled Dhunjibhoy's hopes. Organotherapy was applied at Ranchi until at least 1935. Material from the thyroid gland 'was found to be very useful as "Activating agent" in acute melancholia and stuporous cases'.[72] Liver appears to have done some good in the case of anaemic patients who were fed half a pound to one pound of it per day for a period of six months or more 'throughout the year' in 1931.[73] The raw liver was minced and mixed with cooked food such as curries and apparently it was 'relished and digested by the patients'.[74] Dhunjibhoy did not specify from what kinds of animal the organs were derived. Given that pig and cow were problematic for Muslims and Hindus respectively, attention to the sourcing of the fairly large quantities of liver and brain required would have been paramount. From 1932 onwards there was a shift to the prescription of what would now be called vitamin tablets and food supplements, for example, Colloidal Calcium with Ostelin D, Metatone, Incretone, Haliverol, Calcinol, and Calcium Gluconate.[75] These were listed under the heading of glandular therapy. The results were 'encouraging', particularly in the treatment of 'anaemic conditions' and 'specially in women'.[76]

From today's perspective, organotherapy may be considered a somewhat bizarre interlude in the treatment of mental disorders on the basis of current knowledge about hormones and vitamins. However, it is important to consider that it would have been difficult to differentiate the physiological and mental effects of particular substances. What is more, theories of the toxic and auto-toxic causation of mental illness were prominent during the late nineteenth and early twentieth centuries. As Noll has argued in regard to Kraepelin's use of organotherapy, it was 'rationally derived from' and fitted in with one of the main aetiological paradigms during this period.[77] Indeed, it still fits in today with the rationales of complementary therapies, for example, which employ organomedicine at homoeopathic potency.

A more obscure procedure used at Ranchi in 1928 was 'dermatographia'. Nowadays this term describes a largely idiopathic skin condition in which light scratching leads to raised, red lines. In the 1920s, dermatographia was understood as a diagnostic aid in the identification of dementia praecox, following a court trial in a murder case in Los Angeles in which the accused had set up a defence of insanity. Dhunjibhoy tried this on 50 'cases of dementia praecox with clear skins'.[78] He found that the scratch marks 'grew red and remained so for four to five hours in some cases, and more than 24 in other'. In the control group of patients suffering from other mental diseases 'the scratch marks faded away quickly'. Dhunjibhoy suggested that the 'experiment seems to prove that dermatographia is a reliable sign in the diagnosis of dementia praecox'.[79] He may not have been too sure about this, as there is no further reference to the use of dermatographia for diagnostic purposes at Ranchi. The assumption that mental illness was more than skin deep but could be made to reveal itself by prodding and scratching at the surface clearly held some appeal. Rorschach diagnostics, which were tried at Ranchi only in 1937 on 'two educated patients suffering from Schizophrenia' were considered by critics no less based on conjecture and on the hope that deep-seated complexes could be made to come to the surface by means of visual stimuli.[80]

Another treatment that was discussed controversially at the time and apparently discontinued after a one-year trial at Ranchi in 1936 involved the application of 'Lowenstein's skin tuberculin' or Dermotubin.[81] Dhunjibhoy had met the bacteriologist and pathologist E. Loewenstein in Vienna in 1935 prior to his emigration to the United States. Loewenstein had postulated that schizophrenia was 'due to the presence of tubercle bacilli in the blood and Cerebro Spinal Fluid' and suggested treating schizophrenics with skin tuberculin.[82] Researchers in England rejected Loewenstein's theory as mere conjecture and Dhunjibhoy, after acknowledging both sides of the argument, decided not to pursue this particular treatment – but not without thanking 'Herr Professor and Frau Dr Lowenstein for the kindness and help' he had received from them during his visit to Vienna.[83] Scientific networks and personal relationships across continents had an important role in the kinds of treatment tested and applied at Ranchi. However, it appears that at least in some cases, such as that of tuberculin therapy, personal feelings and friendship towards the method's originator did not affect Dhunjibhoy's assessment of the wider evidence available. Evidently scientific publications enabled psychiatrists to access a wide range of views.

The Shock Therapies

Sulfosin therapy

Immediately on return from his extended leave in August 1930, Dhunjibhoy trialled on 100 of his patients Sulfosin therapy as developed by Knud Schroeder in Denmark just one year before. In 1928, the psychiatrist Takase Kiyoshi of Japan had applied intramuscular injection of sulphur in 74 cases of general paralysis of the insane (GPI) and *tabes dorsalis*, showing that it was similar in effectiveness to Julius Wagner-Jauregg's malaria fever therapy that was at the time recommended for these conditions. Dhunjibhoy used Schroeder's formula (a 1% solution or suspension of sulphur in olive oil) and applied it to patients he had diagnosed with a range of mental disorders, such as manic depressive psychosis, dementia praecox and epilepsy.[84] The aim was to raise patients' body temperature (to an average of 102°F or 39°C degrees, and occasionally 105°F or 41°C), as improvements in and even recovery from mental illness were expected to ensue in a similar manner to what had been observed following application of malarial plasmodia in the treatment of tertiary syphilis. The results were 'quite encouraging' and Dhunjibhoy considered application of the method in 'all fresh admissions'.[85] He noted that the outcome was better 'in early cases of psychosis as well as in psychoneuroses', noting that 'even in chronic cases' the effects were 'not discouraging'. By 1933 he had trialled the new method in 215 cases of various disorders,[86] making it a 'routine treatment' in new admissions from 1932 onwards.[87] He also experimented with sulphur injections in the case of skin diseases (such as impetigo and eczema).[88]

Dhunjibhoy published articles on his trials in both *The Lancet* and the *Indian Medical Gazette* and received 'many letters from private practitioners in India making enquiries about this therapy with a view to try[ing it] on their cases'.[89] He was clearly the pioneer for this treatment in India and in 1933 was 'glad to note' that the neighbouring mental hospital 'also now adopted this treatment' under the superintendence of its European medical superintendent, Berkeley-Hill.[90] Recognition was forthcoming also from Europe as 'Dr. Knud Shroeder of Denmark, the originator of Sulphur treatment in mental disorders sent [Dhunjibhoy] a letter of congratulation on [his] success with this therapy on the publication of [his] first article on the subject in Lancet of 1931.'[91] Dhunjibhoy continued this particular treatment method, refining it over the years, so that by 1937, when more than 500 cases had been treated, Sulfosin was given in three strengths (one, two and three per cent solutions).[92] It had become the 'sheet anchor' at Ranchi 'for highly excited and non-co-operative types of patients'.[93] According to Dhunjibhoy, at the International Fever Therapy Conference in New York in 1937 'the trend of the discussion was in favour of this therapy specially as it was considered the cheapest and the safest form of fever therapy'.[94] Dhunjibhoy reiterated the advantages, pointing out that Sulfosin 'as a fever creating agent is equal to other active and passive (Physical) methods but holds the advantage of being safe, easy to measure and employ, and above all most inexpensive'. Staff was able to 'prepare fresh solution for our work in the hospital and it costs less than 1/12 of an anna per dose'.[95]

Insulin coma and Cardiazol shock therapy

Cost was, of course, an important factor in all public institutions – in India as much as in Britain and across the world. It was the high cost of particular treatments rather than lack of interest or knowledge that made it impossible for Dhunjibhoy to pioneer some of them. For this reason insulin coma therapy, which had been developed by Sakel in Vienna in 1934 for the treatment of schizophrenia, was not one Dhunjibhoy could have pursued at Ranchi.[96] The procedure required repeated application at a time when many countries were suffering during the economic depression and the prospect of war hovered over Europe and Asia. Resources for the treatment of mental patients in public hospitals in India were restricted. During Dhunjibhoy's extended overseas travels in 1935 insulin coma therapy was widely discussed as the panacea for the treatment of schizophrenia. He pointed out on his return to India that his journeys had not only advanced his knowledge and expertise but 'incidentally have also brought an International recognition to the Ranchi Indian Mental Hospital'.[97] However, insulin coma therapy was not to be one for which Ranchi would become known during Dhunjibhoy's time at the hospital.[98] He did report that 'Two methods of shock treatment, Insulin and Cardiazol have proved to be of therapeutic value', but it was the latter only that he was able to implement in Ranchi immediately on his return.[99]

Like insulin, Cardiazol was very expensive. However, on application to the manufacturers in Germany, the firm Messrs. A. G. Knoll of Ludwigshafen am Rhein agreed to provide Dhunjibhoy with a 'free supply of Cardiazol powder' for initial experiments.[100] Subsequently the firm 'specially reduced their prices to enable [him] to give this treatment to a large number of patients'. But, even with this reduction a 'full course of this treatment would cost Rs.15 per patient – a cost which appears to be almost prohibitive for a hospital of our size'. It was only when the manufacturers agreed to produce Cardiazol in 'ready-made injection form' and as a powder in India that this new shock treatment could be afforded at Ranchi.[101]

Dhunjibhoy had visited Budapest in 1935 and been invited by his 'friend and colleague Dr. Ladislaus v. Maduna, M.D., of the Royal Hungarian State Mental Hospital to see this novel treatment of Schizophrenia evolved by him'.[102] He had the opportunity to observe that Cardiazol produced 'typical epileptic-form attacks in the patient after injection like that of major epilepsy'.[103] He was 'so impressed with all that [he] saw' that he decided to try it at Ranchi. He 'selected 12 typical cases of Schizophrenia for experiment' and felt 'encouraged by the results' as three of the patients recovered sufficiently to be discharged, while another four were categorised as 'improved'. The treatment appeared to work not only in newly admitted cases but also in those of longer duration: the patients in the trial were mainly 'old chronic cases and have been in the hospital without any improvement for the last 4 years and more'.[104]

In 1937, Dhunjibhoy treated another 42 patients diagnosed with schizophrenia (31 men and 11 women), injecting the prescribed large doses of the drug (0.5 to 1 g).[105] A sequence of up to 20 to 30 of these shocks proved 'very beneficial in some Schizophrenic cases'. Although Dhunjibhoy observed that '[s]ome recover, others put on great improvement and on some it has no effect', he concluded that 'the experiments can be called encouraging', with 31 per cent of the 42 cases having apparently gone into 'full remission (complete recovery)', 36 per cent 'improved' and 33 per cent remaining 'stationary'. At this stage it was not clear to practitioners in which particular cases Cardiazol was most effective. Following the view of most of his peers, Dhunjibhoy's evaluation was that it was a treatment that 'appears to be safe in selected cases and is well worth a trial in all types of Schizophrenia and more so in Katatonic and Hebephrenic varieties'. His statistics seem to substantiate this judgement.[106]

Dhunjibhoy was in agreement with many of his peers in America when he pointed out that the treatment was 'free from any dangerous complication and does not require such constant medical and nursing supervision nor involve any grave risk as in the case of Insulin treatment of Schizophrenia'.[107] He concluded that he 'would certainly give this treatment preference over the Insulin Therapy'.[108] It seems likely though that Dhunjibhoy would have trialled insulin coma therapy, too, had it been made available to him at a reasonable cost. Keeping his options open, he was more careful in his differential assessment of the two treatments a year later: 'There can be no question that Cardiazol therapy offers a highly successful adjunct to the Schizophrenic patients far superior to any other treatment with the possible exception of Insulin therapy'.[109] Dhunjibhoy echoed contentions prevalent at the time:

> It is too early as yet to make any positive statement as to the permanence of the remissions or curative effect of the treatment. Many cases that show early improvement have relapsed after a time to their former state. However, Cardiazol has considerably changed the bleak outlook of Schizophrenia.[110]

This view was shared by many clinicians at the time. It would also be criticised by many, mostly with the benefit of hindsight, during the 'anti-psychiatry' decades of the 1960s and 1970s and, more recently, by historians of psychiatry. During the 1930s, however, clinicians tended to clutch at straws and were hopeful that at least some varieties of mental illness could be alleviated if not cured. As Dhunjibhoy pointed out: 'Many patients who might have been chronic institutional cases, can now at least be so improved as to return home and take part in their former activities.'[111]

By 1938 he had administered over 2,000 Cardiazol shocks 'without any fatal or serious injury' and 'achieved 40 per cent remission'.[112] Although the treatment had originally been intended for cases of schizophrenia, Dhunjibhoy decided to experiment with it also in cases of 'Manic Depressive Psychoses, Paranoid reactions, Psycho-neurotics, Ganja insanity, etc.'[113] There was always a chance that a practitioner might stumble across a new insight. As in the case of Sulfosin, Dhunjibhoy was the first to introduce this treatment in India and to carry out experiments with this drug on such a large scale. Again he duly published the results of his trials in the *Lancet* and the *Indian Medical Gazette* in 1937.

Malaria shock therapy

Malaria shock therapy was rarely used at Ranchi. Given Dhunjibhoy's otherwise innovative inclinations and preference for physical therapies, we could expect to see this treatment practised, particularly as malaria shock had been well known and applied all over the world for many years. It was first used on patients suffering from GPI by Julius Wagner-Jauregg in 1917 and was based on his earlier observation, during the 1880s, that a raised body temperature led to the relief of symptoms from psychoses.[114] On those few occasions when malaria therapy was administered at Ranchi, it was not in cases that would necessarily have involved GPI. In 1929, for example, Dhunjibhoy reported that malarial therapy was applied to a small number of patients and that 'appreciable beneficial effects have been noticed in a few cases of Mania'.[115] In 1928, six cases were treated with 'indifferent results'. In 1929, seven inmates were reported to have been treated with malaria therapy, and two 'showed marked improvement'.[116]

It was not until 1934 that Dhunjibhoy listed GPI, for the first time, as one of the principal forms of insanity and mentioned the testing of cerebro-spinal fluid (CSF) by the Wassermann procedure, in addition to blood samples. He then also specified for the first time the kind of treatment received by those who had tested positive in routine Wassermann tests. 'Neurosyphilis cases were treated with Tryparsamide', he reported.[117] He 'found this drug very helpful in General Paralysis of the Insane and other Neurosyphilitic cases in combination with Salversan or Malaria'.[118] Pacheco recommended a treatment that was quite different from that suggested by Dhunjibhoy, this being the 'injection of the patient's own serum which has been salvarsanized, into the spinal canal', also known as the Swift-Ellis method. He claimed that this was more effective than 'the usual methods adopted universally, i.e. injections of arsenical preparations and a course of malarial therapy'. In other words, Pacheco saw both Dhunjibhoy's diagnostics and his therapeutic approach as outmoded and 'shown by research workers in Europe recently to be somewhat disappointing and uncertain'.[119] In his first attempt to specify the treatment for neurosyphilis, Dhunjibhoy had referred to Tryparsamide, 'in combination with Salversan or Malaria'.[120] Pacheco faulted him on this, asserting that the Swift-Ellis method showed 'more favourable' results and that 'malaria need not be used and its attendant risks thus avoided'.[121] Pacheco did not mention that the Swift-Ellis procedure was by no means new, having been proposed as early as 1912. It had also proven efficacious only in some forms of neurosyphilis, not in GPI. The procedure also involved intrathecal injection (injection into the spinal canal), which many considered not without risk even in the 1930s.

Dhunjibhoy pointed out an important issue that confirmed the observation of many in India, that 'it is nearly always difficult to successfully re-infect those who have had previous attacks of Malaria and such is very common in India where Malaria is almost endemic in most parts'.[122] Even in 'the Western countries', Dhunjibhoy went on, it was 'a common experience with all those working with Malarial Therapy' that they found 'great difficulty in re-infecting patients with Benign Tertian who have already had a full course of it'. However, in contrast to his elaborate comments on many other treatments, Dhunjibhoy did not expand any further on this, nor did the Pacheco episode seem to have led him to engage in experimental trials. He would have been in a most advantageous position to have done so.

The hospital statistics from 1935 onwards remain uneven, occasionally identifying GPI but omitting it for the majority of the time. Admittedly, by the mid-1930s malaria therapy in GPI had lost its previous lustre, not least because Tryparsamide and Salversan became more widely used. The latter had been used at Ranchi, too, since the late 1920s. One further reason for the omission of malaria therapy as a sheet anchor of treatment may have been that in a place where malaria was endemic and a high percentage of patients were infected with it, re-infection with the plasmodium necessary for malaria fever therapy was difficult to achieve, as Dhunjibhoy had pointed out in 1936. He may well have been right in his decision to avoid malaria therapy, but his insistence on GPI being rare despite some indications to the contrary, and his problems in getting a clear and well-grounded line on its prevalence, is difficult to fathom.

By 1937 Dhunjibhoy's very brief period of attention to GPI and malaria therapy had come to an end. He still reported (only small) numbers of syphilitics in his statistics, despite a significant number of Wassermann positives. Wassermann investigations again became focused on the less accurate blood results as opposed to CSF samples (182 for the former, 35 for the latter). Only brief reference was made to treatment, without any specific details: 'Trypersamide combined with Salversan was found much more effective in the treatment of General Paralysis of Insanes than Malarial Therapy.'[123]

It may well have been the case that Dhunjibhoy was aware of epidemiological factors such as the endemic nature of malaria in the region and hence considered malaria shock therapy unsuitable treatment when other options were available. We could also speculate that lingering cultural stereotypes of different races' predispositions as well as perhaps certain unease about getting involved in discussions about sexual disease among Indians might have been Dhunjibhoy's blind spots. This would not detract from his other achievements, but it does alert us to the possibility that other factors than those related to scientific research are implicated in the choice of treatments to be pursued.

Justifying the Need to Shock and Sedate

Generally though, Dhunjibhoy was clearly in touch with local and international developments in therapeutics – not only in implementing novel treatments but also in dealing with ensuing controversies. In 1939 he highlighted some of the emerging, contemporary concerns about shock therapies such as insulin and Cardiazol treatments. He dealt with these from a pragmatic perspective, putting forward arguments that might be seen by some to have the ring of evasive apologetics.

> From the dim past mental patients have been subjected to various forms of treatment with the object of creating a shock to their central nervous system; some of these methods were no doubt barbarous in the extreme. In more recent times Shock Treatment has been greatly elaborated. Insulin, Cardiazol, Triazol, etc., have all had their turn and even these have had their risks and terrors. However, in the present state of our knowledge of mental diseases any treatment that gives encouraging results must be tried with a hope of cure or amelioration of the patients' mental conditions, and the shock therapy in spite of its being expensive and highly specialised no doubt gives encouraging results and is worth trying.[124]

Dhunjibhoy produced this statement in the same year that he implemented another treatment that was considered controversial: sub-shock nitrogen gas inhalation in schizophrenia. This was a spin-off from research into insulin coma and Cardiazol shock therapy. Patients were made to breathe mixtures of nitrogen and oxygen, with the latter being gradually decreased from 20 per cent to a minimum of 9 per cent, inducing 'gradual anoxia with sleepiness'.[125] Coma and seizures could be severe side-effects, but Dhunjibhoy did not report any. When 'given to highly excited patients for five minutes the patients not only quietened down in their excitement but were also able to sleep for hours'.[126] A number of patients remained 'quiet after this treatment for some days'. The procedure apparently had its advantages, as Dhunjibhoy was quick to point out: 'Our success with Nitrogen Gas Inhalation in excited cases was so great that for some time we temporarily closed down our Hydrotherapy Wards and all old and new highly excited patients with marked insomnia were submitted to this treatment.'[127]

This statement attests to Dhunjibhoy's ability to keep his hands on the pulse of scientific development. The originator of the procedure, Dr G. Edward Hall from the Department of Medical Research at the Banting Institute of the University of Toronto, where, incidentally, insulin had been discovered, wrote to Dhunjibhoy, telling him that 'This work of [his] should be continued.'[128] However, as in the cases of insulin and Cardiazol, physical therapies were not unanimously favoured. Clinicians with a psychoanalytic background, in particular, did not always appreciate them. At the time, a certain psychoanalytic fad prevailed in Calcutta, the cosmopolitan centre closest to Ranchi.[129] Like his colleagues in America who practised shock and other physical therapies, Dhunjibhoy too needed to pre-empt and respond to potential criticisms.[130] It is likely that we owe some of Dhunjibhoy's lengthy reflections to this need to justify certain practices. As far as nitrogen gas inhalation treatment was concerned, it seems that Dhunjibhoy's enthusiasm was met with a more sober approach the following year, under the leadership of Das. The procedure had been tried again on 47 excited inmates in 1940, but as 'only 11 patients showed slight temporary improvement', Das concluded that 'we have yet to be convinced about the distinctive efficacy of this treatment'.[131] The alternative option of hydrotherapy increased somewhat that year, from 108 patients in 1939 to 125 in 1940. The numbers of water therapy applications was however considerably lower than it had been before Dhunjibhoy had glimpsed 'a ray of hope' that patients 'not only quietened down in their excitement but were also able to sleep for hours' following nitrogen shock treatment.[132] Whether the people who were submitted to gradual oxygen deprivation for five minutes every alternate day, from between one week up to three months, shared this optimism can only be guessed.

Psychoanalysis

Unlike in the case of insulin coma therapy, the very restricted use of psychoanalysis-based diagnostics and therapy was not primarily constrained by cost. Dhunjibhoy had visited psychoanalysts of different stripes in Austria and Switzerland during his travels. He had been introduced to Freud in Berlin and attended lectures by Jung and Schmideberg. He was not averse to psychoanalytic methods and trialled them during his early years at Ranchi. During the period 1927–29, for example, he treated four patients 'with suggestions under hypnosis with satisfactory results.'[133] In 1934 one of 'two early cases of Psychoneurosis' was discharged during the year as 'recovered', while the other was expected to be 'fit for discharge in early part of 1935'.[134] He had also reported one very successful case in 1930, when a patient was admitted from Calcutta who had 'a case of complete paralysis of both legs with mental excitement' who 'was brought into the hospital on a stretcher'.[135] He reported,

> On examination the case was diagnosed as a case of 'conversion hysteria' and the patient, who was treated as a case of paralysis of the legs from three months outside, was made to walk within eight days of his admission and was discharged cured within two months, and he went to Goa – his native place – which is a distance of 1,500 miles from Ranchi on his own.[136]

Implying that the patient went home on foot, this was a spectacular cure, achieved with the help of Rev. A. C. Chatterji, the Church of England Chaplain who also provided a regular church service for Christian patients in the mental hospital. The Reverend had been 'kind enough to give religious suggestions to [the] above stated patient'.[137]

Ranchi provided for about 1,400 inmates. A couple of recoveries and one spectacular success over a period of six years show that psychoanalysis and religious suggestion were not routine. Rorschach diagnostics were trialled in 1934 in one hospital and on two of his private patients, and in 1937 on 'two educated patients suffering from Schizophrenia'.[138] Dhunjibhoy explained that 'no other suitable cases were available' and that the ink blot tests were 'very complex and require a lot of time and patience both of the Doctor and the patient and can only be usefully employed in those border line cases which are well educated and are willing to co-operate'.[139] Similar caveats were applied to psychoanalysis and hypnosis.

From its inauguration, Ranchi provided for people who were considered too dangerous to be kept at large. The local government official noted in the triennial report for 1927–29 that 'of the total number of male patients, nearly half have every year been criminals', and that in those circumstances the 'curative treatment must obviously be carried on under serious disadvantages'.[140] The shortage of accommodation was severe and those considered 'incurable but harmless' were discharged 'to the care of friends and relatives'.[141] Admissions were 'confined rigidly to dangerous patients'. Magistrates were instructed to 'avoid' sending harmless mentally deranged people to Ranchi. Clearly, Dhunjibhoy's patients were a select group less amenable to psychoanalytic methods. On occasion of the spectacular recovery of the case of 'conversion hysteria' related previously, Dhunjibhoy mused:

> We rarely see such early cases admitted into this hospital. We are only called upon to treat all chronic cases whose relations and friends have kept them in their homes for years under treatment of every one but a psychiatrist, and are only sent to us when they become unmanageable and dangerous at home. This is further aggravated by the present unavoidable congestion of the hospital with the result that cases are allowed to remain in jails or houses untreated until such time accommodation is available.[142]

Given this context, physical and drug treatments were the methods of choice. It is indeed remarkable that Dhunjibhoy managed to run the institution so successfully. As he pointed out:

> In spite of all these difficulties I am happy to be able to report that our percentage of cure to so-called 'new admission' as well as to average strength of the total population, can proudly be looked upon as extremely reasonable and good.[143]

Western and Indian Tubs: Hydrotherapy

Water treatment that helped to calm down excited patients had been an important feature in mental hospitals in many parts of the world. It had a long history in Europe and had been raised from heterodox to mainstream and even scientific status in Germany in particular.[144] In a hot country, immersion in tepid baths was particularly successful in reducing excitement in patients. It had been used in India throughout the nineteenth century, especially in the case of European and higher-class Eurasian patients who benefited from confinement in better-equipped institutions with a superior water supply.

From the inauguration of Ranchi hospital Dhunjibhoy had stressed the importance of appropriate hydrotherapy facilities. He introduced water therapy at Ranchi just one year after the hospital was opened, in 1926, when 12 bath tubs were in use, sometimes six of them at a time. Dhunjibhoy reported:

> Hydrotherapy is very useful in highly excited cases and in some cases it works wonders. A few cases of Manic Depressive Psychosis which did not respond to any other treatment, even to prolonged powerful sleeping dr[a]ughts, readily responded to hydrotherapy. [In 1926] 22 patients were given this special treatment. The minimum immersion was 3 hours and maximum 8 hours. While immersed, patients can read, smoke and take nourishment and on returning to bed after a few hours of immersion, fall into a natural sleep.[145]

As no dedicated premises were available for the procedure and patients had to be 'given baths in the cells of the infirmary wards which are not at all suited for this kind of treatment', he suggested the erection of a special ward.[146] The number of patients undergoing water therapy increased steadily, despite the use of newly developed sedatives and hypnotics. By 1931, 102 patients were treated. Dhunjibhoy reported:

> It is a very active therapy department and is worked to its fullest capacity at all times [...] 10 continuous baths have been in operation daily and were chiefly instrumental in allaying excitement and insomnia in highly excited and boisterous cases. There was a great rush on the baths during the year as we had 132 admissions and most of them were chronic refractory cases.[147]

It seems that the procedure was highly successful. Dhunjibhoy even felt it 'necessary that some reference should be made here to the results which were obtained' and noted that 'in [a] good many cases', many of which involved psychotic patients, the results were 'astonishing'.[148] This strongly positive assessment contrasts with the more tepid appraisals of the effects of Nembutal, Soneryl, Somnifene and Hypnol. All were tried that same year, but found only to produce 'encouraging results' and therefore were considered to be merely 'worth trying'.[149] The number of hydrotherapy treatments had increased to 308 by 1933, dipping down to 222 in 1935, and 120 in 1937. The sorely missed improved facilities were not granted for many years by the cash-strapped provincial authorities on account of the poor economic situation in the wake of the First World War. Dhunjibhoy saw the need to adapt the system to Indian requirements:

> The bath tubs with continuous automatic flow of water as used in the West are very expensive and probably unsuitable for our work in India, so I had to invent a cheap bath tub for this treatment more or less on the same style as those used in the West with modifications suiting the Eastern environment.[150]

Clean water was a problem in a place like Ranchi and Dhunjibhoy's practical solution seemed to make much sense. Prolonged bathing required considerable quantities of water. In 1938 the 'average hours of immersion per patient were 253.92 hours' (nearly 11 days), and 160 men and 29 women had been given this treatment.[151] News of Dhunjibhoy's cost- and water-saving invention spread and he reported: 'As our bath tubs have proved very satisfactory, easy to manipulate and cost little, they were copied by some hospitals, jails and private practitioners in India who were supplied free of charge with the plans of our tubs on request.'[152] One institution even placed an order with Dhunjibhoy for the tubs, so that he had to 'make it clear that we do not sell these tubs, but I have no objection to supply the plan of the tub free of charge to any one who applies for it as the tub can be easily made anywhere'.[153]

In 1940, when the average period of immersion had decreased to four days, Das too sang the praises of this treatment while noting the continued absence of dedicated facilities.

> As in the past years, this therapy was more extensively given throughout the year [...]. The average hours of immersion per patient were 95 hours. This was found to be the

best and the safest method of treatment of the excited condition of the patients and also for insomnia. Unfortunately, on account of financial stringency, we are still without a properly equipped Hydrotherapy Ward for this most important branch of therapy in a Mental Hospital.[154]

Considerable emphasis has been placed in recent historical writing on the importance of drugs and shock therapies in mental hospitals during the 1920s and 1930s. In order to get a more balanced view of how these figured within the wider spectrum of therapeutic interventions, more mundane methods need to also be considered alongside the range of drugs-based interventions. One of the less conventional therapies that featured at Ranchi was a modified kind of song and dance therapy.

Dutt's *Bratachari*

During his visit to Britain in 1935 Dhunjibhoy had attended a 'striking demonstration of physical exercises combined with musical rhythm in one of the London County Council Mental Hospitals'.[155] He felt that these might be beneficial also to patients in India. In Britain, he observed, the 'physical exercises in Margaret Morris Movement classes are set to Schubert marches and Waltzes which are played either on Piano or on Gramophone records'. However, in mental hospitals he considered it 'more important to get a response from patients than to educate their musical taste'. Therefore, 'any music is beneficial which appeals to them'. When he attended a 'demonstration of the Bratachari Movement in Calcutta under its versatile founder and leader', G. S. Dutt, Dhunjibhoy was 'much impressed' and found that it had 'many points in common' with the Morris approach yet was 'more suitable for [his] patients than the Margaret Morris Movement'.[156] He introduced it at Ranchi. A staff member was specially selected for training and attended the eighth All-Bengal Bratachari Training Camp held in Calcutta for six weeks in 1938.[157]

Dance therapy is nowadays a normal part of occupational therapy practices in institutions, yet at the time it was still a novelty, especially in a public mental hospital.[158] Its underlying rationale was however similar to current considerations. As Dhunjibhoy put it:

> In mental patients the participation in such exercises provides a strong mental stimulus sustaining the patients' interest when treatment has to be continued over a long period and makes co-operation between patients habitual. The knowledge that they are a part of a group and not separate units tends to take their minds off their troubles and helps the self-conscious to forget themselves.[159]

Perhaps not altogether incidentally, the wider agenda of the Bratachari movement fitted in with Dhunjibhoy's internationalist outlook. Dutt aimed at breaking down social barriers of caste, religion, sex and age among its practitioners, accentuating feelings of Indian national pride and consciousness within the context of world citizenship. Dutt was an Indian Civil Service officer and had been renowned in Bengal not only for his revival of folk dance and culture, but also for his brave criticism of British actions, such as the firing at a crowd of protesters by police, or his refusal to deal with protesters who had followed M. K. Gandhi's call for a *satyagraha* against the Salt Act. Dutt was an Indian nationalist with an internationalist outlook, who fought against communalism and social hierarchies that separate individuals from each other.

Dhunjibhoy's involvement with Dutt does not necessarily imply that he, too, was interested and engaged in wider politics. He was primarily preoccupied with his professional work and, like everybody else, Dhunjibhoy knew that staff employed by the British who got involved in nationalist politics faced dismissal and were imprisoned. In 1939 he reported: 'Remedial classes were regularly held every evening and some patients were trained in the Bratachari dance along with some of the attendants.' Apparently, patients took 'a great liking' to it. Dutt attended a demonstration 'given by [the] patients' in 1939 and congratulated them 'for the good start', advising them 'to keep it up'.[160]

Feasts and Religious Therapy

According to Dhunjibhoy's daughter, her father was conscious of the importance of religion to patients from the varied communities within Ranchi's catchment areas. He made sure that religious festivals were celebrated and facilities for prayer were made available. At the previous institutions, too, attention had been paid throughout the nineteenth century to patients' religious feelings and sentiments. This became even more pronounced during the 1920s and 1930s when the politics of communal strife in India were ideologised in religious terms. Not surprisingly therefore, from the hospital's inauguration the standard comments in the reports, under the heading 'feasts', read as follows:

> Feasts were given to all patients during the Pujah and Holi festivals. Special feasts were given to Hindu, Muhammadan and Christian patients during their respective festivals. Patients' religious feelings and sentiments are respected as far as possible and many are encouraged to observe fasts on religious grounds if they so desire and a special diet is arranged for them.[161]

Some communities must clearly have felt a need for more extended and regular religious engagement, as new arrangements were reported in 1931 under the rubric 'attention to patients' religion':

> *Hindus* More than 800 patients attended the Durga Puja which was celebrated with much pomp by the staff and public of Kanke outside the hospital.[162] The Hindus often attend the *Kirtans* [devotional chants with music] whenever a Pandit calls at Kanke.[163]
> *Muhammadans* on request of Muhammadan patients a small spare room was converted into a mosque for their prayers and a maulavi [Sunni religious scholar] who happens to be on our staff conducts the usual Jumma [Friday prayer] and other prayers regularly.[164]

For Christians too arrangements were made 'on request from the Roman Catholic patients' with the Rector of the Roman Catholic Mission, Ranchi, for holding 'regular divine service for the patients belonging to the Church of Rome which hitherto did not exist'. For those belonging to the Church of England, the Reverend A. C. Chatterji had held services throughout the year. 'During X'mas', Dhunjibhoy noted, 'elaborate arrangements were also made for special church service and the festivities of the season were enjoyed by a large number of patients including non-Christians'.[165]

Attention to patients' religion increasingly became better organised and varied. By 1934, 'the learned Pandit and a highly qualified Maulvi were engaged on [a] small honorarium to give religious discourses to patients; religious songs and community singing are encouraged on these occasions'.[166] From the following year, the 'main religious communities had weekly services or instructions imparted to them' and it appears that the 'patients of each denomination were always keen on and regular in attendance'.[167] Religious expression had become an important aspect of hospital life. It was styled 'religious therapy' from 1937 onwards and justified in reference to its arguably closest possible scientific idiom, psychoanalysis: 'in some patients this therapy was found to be of particular benefit in adjusting their mental conflicts.'[168] The definition of what constituted therapy was clearly fluid and context specific. This was the case also in regard to patients' employment in the kitchens and gardens of the hospital.

Work and Occupational Therapy – 'useful both to the patients as well as to the State'[169]

In contrast to the gradual reframing of religious engagement as therapy, work was considered therapeutic from the very beginning. Dhunjibhoy noted in 1926: 'Work is a pleasant pastime and is undoubtedly curative.'[170] He went on to explain that the 'spotless cleanliness found in this large hospital, the pride of the staff and wonder of the visitors, is largely the result of the help of willing patients'.[171] He was also aware of the monetary benefits of patients' labour, stating: 'So far we have been dealing with work of definite economic value for, besides benefiting the patients, it helps finance.' Patients' labour was basically free, apart from 'small monthly rewards which are collected and with which [patients] are allowed to buy any useful articles they desire from the shops at Ranchi'.[172]

Issues of exploitation and power can arise whenever vulnerable people are not fully recompensed for the value of their labour. That not all inmates willingly joined into this particular kind of therapy is in fact clear from another one of Dhunjibhoy's statements:

> When persuasion has been applied to every fit patient to induce him to engage in useful service (compulsion is barred), there is a remnant who refuse to bestir themselves, some are lazy, others obstinate and others perverse.[173]

It is difficult to assess where the line between persuasion and compulsion was drawn. The only cases explicitly exempt from work were the 'sick, old and infirm and refractory patients'.[174] This made it possible for about 50 per cent of the hospital's population to be employed in activities such as 'gardening (vegetable and flowers), house-hold work, carpentry, smithy, basket making, nursing, joss stick making, weaving, tailoring, cleaning of rice and dal, cutting of vegetables, clerical'.[175]

From 1927 onwards, even more 'vigorous efforts' were made to 'carry out occupational therapy in its various branches'.[176] Dhunjibhoy was 'happy to record much improvement and success achieved in this direction'. This was the year when the 'garden scheme' was taken up 'in right earnest', with a view to making the hospital self-supporting 'as far as the supply of vegetable[s] is concerned'.[177] 'Great success' was achieved, Dhunjibhoy gratefully acknowledged, due to efforts of the garden manager, Babu Jaggannath De, as well as, presumably, the on average 136 patients employed every day in the vegetable garden. Self-sufficiency was attained, as the 'full requirement of the hospital of vegetables was supplied' by the garden, which amounted to 8 to 10 *maunds* (299 to 373 kg) a day throughout the year. The total value of 'vegetables and other spices' supplied to the hospital was Rs.17,342-8-0,[178] a sum more than four times the cost of medicines that year.[179] Towards the end of the year 'surplus vegetables' were sold to the staff and public at the market rates. Horticultural activities were extended and included the planting of 'various fruit trees such as bananas, guavas, peaches, papayas, mangoes etc.'[180]

Patients' employment at Ranchi was also seen as a success by international bodies. In 1928, when the number of working patients had 'gradually increased', Dr Yves M. Biraud, a representative of the Health Section of the League of Nations, had visited the institution and commented in very positive terms.

> We were most interested to see the work which you are carry[ing] out at this hospital and especially that of your occupational treatment. We were also struck by the efforts which you are making to utilize the labour of your patients towards the supplying of the needs of the Institution. Public Health Officers regard such work as distinctly beneficial to the community as it enables public funds to be utilized for purposes of prevention as well as for curative measures.[181]

While Dhunjibhoy was clearly proud of this assessment, he had also been made aware of the lack of specialist staff at Ranchi. During the 1920s, occupational therapy became professionalised. Dhunjibhoy noted: 'This institution is not fortunate enough to possess the services of occupational therapists for both the [male and female] sections of the hospital.' However, he added, 'the patients quietly carry on very useful work'.[182] A few years later, when labour therapy had been extended further, he was more assertive and defensive: 'It is a mistake to suppose that occupational therapy is impossible without the employment of a few costly and highly trained occupational therapists.'[183] Dhunjibhoy was at pains to turn a deficiency into a virtue. He had also become attuned to relevant professional and managerial jargon. His report of 1928, in particular, raises more questions than it apparently answers:

> Patients are principally occupied in remunerative work which is mainly directed towards remoulding the more primitive manipulative capacities and which makes very little demand on the more complex mental processes at the same time. The patients are

chiefly engaged in gardening, weaving, cane and bamboo work, smithy, carpentery [sic], tailoring and miscellaneous domestic works, while some are engaged also in mending clothes, cobbling, lace-making, knitting, office work, etc. So that the patients' labour is fully utilised towards supplying the needs of the hospital, which apart from its therapeutic effect on patients themselves, serves to keep down the rates of the institution.[184]

The total income from the garden alone that year amounted to Rs.28,624.[185] The annual average cost per patient was calculated at about Rs.418 (calculated on a total of 1,367 treated during the year).[186] In 1929 about one tenth of the patient population was employed in gardening. Dhunjibhoy considered it the 'sheet-anchor of our treatment in this hospital'.[187] The scope of work was soon extended further, with new therapeutic rationales being provided by reference to contemporary doctrine on work therapy:

> While employing out-of doors is recognised as being of the greatest value, there are many patients who cannot or will not take part in work of the hospital garden or even in domestic occupations and for them provision has been made by the establishment of occupational classes where instructions in various arts and crafts are given by experienced instructors.[188]

The logistics of employing patient labour were complex in Indian mental hospitals as superintendents had to overcome not only patients' personal idiosyncrasies but also sentiments of caste and social standing. The observation that, however deranged patients may have been, they were still frequently sensitive to caste prescriptions, had been made throughout the nineteenth century. To circumvent any such problems in his push to engage evermore patients in useful work, Dhunjibhoy adapted the range of activities:

> The variety of occupations provided is such that there are few patients for whom some congenial form of occupation cannot be found, and the good results both in the contentedness of mind and the consequent improved bodily conditions of the patients as well as the high quality of the articles produced give a return entirely out of proportion to the small initial and recurring cost.[189]

Efforts were also made to engage the 'refractory' and 'turbulent' who had previously been considered exempt from work. The professed aim was to 'make them happier and more tractable'.[190] According to Dhunjibhoy, the 'experiment' had shown that 'practically every ambulant patient can be employed and is infinitely better and more easily controlled when he is employed'. Apparently those in charge of such 'turbulent patients' had noticed that they develop 'a good appetite, eat well and look much fitter and better than before and have put on weight'. One factor may have been that they escaped the various drugs that were dispensed. They even slept better at night, 'which they never did before without hypnotics'.[191] Dhunjibhoy reconfirmed this in 1936, when he noted that the 'number of hypnotic draughts given at night is considerably reduced'.[192] However critical our perspective on work therapy may be, the fact that patients so employed were spared continued sedation and shock treatments may allow us, to an extent, to see it in a less negative light. As with hydrotherapy, it constituted a way for patients to experience daily life without the haze induced by medication. What is more, they may have enjoyed the 'extra gifts' such as 'cigarettes, tobacco and other comforts of life' and their share in the sum of Rs.600 which was annually divided among 'hardworking patients'.[193] Dhunjibhoy noted that 'patients look forward to this reward and spend as they like and some of them even send this money to their family at home'. In those cases, engagement in work may have empowered patients.[194]

Looking back on the experiment of making refractory patients contribute to their own upkeep, Dhunjibhoy mused the following year that his only regret was that he had not tried it earlier. He gave the example of ward no. 11, in which patients considered to be highly excited were kept:

> The whole atmosphere [...] is now completely changed. This was a noisy, dirty and destructive ward before and since the introduction of active outdoor garden work every patient on an average has put on 2 to 3 lbs. in weight, they sleep better, there is no noise in the night or day and no sleeping draughts are now required.[195]

There was also external acknowledgment of the standard of work achieved by patients, as when the occupation therapy department was awarded four first prizes in 1934 in a local exhibition for their lace, baskets, *durries*, and *galichas* and *asnies*.[196] The following year, they secured nine first prizes and one second prize. At a local flower show in 1936, the hospital won 'a beautiful Silver Cup for the best roses grown in Ranchi and 3 First Class certificates for the Annuals and other flowers'.[197] Pacheco provided a review of the varied activities in which patients were employed by 1935. Apart from gardening, arts and craft, carpentry, smithy and the like, they were occupied in the kitchens, and each ward had 'a batch who help[ed with] general ward work'.[198]

Pacheco was a believer in professional OT expertise. He argued that the 'need for a trained occupational instructress' was 'keenly felt' in the female section. In his opinion, without 'a qualified and enthusiastic worker' it was very difficult to 'train patients or stimulate their interests from lethargy and indolence to useful and helpful occupation with a view to rehabilitation'.[199] His views differed somewhat from Dhunjibhoy's in regard to what kind of patient could be employed in agriculture. According to him only 'mild states of excitement' could be allayed by outdoor work. His work enforcement methods may have been harsher and even culturally insensitive. He reported: 'Even though a large number of the patients are agriculturalists to whom this work is suited, those who are not, are also sent.'[200] Like any other treatment, work therapy was subject to varied styles of implementation and, potentially, abuse.

In 1935, the cultivated area was increased by another 20 acres and dedicated to *paddy*, of which 89 *maunds* (a little over three tons) were produced. Fish that had been stocked in the large tanks or water reservoirs supplied the hospital with three *maunds* and 36 *seers* (146 kg) of high-quality protein, while the poultry farm provided 2,942 eggs.[201] The hospital had clearly diversified into an adjunct agricultural enterprise and prevention of idleness became a new catch phrase used by Dhunjibhoy on his return from Europe in 1936.

He had visited the 'famous occupational therapy centres in Europe and England', such as the Devon Mental Hospital at Exminster, which had 'a great name', as well as 'the famous Santpoort Hospital in Holland and in Germany the famous hospital at Gutersloh [Gütersloh]'.[202] His contention was: 'Occupation is recognised as an important therapeutic agent and has been defined as the organisation of suitable employment for the purpose of combating idleness.' This shift of emphasis fitted in with the increased level of activity at Ranchi and also had some affinity with contemporary schemes in Germany, particularly those that promulgated forced labour. Dhunjibhoy did try to emphasise positive aspects such as the breaking up of the 'routine institutional life of the Hospital', its relief of 'monotony' and the 'busy activity with resulting cheerfulness and hope of recovery'. To what extent involvement in work became itself part of the dreaded 'routine institutional life of the Hospital' is difficult to judge, not least in view of some ambiguous statements by Dhunjibhoy to the effect that occupation may for some patients mean 'tearing coir for mattresses as a contrast to tearing up their own clothing'.[203] By 1937, 80 per cent of patients were employed in what Dhunjibhoy called an 'intensive system'.[204] He may have faced some criticism as he kept stressing that patients were allowed to choose their own occupations, reasserting that he was 'confident that "picking threads" out of rags is much better for [the introspective type of patient] than sitting about and "day-dreaming"'.[205]

All activities that the mentally ill engaged in harboured a certain risk of accident and injury. Given the intensity of the work regime pursued at Ranchi, it is surprising that the reported incidence of these was relatively low and that no fatalities occurred. Dhunjibhoy did report some other setbacks that seemed to have affected him as well as his staff and the workers greatly. In 1939, a sudden outbreak of cholera among the poultry led to the loss of 'the beautiful leghorns which were the pride of the patients and staff and this incident broke our heart'.[206] To make things worse, 'another depressing incident' occurred that year when the plantation of 5,000 papayas was affected by 'curlyleaf' disease. There was no remedy, and Dhunjibhoy concluded sadly: 'The patients miss their papayas very much as they enjoyed eating this most delicious fruit from our garden for the last 14 years.' Alas, the plan was now to grow pineapples instead, as apparently 'Ranchi soil is suitable for growing beautiful pineapples'.[207]

The reports on work therapy at Ranchi provide evidence of what seemed to be authentic therapeutic concern for patients' empowerment and physical and mental wellbeing, along with traces of exploitation of patients' labour. Given the wider context within which OT was discussed during the 1920s and 1930s it may not surprise us to find both aspects represented at Ranchi to varying degrees. However, any treatment needs to be assessed in relation to patients' happiness and an institution's success as formally measured in its mortality and morbidity rates. Judging from the latter, on balance, patients may have fared well at Ranchi, in comparison to other institutions in India and Britain – even if some were set to pick coir and threads and all had to forgo their papayas for pineapples for a while.

Diet – 'one of the most important methods of mental treatment'[208]

The impetus for setting up a 'garden scheme', facilitated by patient labour, sprung from the felt need to 'make the hospital self-supporting'.[209] This was seen as necessary, not least because Dhunjibhoy had noticed on his arrival in 1925 that 'articles of diet are very expensive' in the provincial town of Ranchi and, 'more so', at the village of Kanke, where the institution had been built.[210] At the old institutions the cost of diet per head was 6 annas, whilst at Ranchi it was 9 annas. 'Conferences' to deal with this were therefore convened in 1925 and 1926.[211] Following their recommendations, the place was self-sufficient within a year in regard to vegetables, one of the staple foods, alongside rice, *atta* (chapatti flour), *dal* (lentils), mutton, fish, milk and potatoes. Patients' diet was an important aspect of hospital management. It was also a crucial factor in hospital mortality rates as tragic evidence from early nineteenth-century Indian lunatic asylums has shown.[212] Increased death rates were directly related to poor dietary regimes.

By the early twentieth century, adequate food provision was seen to require a scientific approach. Ranchi's diet scales had to be discussed with the chemical examiner to the Government of Bengal, Rai Bahadur Dr Chuni Lal Bose, who analysed them for the 'requisite quantities of protein, fat and carbohydrate' in 1927 and again in 1928.[213] His earlier 'scientific survey of the diet' had shown that it was 'a little deficient in its fat constituents'.[214] It was duly adjusted by immediately adding 'half a chatak [30 grams] of good ghee per head per diem' – a quantity that is currently considered the maximum recommended for an average, sedentary adult. Further improvements were made the following year, with the result that during the three years from 1927 to 1929, patients' average weight had increased significantly by 1.32 lbs. in men and a startling 6.39 lbs. in women. If this figure was indeed correct, the gender differential would again highlight existing disparities in the provisions available to mentally ill men and women prior to admission to Ranchi.[215]

As in other institutions, the reports from Ranchi hospital referred to the importance of diet and the attention given to it. Dhunjibhoy's statement of 1926 put the main considerations into a nutshell. He argued:

> Diet is considered one of the most important method[s] of mental treatment; the better the diet the greater is the hope of recovery. The diet of this hospital is worked out with the greatest care as it effects the well-being and happiness of so many people and is chiefly based on vitamine and caloric value [*sic*]. The majority of patients are fed a great deal better than in their own homes. This can be well ascertained from the weight charts of the patients which show a general increase in weight of the inmates of this hospital during the year under review.[216]

This formulation had become more or less the standard in all institutions and may not necessarily reflect the actual quality of provision at Ranchi. There was also ample scope for food scams, with store managers and accountants conniving in the diversion of patients' victuals for personal profit. However, given that patients were weighed monthly and those who 'lose weight [were] segregated in the Infirmary with a view to ascertaining the cause and [were] fed on special diet until they regain[ed] their original weight', the situation at Ranchi may have been as good as the rhetoric suggested.[217]

Other aspects of patient care were also superior to those in the old institutions and in other provinces. Appropriate attention was paid to inmates' clothing and bedding.

Each patient had his or her own iron bed with coir mattress, a bed sheet, three blankets and one pillow.[218] A mosquito net was also allocated, but seems to have been 'given when necessary' only. Women had saris, blouses (cotton and woollen), frocks and chemises while men had *dhotis*, *kurtas* (cotton and woollen), *jangias*, and shoes. It may not have been worth mentioning these items were it not for the fact that, as Dhunjibhoy pointed out, 'the majority of the patients of the old hospitals used to roam about without clothes'.[219] Ranchi therefore broke with custom when staff enforced the rule that every patient was to wear clothes. According to the superintendent there was 'little trouble' required to enforce this. The situation was more difficult in regard to beds, as patients had not been supplied with any in their former institutions and therefore 'refused to lie on beds at first'. However, 'later they appreciated them so much', Dhunjibhoy noted, that 'the staff had to pull the patients out of beds in the morning as they refused to get up'.[220]

One aspect of patient care that has been discussed contentiously in the historical literature is artificial or forced feeding of patients. This was done as a matter of routine at Ranchi in cases when patients refused food. Some patients were 'spoon-fed by nurses and attendants' and others who 'exhibited active refusal to food' were provided with nutrition 'by tube either per nose, mouth or rectum'.[221] Dhunjibhoy was clearly aware of how controversial this procedure was. He frequently commented on its beneficial effect, as if trying to pre-empt potential objections. He argued: 'The general belief is that nasal feeding is detrimental to general health but the experience proves the contrary; in fact, I have seen patients thriving better on nasal feeding than on forced or coaxed spoon feeding.'[222] One patient had been on nasal feed for the last six years, and, he noted, 'looks a picture of health'. That year, in 1938, the number of nasal feeds reached a high of 2,771. The following two years the figures declined to 1,718 and 1,943 nasal feeds respectively.

Sports and Entertainment – 'helps enormously towards socialisation and rehabilitation of patients'[223]

Patients' entertainment and social events were the least controversial aspects of hospital life, pleasing the hospital committee, visitors and inmates alike. They figured prominently and there was a wide range of them, including music, games, sports, dances and reading. Generally, much 'greater freedom' was given to the patients 'than was allowed in the old hospitals' and 'no difference' was made between 'criminals' and 'non-criminals' as 'All [were] treated as patients'.[224] Patients were also 'sent for motor drives in the hospital Char-a-banc four times a week from the male section and twice a week from the female section' and even allowed to shop at Ranchi.[225] In 1929, about 200 patients were driven to Ranchi to go to a circus and 'during the fine weather' some of the patients 'were taken out to the nearest hills, riversides, gardens, etc.' for picnics.[226] Parole was introduced as early as 1926 and 'dependable and non-dependable' patients were 'allowed to go out for their morning and evening walks' – the latter escorted by staff.[227] This was important for a mental hospital 'run on modern methods', Dhunjibhoy pointed out. 'None of the patients granted parole abused the privileges' and 'the effect on the health of patients [was] striking'.[228]

The tidy sum of Rs.2,000 was earmarked in the hospital budget for periodicals and books in some of the relevant languages (Bengali, Urdu, Orya, Hindi and English). These enabled literate patients – who constituted 'no insignificant part of the population' – to engage in reading.[229] No library facilities to speak of had been available at their previous institutions. Donations were solicited from publishers, so that newspapers and magazines, too, could be perused by staff and patients. Among them were, in 1925, for example, *The Statesman* (2 copies), *Amrita Bazar Patrika*, *Bengali*, *Forward*, *Searchlight*, *Bangabasi*, *Hindi Bangbasi*, *Hitabadi*, *Basumati*, *Bharatbarsha*, *Manasi O Marmabani*, *Prabasi*, *Bangabni*, and *Kallol*.[230] Some of these were of nationalist orientation, others had gained a reputation for their critical and high-quality literary outlook. Given the tense political atmosphere, it is perhaps surprising that colonial authorities allowed these publications to continue on throughout the 1930s.

Football, tennis, badminton and croquet could be 'enjoyed by those patients who [were] able to play these games and those who [were] not sufficiently expert to play enjoy[ed] watching all these games'.[231] In 1927, 30 garden benches were bought to make it possible for patients 'to sit in the open while witnessing games, etc.'[232] By 1929 matches were played regularly with other clubs, such as the Ranchi Public Health Department Football Association, the Accountant-General, Bihar and Orissa Office Football Association, the United Football Club of Kanke, the Young Star of India, Kanke, and the Christian Boys' Football Club Ranchi.[233] Furthermore, Dhunjibhoy could proudly report: 'It is gratifying to note that in all the matches the Hospital team won.' The same year, the patients' hockey team entered into the Chota Nagpur Hockey Cup Competition Tournament and played two matches.[234]

There were also developments in regard to women's sports. Dhunjibhoy noted that 'the female patients, who had never played such games as tennis and badminton have taken to them very seriously and shortly we shall be able to promote matches between the two sections' (men's and women's).[235] The latter remark is particularly surprising within the Indian context, where seclusion of women was widespread. Dhunjibhoy was clearly ahead of his time as far as the participation of women in mixed sex events was concerned. How colleagues, staff, patients and their families responded to these innovations is difficult to ascertain. The emphasis on sport was further increased by the introduction of athletics by Dhunjibhoy's first assistant superintendent, P. C. Das. By the early 1930s only cricket was missing as a regular activity. This was duly rectified when Pacheco filled in as a locum in 1935 and set up 'a fairly efficient team'.[236] The introduction of specific activities appears to have been driven by senior staff's own sporting interests.

Indoors, games were provided, including cards, chess, *satranj*, *carrom*, ludo and ping pong. It is not clear though if patients were engaged in many of these, as Dhunjibhoy mentioned that 'staff forms the back-bone of the indoor and outdoor games'.[237] There was also the in-house 'Kanke Dramatic Society', made up of 'staff and a few sane patients', who provided 'excellent amusement for the patients'. Patients appear to have been actively involved to a certain extent, as Pacheco reported in 1935 that the 'patients themselves staged eight dramatic performances with a high standard of histrionic ability'.[238] Local clubs, too, contributed to patients' entertainment, such as the Ranchi Nari Samity (Women's Association) in 1926, when it performed 'Prahlad', a Hindu devotional play.[239] The same year, the 'Jatra Party' of Mukunda Das (1878–1934), a travelling theatre company, toured Ranchi and was 'invited to give two performances to the patients'.[240] This is intriguing, given that the group's full name, which Dhunjibhoy did not mention in his report, was the 'Swadeshi Jatra Party'. As the name suggests, it combined traditional religious-mythical themes with socio-political issues such as colonial exploitation, patriotism and feudal and caste oppression. It is not clear what the content covered in the mental hospital plays was, nor do we know if the superintendent was criticised for having organised this event. Dhunjibhoy merely noted: 'The patients enjoyed the performances immensely.'[241]

Apart from such occasional events, routine musical entertainment was also established in 1926. A musician performed for the men four times and the women twice a week. This arrangement was highly successful as, according to Dhunjibhoy, the musician was 'very popular with the patients and they look forward to his concert every evening and many of them join in the singing'.[242] In 1927, the hospital acquired the 'latest gramophone machines and a large stock of most up-to-date Bengali, Hindi, Urdu, Oriya and English records'.[243] An '8 valve Radio set with loud speaker' was installed in the male compound in 1929 and patients were reported to 'enjoy immensely' listening to 'Calcutta and Bombay music both instrumental and vocal'.[244] Dhunjibhoy frequently repeated his contention that 'a mental hospital without a Cinema machine is never considered "Modern"' and argued that the 'claims for a Cinema machine as one of the most valuable forms of psychotherapy is undisputed'.[245] He clearly used his report to canvas support for particular innovations. This was a successful strategy, as 'the benign Government' at last sanctioned the purchase of such an apparatus in 1931. The 'Reference Clerk of the hospital', Babu Durga Charan Sarkar, received training by the cinema company's mechanic in operating it and, by 1933, 47 shows could be 'witnessed by crowded houses with happy faces'.[246] Previously, Indian films had been 'exhibited to the patients by the Ranchi Cinema House'.[247] In the mid-1930s, due to the worldwide switchover to talkies, it became difficult in India too to procure silent pictures and a 'Talkie machine' was eventually installed in 1939. The next year, 58 'talkie shows' were organised and English, Bengali and Hindi movies shown, with concessionary rates being offered by the film hire firms.[248] Dhunjibhoy did not fail to reiterate the therapeutic value of the film screenings, pointing out that the talkie machine 'not only provides a pleasant amusement but also helps enormously towards socialisation and rehabilitation of patients'.[249]

The Kanke Dramatic Society continued to flourish too, providing six performances in 1927.[250] Other events included: two dramatic performances by the Kanke Mohila Samity (Women's Association), three magical acts by 'renowned magicians', a 'musical soiree' and three 'Comic Sketches by Professor Chittaranjan Goswami of Calcutta'. Even the Ranchi Bihari Club contributed a one-off theatrical performance – a noteworthy event, given that prestigious and highly exclusive clubs of this kind tended to exhibit elitist English aspirations with condescending attitudes towards Indians. The fact that performances at Ranchi were at times attended by illustrious guests (such as ministers of local self-government departments), may have helped to attract entertainers and outsiders.[251] According to Dhunjibhoy, visitors to these social functions gave 'very great pleasure to the patients who look for outside sympathy and invariably enjoy their presence'.

They also helped to raise funds as, for example, in 1928, when the engineer and industrialist Sir R. N. Mukharji donated a sum of Rs.250 'as a token of [his] appreciation' after attending a musical soiree.[252] That same year about Rs.2,000 had been received in donations by luminaries and members of the local elite, including Raja Baldeo Das Birla (Rs.1,000), A. L. Ojha (Rs.50), Raja Rajendra Narayan Bhanja Deo (Rs.25) and Rai Bahadur D. D. Dhandhania (Rs.100).[253] The mental hospital, its cause and its recreational events clearly attracted attention from the indigenous upper classes.

Dhunjibhoy continued to justify the expansion of entertainment facilities by depicting them as a necessary part of all things modern: 'All modern Psychiatrists are of opinion that the introduction of congenial amusements in mental hospitals is another valuable factor in the treatment of mental conditions.'[254] A number of initiatives came to stay as stable features. A 'concert party' was founded in 1928, made up of attendants who volunteered to be trained in different musical instruments by sub-assistant surgeon D. R. Chaudhuri.[255] The group was to entertain patients twice a week. Staff-led initiatives clearly also had a positive impact on morale, ensuring staff retention. The setting up of the Kanke Employees' Co-operative Society Limited as a savings and money-lending scheme in 1935 would have helped to further increase staff satisfaction.[256]

It could be argued that entertainment, sports and social events should not be dwelled on in a historical analysis of mental hospitals. However, recreational activities were highly valued in contemporary mental hospitals including Ranchi. They constituted an important part of hospital life for those who partook in them and their value was considered comparable to medical intervention. Commenting on what had by then become styled as 'diversional therapy', Das stated in 1940:

> The expenditure in a Mental Hospital under this head as well as 'Occupational Therapy' should be regarded on a standard almost equivalent to that incurred in general hospitals for the purchase of medicines and surgical stores for therapeutic purposes. [257]

Not just medicine, but all matters that were considered relevant at the time require historians' attention. Of course, Dhunjibhoy's insistence that 'recreation' meant, 'literally', 'Re-creation' and constituted a 'most valuable form of treatment', may be considered somewhat overblown.[258] However, he and his medical assistants and locums clearly endeavoured to make life at the hospital more varied and interesting – for themselves as well as for their patients. Subordinate staff, too, seem to have enjoyed these activities, which would have ensured that staff turnover rates, the bane of many mental hospitals in Britain, were kept to a minimum and the quality of social interaction between staff and patients improved. Some of the performances such as the 'musical soiree' in 1928 and the 'Scenes from Shakespeare' enacted by 'Mr Greenberg and Mr Salim' in 1934 provided not only cultural entertainment but also opportunities for socialising between outsiders and the higher grades of the hospital staff. These events demonstrate how those who worked in an institution located in a remote locality tried to create a more attractive work environment for themselves.

Reports of entertainment and leisure activities at Ranchi also helped increase the hospital's reputation among the Indian higher classes. That it was indeed a popular institution is evidenced by the fact that Dhunjibhoy had private patients and that he continually, but unsuccessfully, lobbied the authorities to provide suitable accommodation for paying patients. Last but not least, visiting the mental hospital was one of the activities European and Indian members of the elite liked to engage in to exhibit their charitable disposition. Such motives were of course not at all self-less, as Prochaska has documented so well for Britain during the nineteenth-century heyday of philanthropy.[259] Nevertheless one of the consequences of such engagement by prominent outsiders was that the Ranchi mental hospital came to occupy a firm space in the wider landscape of public health and welfare-related institutions in India.

CONCLUSION

In 1932, Dhunjibhoy proclaimed: 'We introduce all the latest approved Western methods of treatment with due regard to Eastern conditions.'[1] It is clear from the records that he did just that. Finances permitting, he experimented with new treatments as soon as they became publicised in the academic literature, exposing patients at Ranchi to the same benefits and horrors that were bestowed on their counterparts in Europe and North America. From today's perspective, shock therapies and prolonged sedation constitute a woeful chapter in the history of psychiatry. At the time they seemed to provide a glimpse of hope among Western-trained practitioners around the globe, nurturing the belief that modern science and medical technology could effect improvement in some, if not all, types of mental illness. However, despite the emphasis on drug and shock treatments in the official report forms, the 'sheet anchor' at Ranchi was the more mundane, tried and tested hydrotherapy, together with an intense regime of work therapy. These methods, too, could be seen as means to subjugate and exploit patients. Towards the late 1930s in particular there are traces of this. Yet, there is also ample evidence of care and attention being paid to the welfare of patients. The well-established links with the upper echelons of the public, the frequent outings, feasts and nutritious food, and entertainment by external performers, leisure opportunities and the parole procedure for recovering patients indicate that Ranchi's institutional boundaries were permeable, albeit surrounded by a four-metre-high wall. A significant proportion of up to approximately 40 per cent of 'criminal lunatics' would, in England, have been sent to the high-security mental hospital at Broadmoor. The fact that they were accommodated safely, without imparting a prison atmosphere to the whole institution and creating an adverse perception among the public that would have deterred private, paying patients, attests to Dhunjibhoy's ability to strike a balance between control and care. Evidence of patients' own views on this matter are however lacking.

The available information on patients is refracted through the administrative requirements of hospital management. Patients came from a range of communities in the provinces of Bengal, Bihar and Orissa. As a whole, they were a select group. Restrictions were in place with priority given to the reception of the violent and those who had committed criminal acts. Women were significantly under-represented, as were people from the lowest social groups. In terms of the social markers of gender, age, occupation, religion, caste and social class, Ranchi's patient population was not representative of the overall population. Nor of those who suffered from less severe, common mental disorders. Given the acute accommodation pressures on male wards in particular, and the local governments' refusal to extend institutional provision,

Ranchi was not part of a system akin to Foucault's 'great confinement of the insane'. Nor was any mental hospital in India at the time a particularly convenient and logistically and financially feasible way of making invisible the multitude of people who might have been considered as 'undesirables'. Since the late nineteenth century, institution-based mental healthcare had become increasingly seen as a citizen's right and a public good that ought to be provided for by the state. Yet, the measures taken invariably fell far short of such expectations. Governments continued to rely on private initiatives and over-burdened community and family networks for the care of the majority of the mentally ill and intellectually disabled.

The statistical analysis of institutional data highlighted some gendered trends. The extent to which these reflect prevalent gender discrimination prior to admission to or within Ranchi is in some cases difficult to ascertain. It seems likely that gendered trends largely reflected prevalent admission policies and accommodation pressures. Despite patients' apparently severely compromised mental and physical condition on admission, Ranchi's mortality rate was low compared to other Indian mental institutions and public mental hospitals in England and Wales. The main physical life-threatening diseases differed from those commonly treated at Ranchi's infirmary. Airborne diseases figured more in mortality; parasitic and waterborne diseases were more prevalent in morbidity. Neither influenza nor malaria was reported to have led to many deaths, but they were highly prominent among the sick. The standard of treatment of physical diseases at the infirmary, and healthcare in general, must have been sufficiently high to allow a large number of patients to be engaged in work therapy, particularly from the mid-1930s onwards. The low cure rates at Ranchi were a persistent disappointment for Dhunjibhoy. He rightly pointed out that the level of cure, recovery, improvement and temporary remission were difficult to ascertain and predict at the point of an inmate's discharge. The terms used and the varied meanings bestowed on them by doctors presented another complication that made comparison between institutions and assessment of their cure efficiency problematic.

The limited extent to which apparently standardised terminology and conformity of nomenclature can be taken as an indication of uniform conceptualisation and consistent classification practices became clear in regard to diagnostic categories and the presumed aetiology of the different types of disorder. Dhunjibhoy worked eclectically across a range of seemingly discrete if not irreconcilable conceptualisations of particular conditions mooted by psychiatrists in India, Britain, Continental Europe and North America. His diagnostic mindset was flexibly cosmopolitan and transnational and cannot adequately be captured by reference to any single approach, let alone be restricted to 'colonial psychiatry'. The shifts in his own thinking do not dovetail with those of the official nomenclature of annual reports. Nor can they be mapped in a straightforward way onto changing practices at other institutions in India. The plural and changing meanings of diagnostic categories constitute a severe limitation for any inter-institutional comparison as well as longitudinal inner-institutional assessments. The heterogeneity of practices mirrors the difference between terms and meanings, nomenclature and nosology.

Dhunjibhoy was not unique in transcending the referential framework of any particular national style of psychiatric theory and practice. This was common among psychiatrists across the globe. He did however break new ground in the context of the Indianisation of the Indian Medical Service. He had been appointed to the coveted and prestigious senior position of superintendent of a large, newly built institution. Dhunjibhoy's career was facilitated by the British and marked by professional success. Yet he was simultaneously caught up in the hidden and structural racism that persisted during a period that was formally characterised by the reconfiguration of the imperial order as well as the gradual British disengagement from South Asia. Like other Indians in high-ranking positions, he continued to face discrimination from his British colleagues in terms of social status, professional recognition and posthumous tribute. As a Parsi and outsider from Bombay province he also found himself in competition with Indians from the Bihari and Bengali elites in Ranchi's catchment areas. Despite the continued inequities and communal tension during the process of Indianisation, Dhunjibhoy felt, as his daughter pointed out, that he 'owed everything he had achieved to the Army and the British'.[2]

As to Indianisation, Dhunjibhoy's was a success story of sorts. In personal terms, he gained the prestige that went with a senior position in the IMS and he and his family 'lived like minor royalty'.[3] But he also carried the Indian man's burden of having 'an issue with [...] identity':[4] 'He was torn between two loyalties.'[5] His family's burden entailed life with a 'very innovative' man who 'tried to make life bearable for the patients' and may have 'loved the hospital even more than his family'.[6] As his daughter recollected:

> I have seen my father cry only once in my life – the day he said good-bye to the Hospital staff and patients. The mental hospital was his life's work and he had put his heart and soul into it.[7]

NOTES

Introduction

1 Please note that contemporary meaning attributions for particular disease categories, such as mania and malaria will often differ from the way those categories are delineated and understood today. My usage of the terms will mirror the context in which they are being discussed.

Chapter 1   Indianisation and its Discontents

1 K. Ballhatchet, *Race, Sex and Class* (London: Weidenfeld, 1980), 100–111.
2 Ibid., 107. Shortly after this case, the secretary of state, Sir Charles Wood, revealed his Anglo-Saxon elite focus when he recommended that in future examinations for the civil service, 'University men who are gentlemen' rather than merely 'well crammed youths from Irish Universities or Commercial schools' ought to be favoured (Wood to Trevelyan, 1864). However, in public, Wood asserted that the aim was 'to get well-educated young men wherever they are to be found, no matter where or in what manner their education has been acquired'. (110)
3 See P. C. Sen Gupta, Soorjo Coomar Goodeve Chuckerbutty, *Medical History* 14 (1970): 183–91. Although Chuckerbutty had sat his MD examination in London in 1849 (in the first division and as second in order of merit), also being awarded the gold medal for comparative anatomy at University College, the colonial administration did not allow him access to the covenanted medical service on return to India. He had to return to Britain when competitive exams were introduced in 1854, gaining his appointment as assistant surgeon in 1855. Chuckerbutty became, as Sen Gupta points out, 'the first Indian to win by sheer merit his way into this service that had until then been reserved for Europeans only'. (135)
4 Ibid., 184.
5 Hutchins's work focused mainly on the British middle class, omitting the fact that it constituted but a small percentage of non-Indians present on the subcontinent. He thereby contributed to the flawed perception of the British community in India as homogenous, reifying the myth of British rule having been based on the actions of a superior and discrete elite. Although Kipling for example concerned himself with the lower strata of the British in India, elite-focused work continued to dominate British historians' writing up to the 1980s. The elite focus was enshrined particularly well in work such as Philip Mason's [Philip Woodruff] *The Men Who Ruled India* and in much of the Raj literature that focused on the social life and personal turmoil of the (relatively) high and mighty in the face of the 'exotic' and 'alien'. F. G. Hutchins, *The Illusion of Permanence. British Imperialism in India* (Princeton: Princeton University Press, 1967).
6 T. R. Metcalf, *An Imperial Vision* (Berkeley: University of California Press, 1989), 211.
7 Macaulay 1935, in E. Stokes, *The English Utilitarians and India* (Delhi: Oxford University Press, [1959] 1982), 46.
8 Comprador: a Portuguese term, originally employed in relation to household servants in East Asia. Used also to denote indigenous employees of trading companies – also in more recent debates outside East Asia. Concept used in relation to managers, meritocracy and technocracy. P. A. Baran, *The Political Economy of Growth* (New York: Monthly Review Press, 1957).

9 For overview and critique, see F. Cooper, *Colonialism in Question* (Berkeley: University of California Press, 2005); G. K. Bhambra, *Rethinking Modernity* (Basingstoke: Palgrave Macmillan, 2009).
10 Excepting only J. Mills, 'The History of Modern Psychiatry in India: 1795–1947', *History of Psychiatry* 12 (2001): 431–58.
11 V. Hess and B. Majerus, 'Writing the History of Psychiatry in the 20th Century', *History of Psychiatry* 22 (2011): 139–45; 139.
12 For example, see A. Digby and H. Sweet, 'Nurses as Culture Brokers in Twentieth-Century South Africa', in W. Ernst, ed., *Plural Medicine, Tradition and Modernity* (London/New York: Routledge, 2001), 113–29; M. Lyons, 'The Power to Heal', in D. Engels and S. Marks, eds, *Contesting Colonial Hegemony* (London: German Historical Institute, 1994), 202–23; A. Khalid, '"Subordinate" Negotiations', in B. Pati and M. Harrison, eds, *The Social History of Health and Medicine in Colonial India* (Delhi: Primus, 2011), 45–73.
13 For example, see D. Arnold, 'Colonial Medicine in Transition', *South Asia Research* 14 (1994): 10–35; P. Chakrabarti, 'Medicine and Nationhood in British India', *OSIRIS* 24 (2009): 188–211; Y. Guay, 'Emergence of Basic Research on the Periphery', *Scientometric* 10 (1986): 77–94; M. Harrison, *Public Health in British India* (Cambridge: Cambridge University Press, 1994); D. Kumar, ed., *Science and Empire* (Delhi: Anamika Prakashan, 1991); D. Raina and S. I. Habib, eds, *Domesticating Modern Science* (New Delhi: Tulika, 2004).
14 He was made a lieutenant in the IMS on 3 March 1917. This meant that he could be recalled to duty as a military doctor any time. This happened in 1940, when he returned to the province of Bombay to be deployed in Karachi.
15 Anon., 'Naval and Military Appointments', Supplement, *British Medical Journal* 27 (October 1923): 207.
16 Report 1925, 1.
17 Anon., *Journal of Mental Science* 73, 302 (1927): 485.
18 Report 1936, 23.
19 Anon., *British Medical Journal* 3636 (1930): 87.
20 Roshan Dhunjibhoy, a political activist, feminist, eminent documentary filmmaker and journalist, and former director of the Heinrich Böll Foundation, Germany, who had gained much insight into the politics of international development, added her critical observation: 'There was a double standard of payment, in those days, one for the British and the other for the locals. Many foreign NGOs to-day, continue this racist practice.' R. Dhunjibhoy, 2009, personal communication. On the 'grand old dame' of the Heinrich Böll Foundation, see Barbara Unmüßig, Britta Petersen and Jost Pachaly. 2011. 'We Grieve for Roshan Dhunjibhoy'. Heinrich Böll Foundation. Online: http://www.boell.de/worldwide/asia/asia-obituary-roshan-dhunjibhoy-11843.html (accessed 13 June 2011).
21 Report 1921–23, 5.
22 'Proceedings of Council', Supplement *British Medical Journal* 3349 (1925): 90.
23 The remaining six provinces were Punjab, United Provinces, Central Provinces, Bihar and Orissa, Burma, and Assam.
24 R. Jeffery, 'Recognizing India's Doctors: The Institutionalization of Medical Dependency, 1918–39', *Modern Asian Studies* 13 (1979): 301–26; Chakrabarti, 'Nationhood'.
25 Chakrabarti, 'Nationhood', 189.
26 Ibid., 193.
27 Ibid.
28 M. Sinha, 'Britishness, Clubbability, and the Colonial Public Sphere', *Journal of British Studies* 40 (2001): 489–521; 515.
29 M. Sinha, *In My Father's Footsteps* (Delhi: 1981), 24.
30 A. Memmi, *The Colonizer and the Colonized* (Boston: Beacon, 1965), 120.
31 J. Bara, 'Schooling the "Truant" Tribe', *Studies in History* 26 (2010): 143–73.

32 R. Dhunjibhoy, personal communication, 2009.
33 Madras Report 1928, 5; see also Madras Report 1929, 515.
34 Madras Report 1929, Appendix.
35 Madras Report 1928, 5.
36 A. R. Basu, 'The Coming of Psychoanalysis in Colonial India', *Centre for Studies in Social Sciences Occasional Paper* 5 (1999): 36–54; C. Harding, 'The Freud Franchise', in R. Clarke, ed., *Celebrity and Colonialism* (Newcastle: Cambridge Scholars, 2009); C. Hartnack, *Psychoanalysis in Colonial India* (Oxford: Oxford University Press, 2001); S. Kapila, 'Freud and His Indian Friends', in S. Mahone and M. Vaughan, eds, *Psychiatry and Empire* (Basingstoke: Palgrave Macmillan, 2007), 124–52; S. Kakar, *Culture and Psyche* (New York: Psyche, 1997); P. Mehta, 'The Import and Export of Psychoanalysis', *Journal of American Academy of Psychoanalysis* 25 (1997): 455–71; A. Nandy, *The Savage Freud* (New Jersey: Princeton University Press, 1995); T. G. Vaidyanathan and J. J. Kripal, eds, *Vishnu on Freud's Desk* (Delhi: Oxford University Press, 2003); C. V. Ramana, 'On the Early History and Development of Psychoanalysis in India', *Journal of the American Psychoanalytical Association* 12 (1964): 110–34.
37 O. Berkeley-Hill, *All Too Human*, (London: Peter Davies, 1939), 252, 249.
38 Ibid., 336–7. Hubback was held in esteem by members of the Orissan elite, but exhibited in his memoir, as Nayak put it, 'a tone of mild contempt for Indians', considering nationalistic self-assertion as 'an act of petulance on the part of power-loving [Indian National] Congressmen'. J. K. Nayak, 'Hubback's Memoirs', *Telegraph – Calcutta* (29 November 2010).
39 The area in which Ranchi is located has a well-established record of *adivasi* (tribal) revolts. It got separated from Bihar in 2000, when the state of Jharkhand was formed.
40 Berkeley-Hill, *All Too Human*, 111.
41 Ibid., 110.
42 Ibid., 79–80.
43 R. Dhunjibhoy, personal communication, 2009.
44 W. S. J. Shaw, 'The Heredity of Dementia Praecox', *British Medical Journal* 3534 (1928): 566–8 (567). There was the Sir Cowasjii Mental Hospital and a dedicated Parsi ward at the Yeravda Mental Hospital.
45 Ibid., 566, 568.
46 Ibid., 566, 568.
47 A. J. Brock, Correspondence, *British Medical Journal* 3535 (1928): 634–5; 634.
48 H. Devine, 'Review', *Journal of Mental Science* 70 (1924): 453–4; 454.
49 On Geddes, see R. Home, *Of Planting and Planning* (London: Spoon/Chapman Hill, 1997); H. Meller, *Patrick Geddes* (London/New York: Routledge, 1990); C. Renwick, 'The Practice of Spencerian Science', *Isis* 100 (2009): 36–57.
50 W. S. J. Shaw, Correspondence, *British Medical Journal* 3537 (1928): 728.
51 Ibid.
52 H. C. Aspengren, 'Sociological Knowledge and Colonial Power in Bombay around the First World War', *British Journal for the History of Science* 43 (2010): 100–116; 112.
53 J. E. Dhunjibhoy, Letters, Notes, *British Medical Journal* 3555 (1929): 382.
54 Ibid., 382.
55 W. S. J. Shaw, 'Some Observations on the Aetiology of Dementia Praecox', *Journal of Mental Science* 76 (1930): 505–11; 511.
56 J. E. Dhunjibhoy, Correspondence, *Journal of Mental Science* 77, 316 (1931): 294–7; 297.
57 Ballhatchet, *Race, Sex and Class*, 107.
58 A. Guha, 'More about the Parsi Seths', *Economic and Political Weekly* 19 (1984): 117–31; 117.
59 Ibid.
60 For examples, see T. M. Luhrmann, 'The Traumatized Social Self', in A. C. G. M. Robben and M. M. Suarez-Orozco, eds, *Cultures under Siege* (Cambridge: Cambridge University Press, 2002), 158–93.

61 Ibid., 162.
62 R. P. Karkaria, *India: Forty Years of Progress and Reform* (London: Henry Frowde, 1896), 50.
63 H. D. Darukhanawala, *Parsis and Sports* (Bombay: Darukhanawala, 1935), 43.
64 S. F. Markham, *A Report to the Sir Ratan Tata Trustees on Problems Affecting the Parsee Community* (Bombay: Sir Ratan Tata Trust, 1932), xi.
65 Ibid., 45.
66 N. B. R. Kotwal, *A Discourse! The Naked Truth! etc.* (Bombay: Kotwal, 1937), 13.
67 F. Fanon, *Black Skins White Masks* (New York: Grove, 1967), 10.
68 S. F. Desai, *A Community at the Crossroad* (Bombay: New Book, 1948), 74.
69 Guha, 'Parsi Seths', 118.
70 R. Dhunjibhoy, personal communication, 2009.
71 J. F. Bulsara, *Parsi Charity Relief and Community Amelioration* (Bombay: Bulsara, 1935), 33.
72 Guha, 'Parsi Seths', 129.
73 Ibid., 129.
74 Dhunjibhoy, Correspondence, 296.
75 T. M. Luhrmann, *The Good Parsi* (Cambridge, MA: Harvard University Press, 1996), 170.
76 P. A. Wadia, *Parsis Ere the Shadows Thicken* (Bombay: Wadia, 1949), 138.
77 Desai, *Crossroad*, 74.
78 Memmi, *Colonizer*, 140.
79 R. Dhunjibhoy, personal communication, 2009.
80 A. Nandy, *The Intimate Enemy* (Delhi: Oxford University Press, 1983), 14.
81 H. Bhabha, *The Location of Culture*, (London/New York: Routledge, 1994), 86.
82 M. Kureishi, Christmas Letter to my Sister, in M. Shamsie, ed., *A Dragonfly in the Sun. An Anthology of Pakistani Writing in English* (Karachi: Oxford University Press, 1997) 67–8. Kureishi was born in Calcutta in 1927 and studied English Literature at Cambridge. Back in Pakistan she married a Muslim, Abo Kureishi, the brother of cricket legend and writer Omar Kureishi and of Hanif Kureishi's father Rafiushan. She was the aunt of Hanif, who famously introduced the leading character in his novel *The Buddha of Suburbia* (London: Faber and Faber, 1990) with the words: 'My name is Karim Amir, and I am an Englishman born and bred, almost.'
83 Guha, 'Parsi Seths', 130.
84 Ibid., 122.
85 R. Dhunjibhoy, personal communication, 2009.
86 Report 1939, 20.
87 R. Dhunjibhoy, personal communication, 2009.
88 Guha, 'Parsi Seths', 130.
89 R. Dhunjibhoy, personal communication, 2009.
90 Ibid.
91 Ibid.
92 Details are available in the German National Archive in Berlin: Geheimes Staatsarchiv Preussischer Kulturbesitz, Berlin: HA Rep 208 A Nr 96, 1.
93 R. Dhunjibhoy, personal communication, 2009.
94 Ibid.
95 Berkeley-Hill, *All Too Human*, 242.
96 R. Dhunjibhoy, personal communication, 2009.
97 Jeffery, 'Recognizing India's Doctors'.
98 Report 1925, 24. In 1925, the female subassistant surgeon also carried out the duties of the female compounder, as the post had not yet been filled. Ibid., 7.
99 C. Hochmuth, 'Patterns of Medical Culture in Colonial Bengal, 1835–80', *Bulletin of the History of Medicine* 80 (2006): 39–72; 54.
100 Report 1925, 7, 24. Matron: Rs.266, Male Subassistant Surgeon: Rs.120–130, Female Subassistant Surgeon: Rs.150.

101 By 1933, attendants were graded into 1st, 2nd and 3rd grade, being paid Rs.24, Rs.21 and Rs.18 respectively. Report 1933, 47.
102 Report 1925, 8.
103 Report 1926, 2.
104 Ibid., 10.
105 Ibid.
106 Ibid.
107 Report 1927, 4, 6.
108 Report 1928, 10.
109 Report 1929, 16; Report 1931, 18.
110 Report 1931, 18.
111 Ibid., 15.
112 Ibid., 19.
113 Report 1937, 25.
114 Report 1939, 20.
115 Report 1940, 15.
116 Ibid.
117 Report 1926, 2.
118 Ibid.
119 Jamadars were paid Rs.30 per month. The pay for the attendants/keepers fluctuated between Rs.18 and Rs. 4.
120 The outpatient department is mentioned for the first time in 1931: 'Approximately 9,347 cases were treated as outdoor patients for minor ailments such as ulcers, slight injuries, headaches, constipation, etc.' Report 1931, 7.
121 Report 1930–32, 23; Report 1933, 21; Report 1934, 21.
122 The Kanke Employees' Co-operative Society Limited had 335 members by 1936. Local moneylenders had charged interest for loans at the rate of two to four annas per rupee per month on small loans. Report 1936, 23.
123 Report 1938, 20; Report 1931, 15.
124 Report 1931, 19.
125 Report 1930, 18.
126 Report 1930–32, 24.
127 Report 1934, 22.
128 Report 1935, 19.
129 Report 1936, 23.
130 However, there is evidence that Mapother disliked Dhunjibhoy as a person.

Chapter 2   The Patients: The Demographics of Gender and Age, Locality, Occupation, Caste and Religion

1 A. T. Scull, *Museums of Madness* (1979) (Harmondsworth: Penguin, 1982), 13.
2 For example, see the work of P. Bartlett, A. Cellard and M. Thifault, E. Dwyer, R. Fox, J. Hughes, J. Moran, R. Porter, A. Suzuki, N. Tomes and D. Wright. See also Scull's later work.
3 J. H. Mills, *Madness, Cannabis and Colonialism* (Houndsmills: Macmillan, 2000), 6, 112.
4 Ibid., 2.
5 F. Groenhout, 'Loyal Feudatories or Depraved Despots?', in W. Ernst and B. Pati, eds, *India's Princely States* (London/New York: Routledge, 2007; New Delhi: Primus, 2010), 99–117; 103.
6 S. Kapila, 'Masculinity and Madness' *Past and Present* 187 (2005): 121–56; 156.
7 See the case of Devie Singh, claimant to the *gadi* (throne) of Ghadvi in the Dangs: W. Ernst, 'Mad, bad and/or subaltern?', paper presented at the Situating the Subaltern in South Asian Medical History Workshop, University of Warwick, 2009.

8 For example, see musical healing at Tajuddin Baba's *dargah*: J. Newell, 'Unseen Power', *The Muslim World* 92 (2007): 640–56.
9 For example, see B. V. Davar, *Mental Health of Indian Women* (New Delhi: Sage, 1999).
10 I. Illich, *Medical Nemesis* (New York: Random House, 1976), 5.
11 For the eighteenth century, for example, see J. Andrews, 'In her Vapours ... [or] indeed in her Madness?', *History of Psychiatry* 1 (1990): 125–43; R. Porter, *Mind-Forg'd Manacles* (London: Athlone, 1987).
12 Report 1925, 9.
13 Two provincial governments administered these three regions: the government of Bengal and the government of Bihar and Orissa. Following the Government of India Act of 1935, Bihar and Orissa were governed separately from 1937 onwards.
14 Report 1924–26, 1.
15 On the colonial situation, see S. Sen, *Women and Labour in Late Colonial India* (Cambridge: Cambridge University Press, 2006); G. Forbes, *Women in Modern India* (Cambridge: Cambridge University Press, 1996); S. Kak and B. Pati, eds, *Exploring Gender Equations* (New Delhi: Nehru Memorial Museum, 2005). On the situation in the postcolonial period, see: T. V. Sekher and Neelambar Hatti, eds, *Unwanted Daughters* (Jaipur/New Delhi: Rawat, 2009).
16 For example, see R. Porter, 'Foucault's Great Confinement', in A. Still and I. Velody, eds, *Rewriting the History of Madness* (London/New York: Routledge, 1992), 119–25.
17 A. Scull, *The Most Solitary of Afflictions* (New Haven: Yale University Press, 1993), 287. On the debates surrounding this issue, see A. Scull, 'Psychiatrists and Historical Facts', *History of Psychiatry* 6 (1995): 387–94.
18 Report 1933–35, 10.
19 Ibid.
20 Ibid.
21 Ibid.
22 Report 1930–32, 2.
23 Report 1939, 2.
24 Report 1927–29, 3.
25 Ibid., 2.
26 Ibid.
27 Ibid.
28 Ibid.
29 Ibid., 3.
30 Data refer to the period from 1929 to 1939.
31 On the Indian Lunacy Act 1912, see O. Somasundaram, 'The Indian Lunacy Act 1912', *Indian Journal of Psychiatry* 29 (1987): 3–14.
32 Report 1930–32.
33 R. Eager, 'Review of Report of the Board of Control for 1937', *Journal of Mental Science* 85, 355 (1939): 293–4; 293. The numbers in specialist hospitals in the US, such as Ionia State Hospital for the Criminal Insane in Michigan, totalled about 650 in 1930. See E. Pilcher, 'Relation of Mental Disease to Crime', *Journal of the American Institute of Criminal Law and Criminology* 21 (1930): 212–46; 214.
34 Report 1927–29, 6.
35 This issue is highlighted also by Busfield in relation to her analysis of gender and mental illness: 'I also note that the epidemiological data often tell us more about psychiatric practices and the mental health services than they do about gender differences in mental health problems.' J. Busfield, *Men, Women and Madness* (New York: New York University Press, 1996), 9.
36 Ibid., 22.
37 Data from 1926 to 1939.
38 Eager, 'Review', 293; Pilcher, 'Relation', 214.

39 Pilcher, 'Relation', 214.
40 Ibid., 246. The four other institutions were Central State Hospital for the Criminal Insane, Waupun, Wisconsin; Lima State Hospital, Ohio; Bridgewater State Hospital, Massachusetts; Farview State Hospital of Waymart, Pennsylvania. In total, there were eight institutions of this type in the US.
41 See Busfield, *Men, Women and Madness*, 30. On the impact of changes in women's domestic role in the postwar period and on the predominance of women in mental hospital populations, see W. R. Gove and J. F. Tudor, 'Adult Sex Roles and Mental Illness', *American Journal of Sociology* 78 (1972): 812–35. The over-representation of men in Western institutions during this period was also linked to the prevalence among male populations of the now-rare neuropsychiatric disorder 'general paresis of the insane' or GPI; see Busfield, *Men, Women and Madness*, 127. GPI was however rarely acknowledged as a disorder common among Indian patients.
42 Report 1930–32, 9.
43 Ibid., 8. The table presented here is a condensed version, omitting gender-specific detail.
44 A. Mohanty and N. Hazary, *Indian Prison Systems* (New Delhi: Ashish, 1990), 49.
45 The classifications were in place until after Independence. For example, see *Orissa Jail Manual* (Cuttack: Orissa Government, 1964), quoted in Mohanty and Hazary, *Indian Prison Systems*, 49.
46 P. K. Sen, *Penology Old and New* (London: Longmans, Green, 1943). One of the classic works on penology in India, Sen's book made much of the overlap of ancient law with modern legal lore. The book was based on Sen's Tagore Law Lecture of 1929 and included a foreword by Sir Maurice Gwyer, Vice Chancellor of Delhi University from 1938 to 1940 and Chief Justice of India from 1937 to 1943.
47 Report 1930–32, 9.
48 O. Walsh, 'Race, Religion and Irish Insanity', in J. Melling and B. Forsythe, eds, *Insanity, Institutions and Society* (London/New York: Routledge, 1999): 223–42; 225.
49 Report 1933–35, 7. The other 'crimes committed' by people admitted in 1935 were: 20 murders, 5 culpable homicides, 15 hurt and grievous hurt, 3 attempted suicides, 0 dacoity (armed robbery by a group of highwaymen) with murder, 15 petty offences, 0 harbouring an offender.
50 The blowing up of railway lines is still pursued by Naxalite rebels in the Jharkhand region. For example, one such incident occurred during this author's research period at Ranchi in August 2009.
51 Report 1927–29, 6.
52 Report 1924–26, 5.
53 Ibid., 4–5.
54 Ibid., 4 (emphasis in the original).
55 Report 1940, 6.
56 Pilcher, 'Relation', 246.
57 Report 1930, 19.
58 Ibid.
59 There existed however a perceived overlap between idiocy or imbecility and criminality, as suggested in Fernald's contention of 1912 that every intellectually disabled person 'is a potential criminal'. This issue will be discussed further in the chapter on treatments. See D. A. Wolfe and E. J. Mash, eds, *Behavioral and Emotional Disorder in Adolescents* (New York: Guildford, 2006), 385.
60 Report 1938, 7.
61 Ibid., 8.
62 Sen, *Penology*.
63 Report 1938, 6.
64 Report 1937, 8.

65 Ibid., 9. Dhunjibhoy's suggestions are discussed fully in the chapter on treatment.
66 Report 1936, 7.
67 Ibid.
68 Busfield, *Men, Women and Madness*, 23–4; W. R. Gove and T. R. Herb, 'Stress and Mental Illness Among the Young', *Social Forces* 53 (1974): 256–65.
69 Busfield, *Men, Women and Madness*, 21–30.
70 Ibid., 25.
71 At St Andrews, age cohorts are grouped into ten-year groups, i.e., 25–34, 35–44 etc. S. Cherry, *Mental Health Care in Modern England* (Woodbridge: Boydell, 2003), 186–7.
72 Ibid., 187.
73 A. E. Porter, *Census of India, 1931*, vol. V (Calcutta: Central Publication Branch, 1933), 36; W. G. Lacey, *Census of India, 1931*, vol. VII (Patna: Government Printing, 1932), 30.
74 For example, see Report 1930, 19.
75 For example, see S. Bandyopadhyay, 'Caste in the Perception of the Raj', *Bengal Past and Present* 104 (1985): 56–80; S. Bandyopadhyay, *Caste, Culture and Hegemony: Social Dominance in Colonial Bengal* (London: Sage, 2004); S. Bayly, *Caste, Society and Politics in India from the Eighteenth Century to the Modern Age* (Cambridge: Cambridge University Press, 1999); L. Carroll, 'Colonial Perceptions of Indian Society and the Emergence of Caste(s) Associations', *Journal of Asian Studies* 37 (1978): 233–50; L. Carroll, 'Caste, Social Change, and the Social Scientist', *Journal of Asian Studies* 35 (1975): 63–84; A. A. Yang, *Bazaar India* (Berkeley: University of California Press, 1999).
76 B. S. Cohn, 'Notes on the History of the Study of Indian Society and Culture', in M. Singer and B. S. Cohn, eds, *Structure and Change in Indian Society* (Chicago: Aldine, 1968), 3–28; 24.
77 Goalas were often referred to as belonging to the Yadav caste, as in Bihar Goalas use Yadav as their surname.
78 For example, on caste and the census, see B. S. Cohn, *Colonialism and Its Forms of Knowledge* (Princeton: Princeton University Press, 1996); S. Bandyopadhyay, 'Construction of Social Categories', in D. S. Singh, ed., *Ethnicity, Caste and People* (New Delhi: Manohar, 1992), 26–36.
79 W. S. Meyer et al., *Imperial Gazetteer of India*, vol. I (Oxford: Clarendon, 1880–1931), 486.
80 See A. Malhotra, *Gender, Caste and Religious Identities* (Delhi: Oxford University Press, 2002).
81 Abundant literature is available. The 'classics' include A. Beteille, *Caste, Class and Power* (Berkeley: University of California Press, 1965) and *Castes: Old and New* (Bombay: Asia Publishing House, 1969); L. Dumont, *Homo Hierarchicus* (Paris: Gallimard, 1966); M. N. Srinivas, 'A Note on Sanskritization and Westernization', *Far Eastern Quarterly* 15 (1956): 481–96 and *Caste in Modern India* (Bombay: Media Promoters, 1962).
82 On this issue, see Carroll, 'Caste'.
83 A. Sharan, 'From Caste to Category', *Indian Economic and Social History Review* 40 (2003): 279–310; 291n59.
84 Percentage of 'not known' of women's occupation as a percentage of all women admitted: 22.22 per cent in 1924, 34.15 per cent in 1926, 30.19 per cent in 1927–29, 28.44 per cent in 1930–32. Percentage of 'not known' of men's occupation as a percentage of all men admitted: 20.5 per cent in 1925, 19.73 per cent in 1926, 17.46 per cent in 1927–29, 15.95 per cent in 1930–32.
85 Percentage of 'unknown' occupations among women, as a percentage of women admitted: Patna, 0 per cent in 1925; Berhampore, 29.41 per cent in 1925; Dacca, 0 per cent in 1925; Patna, 42.86 per cent in 1924; Berhampore, 43.48 per cent in 1924; Dacca, 22.22 per cent in 1924. Percentage of 'unknown' occupations among men, as a percentage of men admitted: Patna, 15.39 per cent in 1925; Berhampore, 22.69 per cent in 1925; Dacca, 8.20 per cent in 1925; Patna, 24.49 per cent in 1924; Berhampore, 28.8 per cent in 1924; Dacca, 9.55 per cent in 1924.

  Note: The numbers for women admitted are low, e.g., 5 for Berhampore in 1925 (of 17), 3 (of 7) for 1924 at Patna, 10 (of 23) at Berhampore and 2 (of 9) at Dacca.

86 Percentage of total admissions (including readmissions) for women: Patna, 10 per cent in 1924; Berhampore, 15.54 per cent in 1924; Dacca, 12.5 per cent in 1924; Patna, 8.78 per cent in 1925; Berhampore, 12.5 per cent in 1925; Dacca, 10.45 per cent in 1925. And for Ranchi: 12.72 per cent in 1925, reflecting average total transferred from Patna, Berhampore and Dacca; 26.89 per cent in 1926; 21.90 per cent in 1927–29; 29.78 per cent in 1930–32.
87 Report 1924–26, 22.
88 B. Pati and C. P. Nanda, 'The Leprosy Patient', in B. Pati and M. Harrison, eds, *Social History of Health and Medicine in Colonial India* (London/New York: Routledge, 2009), 113–28.
89 Lacey, *Census of India*, 135.
90 Meyer, *Gazetteer*, 488.
91 Ibid., 516.
92 The superintendent of census operations for Bihar and Orissa reported, in relation to the census of 1931, that there were 'important differences' between the 1931 definitions and those applied in 1921: 'In 1921 the total population was divided into "actual workers" and "dependants". On the present occasion it has been divided into "earners", "working dependants" and "non-working dependants".' In 1921, against each occupation 'the total number of persons *supported* by it' was shown, i.e., 'both workers and dependants. This time only persons actually *following* an occupation, either as earners or as working dependants, have been shown against it, and no attempt has been made to distribute the non-working dependants between the various occupations by which they are supported.' Lacey, *Census of India*, 55.
93 Report 1933–35, 14.
94 Meyer, *Gazetteer*, 486.
95 For example, see S. Jain and P. Murthy, 'Madmen and Specialists', *International Review of Psychiatry* 18 (2006): 345–54.
96 For example, see R. P. Behal, 'Power Structure, Discipline, and Labour in Assam Tea Plantations under Colonial Rule', *International Review of Social History* 51 (2006): 143–72; J. Sharma, '"Lazy" Natives, Coolie Labour, and the Assam Tea Industry', *Modern Asian Studies* 43 (2009): 1287–1324; N. Varma, 'Coolie Acts and the Acting Coolies', *Social Scientist* 33 (2005): 49–72. For an early twentieth-century account, see J. F. Gruning, *Recruitment of Labour for Tea Gardens in Assam* (Chilong[?], 1900).
97 See J. Bara, *Colonialism, Christianity and the Tribes of Chotanagpur in East India* (London/New York: Routledge, 2007); Sharma, '"Lazy" Natives'; P. Robb, ed., *Dalit Movements and Meanings of Labour in India* (New Delhi: Oxford University Press, 1993); C. Bates and M. Carter, 'Tribal and Indentured Migrants', in P. Robb, ed., *Dalit Movements and Meanings of Labour in India* (New Delhi: Oxford University Press, 1993).
98 Meyer, *Gazetteer*, 471. There is much evidence of economic exploitation, hardship and suffering among coolies, see S. S. Sinha, 'Adivasi Women in Transition', in Kak and Pati, *Exploring Gender Equations*, 175–202; E. V. Daniel, 'The Making of a Coolie', in H. Bernstein et al., eds, *Plantations, Proletarians and Peasants in Asia* (London: Frank Cass, 1992); B. V. Lal, 'Veil of Dishonour', *Journal of Pacific History* 20 (1985): 135–55; V. Naidu, *The Violence of Indenture in Fiji* (Suva: University of the South Pacific Press, 1980); H. Tinker, *A New System of Slavery* (London/New York: Oxford University Press, 1974).
99 Earlier economic historians had pointed out that there was always considerable seasonal migration in the region's labour supply with many working far away from their villages during the nonharvest season. But it is doubtful if they would have been referred to as 'coolies'. In Assam's case, after the rise of Gandhian politics, there was a major movement of tea labour back from Assam to the Chota Nagpur/Jharkhand region, which was initially supported by the Congress. In terms of foreign labour, recent studies argue that many labourers did travel back home after their indentured period was over, sometimes only to visit, before returning to their new homes. The latter might not have been possible for poorer people who failed to

make arrangements for the period following expiry of indenture (manumission). K. K. Sircar, 'Coolie Exodus from Assam's Chargola Valley', *Economic and Political Weekly* 22 (1987): 184–93. Hughes notes that about one-quarter of indentured Indian workers in Natal, South Africa, opted to return to India after five years. H. Hughes, 'The Coolies Will Elbow us out of the Country', *Labour History Review* 72 (2007): 155–68 (158).

100 On the effect of the Great Depression on Indian coolies, see C. Bayly and C. Harper, *Forgotten Wars* (London: Allen Lane, 2007); Hughes, 'The Coolies', 155–68. Daniel shows how this term came to be used in a dehumanising way in relation to Indian labourers in varied colonial contexts. Daniel, 'Making of a Coolie'.

101 Excluding those of 'cultivator', 'cooly', 'beggar', 'prostitute', 'unknown', 'no occupation', 'housewives' and 'dependants', which together accounted for 4 per cent, 10 per cent, 23 per cent and 17 per cent in 1925, 1926, 1927–29 and 1930–32 respectively.

102 Note: some of these may have been readmitted.

103 'Service' did not refer to 'domestic service', i.e., 'servants'. This group was listed separately.

104 S. Sarkar, *Writing Social History* (Delhi: Oxford University Press, 1997), 172.

105 'Cranny' was defined in the *Hobson-Jobson*: 'In Bengal commonly used for a clerk writing English, and thence vulgarly applied generically to the East Indians, or half-caste class, from among whom English copyists are chiefly recruited. The original is Hind. *karānī, kirānī*.' H. Yule, *Hobson-Jobson* (London: Murray, 1902 [1886]), 273. During the earlier period, 'crannies' were described as 'kranees, or writers, on salaries varying, according to their duties and abilities, from five to thirty roopees.' Ibid., 973.

106 In relation to 'keranis', Sarkar also refers to their subordination to the 'discipline of time', as evoked in Gangopadhyay's play *Kerani-carit* (1885): 'We lose the day's salaries if we reach office a minute late […] half the salary goes on fines […] there is not a single gap in our day's routine.' S. Sarkar, '"Kaliyuga", "Chakri" and "Bhakti"', *Economic and Political Weekly* 27 (1992): 1543–59, 1561–66; 1549.

107 J. Bara, 'Schooling the "Truant" Tribe', *Studies in History* 26 (2010): 143–73.

108 S. Rao, 'Caste and Mental Disorders in Bihar', *American Journal of Psychiatry* 9 (1966): 1045–55. A team of researchers based in Kolkata confirmed Rao's findings in relation to Bengali Hindus presenting at an urban clinic and at the psychiatric outpatient department of a teaching hospital in a rural area during the 1970s. D. N. Nandi et al., 'Demographic Characteristics and Mental Morbidity amongst Different Castes in West Bengal', *International Journal of Social Psychiatry* 29 (1983): 21–8.

109 Jain and Murthy suggest in relation to the mental hospital in the Indian princely state of Mysore: 'Religious, caste and social background [. . .]were representative of the population of Bangalore.' Jain and Murthy, 'Madmen and Specialists', 349. However, the figures they provide relate to religion only and the extrapolation from religion to caste and social background therefore seems based on speculation rather than any more detailed analysis of patients and the statistics relating to them.

110 Meyer, *Gazetteer*, 486.

111 Although caste was also relevant to Muslims in Bengal, it would not always have been applicable to Muslim and Christian patients. On Islam in Bengal and the existence of caste, see A. Roy, *Islam in South Asia* (New Delhi: South Asia Publishing, 1996); R. Ahmed, *The Bengal Muslims* (Delhi: Oxford University Press, 1988). See also N. Bose's work (translated by A. Beteille), in which Muslim reformers' attempts to counteract caste prejudice is discussed and listings of the varied castes predominant among Bengal Muslims are provided. N. Bose, *The Structure of Indian Society* (Hyderabad: Orient Longman, 1996 [1949]).

112 Alternative spelling of *dome*: *dom* or *domb*.

113 The seven 'main classes of Hindus in Bengal', for example, identified in the *Gazetteer*, were: Brahmans of various status; Rajputs, Baidyas and Kayasths; Navasakha and other 'clean' Sudras; Chasi, Kaibartta and Goala; those whom the village barber will shave; those whom

NOTES 219

the regular barber will not shave; eaters of all manner of unclean food, scavengers. Doms, Chamars and Muchis were identified as 'castes of the seventh and lowest class in Bengal; Goalas as the 'subcaste of 4th class'.
114 Bhandopadhya, *Caste*.
115 Carroll, 'Colonial Perceptions'.
116 For a discussion of these issues, see Malhotra, *Gender*.
117 Report 1924–26, 4.
118 Other categories for 'religion' referred to in the census of 1931, for example, were Sikh, Jain, Buddhist, Zoroastrian (Parsi) and 'Others' (including Jews, Kumbhipatia, and 'Indefinitive Beliefs', i.e., 'Agnostics, Atheists and the like'). The categories changed over time. In 1941, they consisted of 'Sikhs, Jains, Parsees, Buddhists, Jews, Tribes, Others'. 'Others' then represented '2 percent and in this omnibus head go all foreigners and minor elements of the Indian population which do not fall within the main divisions'. M. W. M. Yeatts, *Census of India 1941*, vol. I (Simla: Government of India, 1943), part 1, 29.
119 Meyer, *Gazetteer*, 476.
120 Ibid., 471. Practical criteria 'by means of which Hinduism may be distinguished from other religions indigenous to India' were published in the *India Census Report for 1901*.
121 Yeatts, *Census*, 30.
122 Meyer, *Gazetteer*, 471.
123 Ibid. The 'varying extent to which, in different parts of India, ceremonial uncleanness is held to conflict with a man's claim to be considered a Hindu' was held to be another factor.
124 Meyer, *Gazetteer*, 471.
125 Brahmo Samaj, founded in 1828 by Raja Ram Mohan Roy; Arya Samaj, founded in 1875 by Swami Dayananda.
126 Yeatts, *Census*, 28.
127 Ibid.
128 Ibid.
129 Ibid.
130 Ibid.
131 On 'race', see W. Ernst and B. J. Harris, eds, *Race, Science and Medicine* (London/New York: Routledge, 1998); P. Gilroy, *Between Camps* (London: Allen Lane, 2000).
132 The census ratios for eastern Bengal would have been more favourable to Muslim communities. However, it is difficult to judge whether census data for 'Bengal proper' or for the whole province would have been more appropriate for comparison with Ranchi data, as occasionally a whole batch of patients was sent to Ranchi from a specific area, as in 1938, when 11 patients from Tippera were admitted, and, in 1937, 11 patients from Bogra.
133 **Table 2.4.** Gender ratio for selected religious groups, for Bengal, Bihar and Orissa, Census 1941.

	Male	Female
Hindu	50	49
Muslim	43	44
Christian	0	0

134 **Table 2.5.** Percentages for main religious groups calculated for Ranchi, 1928–1939.

	Male	Female
Hindu	65	58
Muslim	29	15
Christian	4	19

135 Meyer, *Gazetteer*, 480.
136 Ibid.
137 Ibid.

138 See for example, Kak and Pati, *Gender*; Sekher and Hatti, *Unwanted Daughters*. On gender bias against girls and the resulting significant difference in weight-for-age statistics: A. Sen, 'Many Faces of Gender Inequality', *Frontline* 18: 22 (2001).
139 Meyer, *Gazetteer*, 480.
140 Ibid., 479.
141 Yeatts, *Census*, 59.
142 Ibid., 51.
143 Meyer, *Gazetteer*, 475.
144 Ibid.
145 Yeatts, *Census*, 51.
146 Report 1939; Yeatts, *Census*, 98.
147 These patients came from Manbhum (1), Palaman (1), Singhbhum (2) and Hazribagh (2) – all in Chota Nagpur.
148 In respect to hospital admissions overall, Ranchi was second only to the large metropolitan area of Calcutta. From 1928 to 1939, 200 patients came from Calcutta and 118 from Ranchi. Other major towns, such as Dacca and Patna, were also prominently represented, but still provided considerably fewer patients.

Chapter 3   Institutional Trends and Standardisation: Deaths, Diseases and Cures

1 D. Tidemalm et al., 'Excess Mortality in Persons with Severe Mental Disorder in Sweden', *Clinical Practice and Epidemiology in Mental Health* 4 (2008): 1–9; 1.
2 Ibid., 1.
3 V. Hansen et al., 'Total Mortality in People Admitted to a Psychiatric Hospital', *British Journal of Psychiatry* 170 (1997): 186–90; 186.
4 W. Hewer et al., 'Mortality Among Patients in Psychiatric Hospitals in Germany', *Acta Psychiatrica Scandinavica* 91 (1995): 174–9; 174.
5 M. Valenti et al., 'Mortality in Psychiatric Hospital Patients', *International Journal of Epidemiology* 26 (1997): 1227–35; 1227.
6 This assessment is based on the author's work on Indian mental hospitals throughout the nineteenth and twentieth centuries. The average percentage of 'criminal lunatics' reported for the 22 mental institutions in British India in 1924 amounted to 30 per cent.
7 Report 1930–32, 3.
8 The estimated mortality per 1,000 of the population (for all age groups) in British India, 1881–91, was 40.6 for males and 38.6 for females (39.6 for both sexes). This compared unfavourably to England and Wales (20.2 for males, 18.0 for females, 19.1 for both sexes). See W. S. Meyer et al., *Imperial Gazetteer of India*, vol. I (Oxford: Clarendon Press, 1909), 515. The 'recorded mean' of deaths per 1,000 in Bengal from 1881 to 1900 fluctuated between 18.8 and 36.6; the 'probable true normal rate' for 1888 to 1891 was estimated at 44.8. See ibid., 512.
9 Based on figures from the annual reports of the Board of Control. See A. W. B. Livesay, 'Decreasing Mortality and Eliminating Phthisis in Mental Hospitals', *British Medical Journal* 1, 3937 (1936): 1246–9; 1247. Michael refers to a death rate of 7.6 per cent in 1940 at the Denbigh Mental Hospital in Wales, remarking that the institution 'had prided itself on the very low rate of death amongst patients in comparison with other establishments'. See P. Michael, *Care and Treatment of the Mentally Ill in North Wales, 1800–2000* (Cardiff: University of Wales Press, 2003), 160.
10 G. K. Tokuhata and V. A. Stehman, 'Mortality in State Mental Hospitals of Michigan, *Public Health Reports* 73 (1958): 750–64.

11 Meyer et al., *Imperial Gazetteer of India*, 513.
12 Ibid.
13 Ibid.
14 Ibid.
15 M. W. M. Yeatts, *Census of India 1941*, vol. I (Simla: Government of India, 1943), Part 1, 51–2. The figures given are crude death rates (CMR) not age-adjusted, standardised mortality rates (SMR). See the debate in the *British Medical Journal* on the relative merit of crude and age-adjusted mortality rates in H. Tunstall-Pedoe, 'Crude rates, Without Standardisation for Age, are Always Misleading', *British Medical Journal* 317 (1998): 475–8 and T. Nakayama et al., 'Clinicians and Epidemiologists View Crude Death Rates Differently', *British Medical Journal* 318 (1999): 395.
16 Report 1924–26, 14–15.
17 Report 1939, 3.
18 Report 1924–26, 14–15. Population/sample sizes: For Dacca, 265 men, 40 women (1924); 276 men, 42 women (1925). For Berhampore, 540 men, 101 women (1924); 574 men, 96 women (1925).
19 For details on overall patient numbers at Ranchi at different periods, see chapter 2.
20 Report 1933–35, 5.
21 Obituary, *British Medical Journal* 5249 (1961): 459.
22 Report 1936, 5–6.
23 Ibid., 6.
24 O. Berkeley-Hill, *All Too Human* (London: Peter Davies, 1939), 244.
25 See Chapter 2 for further discussion of this aspect.
26 Report 1933–35, 9.
27 In 1935, '20 acres more were brought under cultivation for growing paddy'. Report 1933–35, 15.
28 Ibid.
29 Report 1938, 1.
30 Principal Causes of Death, in numbers, 1927–38.
   1927–29 (total of 115 deaths)
      Tuberculosis of the lungs (18)
      Debility (12)
      Pneumonia (10)
   1930–32 (total of 77 deaths)
      All other general diseases (23)
      Tuberculosis (lungs) (11)
      Pneumonia (8)
   1933–35 (total of 104 deaths)
      Pneumonia (no numbers provided)
      T.B. of Lungs (no numbers provided)
      Heart Failure (no numbers provided)
   1936–38 (total of 113 deaths)
      Tuberculosis of lungs (no numbers provided)
      Pneumonia and broncho-pneumonia (no numbers provided)
      General paralysis of insanes (no numbers provided)
   (The terms used in the above table are those provided in the relevant triennial reports.)
31 On the contemporary epidemiology of TB and the national TB programme in England, see J. M. Eyler, *Sir Arthur Newsholme and State Medicine* (Cambridge: Cambridge University Press, 1997). See also, F. Condrau and M. Worboys, eds, *Tuberculosis Then and Now* (London: McGill, 2010).

32 Livesay, 'Decreasing Mortality', 1248.
33 Report 1934, 4.
34 Ibid.
35 See for example, Report 1934, 4.
36 Livesay, 'Decreasing Mortality', 1248.
37 P. Stokes, 'Cancer Mortality in Mental Institutions (Correspondence)', *British Medical Journal* 3337 (1924): 1136.
38 Michael, *Care and Treatment*, 110. Number of deaths: 1914 (18), in 1918 (36).
39 Ibid., 140. No numbers or percentages are provided for this period.
40 Tokuhata and Stehman, 'Mortality in State Mental Hospitals', 760.
41 Hewer, 'Mortality in Patients'.
42 See, for example, A. Hardy and M. E. Magnello, 'Statistical Methods in Epidemiology', in A. Morabia, ed., *A History of Epidemiologic Methods and Concepts* (Basel: Birkhaeuser, 2004); J. R. Matthews, *Quantification and the Quest for Medical Certainty* (Princeton: Princeton University Press, 1995) and V. Farewell et al., '"A memorandum on the Present Position and Prospects of Medical Statistics and Epidemiology" by Major Greenwood', *Statistics in Medicine* 25 (2006): 2161–77.
43 ICD-10 was endorsed by the 43rd World Health Assembly in May 1990 and came into use in WHO Member States in 1994. On ICD see: World Health Organization, International Classification of Diseases (ICD). Online: http://www.who.int/classifications/icd/en/ (accessed 24 November 2010).
44 N. N., 'International List of Causes of Death', *British Medical Journal* 3447 (1927): 200.
45 Ibid.
46 *Manual of the International List of Causes of Death, as adapted for use in England and Wales, Scotland, and Northern Ireland* (London: His Majesty's Stationery Office, 1926).
47 N. N., 'International List', 200.
48 Ibid.
49 K. L. White, 'Contemporary Epidemiology', *International Journal of Epidemiology* 3 (1974): 295–303; 297.
50 See quote at beginning of this chapter. Quoted from WHO, *International Classification of Diseases: Manual of the international statistical classification of diseases, injuries and causes of death*. Ninth revision, vol. I (Geneva: World Health Organisation, 1977), ix, in B. C. K. Choi, *Journal of Epidemiology and Community Health* 56 (2002): 334–5 (335). M. Greenwood, *Medical Statistics from Graunt to Farr* (Cambridge: Cambridge University Press, 1948).
51 G. Risse, 'Cause of Death as a Historical Problem', *Continuity and Change* 12 (1997): 175–88; 175. See also S. Guha, 'The Importance of Social Intervention in England's Mortality Decline', *Social History of Medicine* 7 (1994): 89–113.
52 Risse, 'Cause of Death', 176.
53 Ibid.
54 For a recent reappraisal of the debate see: B. J. Harris, 'The Importance of Social Intervention in England's Mortality Decline', *Social History of Medicine* 13 (2004): 379–407.
55 Not included in Revision 4 of 1929, where 'other diseases of [particular anatomical location]' was used.
56 Report 1939, 4.
57 Report 1933, 8.
58 Ibid.
59 Ibid., 9.
60 Ibid.
61 Report 1924–26, 3.
62 For Dhunjibhoy see: Report 1924–26, 3. For Ainsworth see Letter of 7 June 1926, in Report 1925.

63 **Figure 3.9.** Percentage of infirmary patients admitted on account of malaria, by gender, 1927–1935

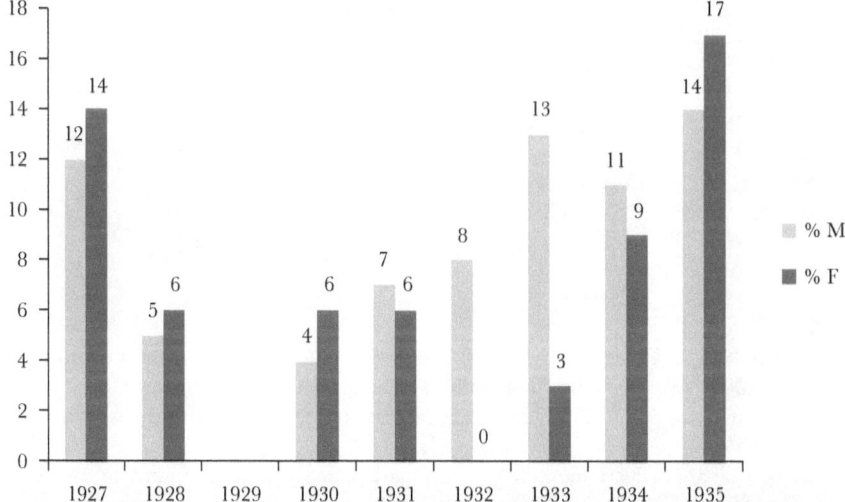

Note: No separate data for male and female patients for 1929 is available. The percentage for men and women combined is four per cent.

64 Report 1925, 6.
65 People in African countries were found to have reservations and fears about sleeping under mosquito nets. See C. A. Baume and M. C. Marin, 'Intra-household Mosquito Net Use in Ethiopia, Ghana, Mali, Nigeria, Senegal, and Zambia', *American Journal of Tropical Medicine and Hygiene* 77 (2007): 963–71; K. J. Njuna et al., 'Trial of Pyrethroid Impregnated Bednets in an Area of Tanzania Holoendemic for Malaria', *Acta Tropica* 49 (1991): 87–96; J. A. Alaii et al., 'Community Reactions to the Introduction of Permethrin-Treated Bed Nets for Malaria Control During a Randomized Controlled Trial in Western Kenya', *American Journal of Tropical Medicine and Hygiene* 68 (2003): 128–36.
66 **Figure 3.10.** Percentage of infirmary patients admitted on account of all other diseases of the respiratory system, by gender, 1927–1935

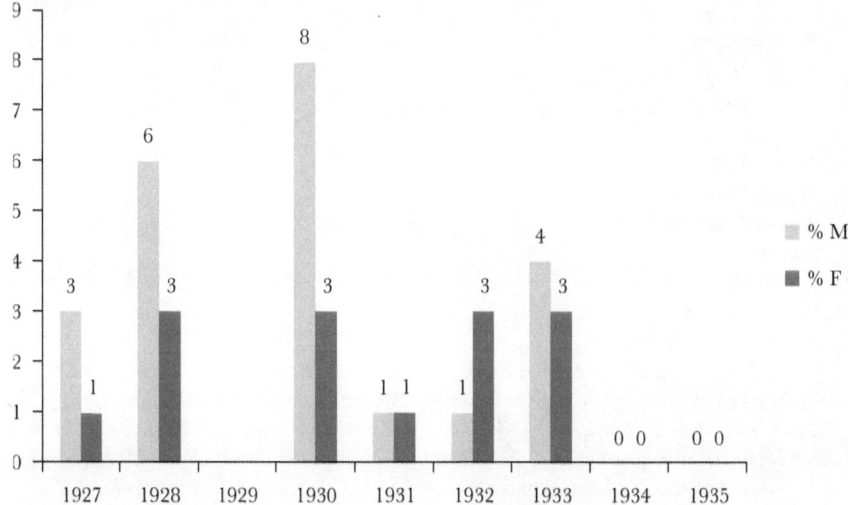

Note: No separate data for male and female patients for 1929 is available. The percentage for men and women combined is three per cent.

67 Report 1927–29, 4.
68 Ibid., 3.
69 Report 1930, 1.
70 Report 1934, 7.
71 Ibid., 4.
72 Report 1925, 2.
73 Report 1936, 14.
74 Michael, *Care and Treatment*, 139.
75 Report 1933, 9.
76 Report 1933–35, 5.
77 Ibid.
78 Report 1933–35, 10.
79 Ibid., 5.
80 Report 1928, 2. On hookworm, see J. Farley, *To Cast Out Disease* (Oxford: Oxford University Press, 2004), esp. 'The First Hookworm Campaigns, 1913–20', 61–74.
81 Hookworm first appeared in 1931 in the reports on illnesses; roundworm in 1933.
82 Report 1931, 6.
83 R. Peduzzi and U. C. Piffaretti, 'Ancylostoma Duodenale and the Saint Gothard Anaemia', *British Medical Journal* 287 (1983): 1942–45; 1942.
84 A. E. Boycott and J. S. Haldane, 'An Outbreak of Ankylostomiasis in England', *Journal of Hygiene* 3 (1903): 95–136. See also A. E. Boycott and J. S. Haldane, 'Ankylostomiasis', *Journal of Hygiene* 4 (1904): 73–111.
85 Farley, *To Cast Out*.
86 E. W. Hook and C. M. Marra, 'Acquired Syphilis in Adults', *New England Journal of Medicine* 327 (1992): 959–61.
87 Michael, *Care and Treatment*, 130.
88 Ibid.
89 Report 1927–29, 10.
90 Ibid.
91 Report 1931, 3.
92 Ibid..
93 Report 1928, 3.
94 Report 1927–29, 7.
95 Report 1934, 10.
96 Report 1927–29, 7.
97 Report 1928, 3, and almost all subsequent reports.
98 Report 1934, 10.
99 Report 1930–32, 14.
100 Report 1933, 12.
101 Report 1927–29, 7.
102 Report 1930, 8.
103 Report 1937, 10.
104 Report 1928, 4.
105 Report 1933–35, 10.
106 O. Anderson, *Suicide in Victorian and Edwardian England* (Oxford: Oxford University Press, 1987); M. MacDonald and T. R. Murphy, *Sleepless Souls* (Oxford: Oxford University Press, 1990); D. Wright and J. Weaver, eds, *Histories of Suicide* (Toronto: University of Toronto Press, 2009); H. Kushner, *Self-Destruction in the Promised Land* (New Brunswick: Rutgers University Press, 1989); J. Staples and T. Widger, eds, 'Special Issue: Ethnographies of Suicide', *Culture Medicine and Psychiatry* 35 (2012).
107 S. York, 'Alienists, Attendants and the Containment of Suicide in Public Lunatic Asylums', *Social History of Medicine* 25 (2012): 324–42. See also A. Shepherd and D. Wright, 'Madness,

Suicide and the Victorian Asylum', *Medical History* 46 (2002): 175–96. See for an exception, on Australia: J. Weaver and D. Wright, 'Suicide, Mental Illness, and Psychiatry in Queensland', *Health History* 11 (2009): 102–27.
108 Anderson, *Suicide*, 403; O. Anderson, 'Did Suicide Increase with Industrialization in Victorian England?', *Past and Present* 86 (1980): 149–73.
109 Shepherd and Wright, 'Madness, Suicide and the Victorian Asylum', 195, fig. 4.
110 Report 1934, 10.
111 Ibid.
112 Report 1930–32, 13.
113 Report 1934, 10.
114 Report 1926, 4.
115 Report 1933–35, 5.
116 Report 1933, 11; Report 1934, 10; Report 1938, 8.
117 Report 1939, 6; Report 1940, 8.
118 Shepherd and Wright, 'Madness, Suicide and the Victorian Asylum', 195; referring to Charlotte Mackenzie, *Psychiatry for the Rich* (London/New York: Routledge, 1992), 194. York, 'Alienists, Attendants and Containment of Suicide', 337 fully references Bethlem resident physician George Savage's report of 1884 of five per cent of patients being likely to make a suicide attempt, while between 20 to 30 per cent were registered as suicidal.
119 Shepherd and Wright, 'Madness, Suicide and the Victorian Asylum'; 194. This issue has now been explored further in York, 'Alienists, Attendants and Containment of Suicide'.
120 Report 1926, 5. The superintendent remarked that the 'staff concerned found negligent in these cases were suitably dealt with'.
121 Report 1933–35, 9.
122 Report 1940, 8.
123 Report 1937, 11.
124 Ibid.
125 It is likely that the term is used here in the colloquial sense of a businessperson. *Marwaris* originally came from Marwar, Rajasthan.
126 It is difficult to engage in retrospective diagnostics. A simple translation of the term would be 'depression' or 'involutional-onset depression'. The involutional years are supposed to be ages 50–65 for males and 40–55 for females. These age cohorts do however reflect the circumstances of life in relation to average life expectancies in Western countries at a particular historical period and are not necessarily applicable to different periods and contexts. See R. P. Brown et al., 'Involutional Melancholia Revisited', *American Journal of Psychiatry* 141 (1984): 24–8.
127 Report 1937, 11.
128 Shepherd and Wright, 'Madness, Suicide and the Victorian Asylum', 179.
129 Report 1937, 12.
130 M. Finnane, *Insanity and the Insane in Post-Famine Ireland* (London: Croom Helm, 1981), 13.
131 Report 1937, 12.
132 Report 1933, 4.
133 Ibid.
134 Report 1934, 4.
135 Report 1936, 3.
136 For example, see Report 1937, 3.
137 Report 1927–29, 2–3.
138 Michael, *Care and Treatment*, 155.
139 Report 1927–29, 3.
140 Although capacity on the male side had already been reached when the institution was opened, up until 1926 the shortfall of beds was not as drastic as in the following years.

In 1926 the maximum number of patients resident in the hospital was 1,172 males (for 1,014 places); in 1927 the figure was 1,197 and by 1929 1,274. See Report 1926, 1; 1927–29, 3.
141 Report 1927–29, 3.
142 Report 1931, 1.
143 Ibid., 2.
144 Ibid., 3.
145 Report 1933, 4.
146 Report 1938, 3.
147 Report 1939, 2.
148 A. Scull, *Madhouse* (New Haven: Yale University Press, 2005). For a critical and balanced appraisal of Scull's assessment of Cotton's work within the context of Cotton's time, see H. Freeman, 'Infectious Lunacy' (a review of *Madhouse*, by A. Scull), *Times Literary Supplement*, September 2005.
149 P. Greenacre, Threnton State Hospital Survey, 1924–26, unpublished manuscript, referred to in A. Scull and J. Schulkin, 'Psychobiology, Psychiatry, and Psychoanalysis', *Medical History* 53 (2009): 5–36; 25. Following 18 months of meticulous research, Phyllis Greenacre identified that the actual rate for New Jersey was in the 40 per cent range.
150 S. Cherry, *Mental Health Care in Modern England* (Woodbridge: Boydell Press, 2003), 214. See also Michael, *Care and Treatment*, 149.
151 Michael, *Care and Treatment*, 149.
152 Report 1938, 3.

Chapter 4   Classifications, Types of Disorders and Aetiology

1 On Kraepelin, see: E. J. Engstrom, 'Nachwort zur Selbstschilderung', in W. Burgmair et al., eds, *Emil Kraepelin* (Munich: Belleville, 2000), 73–97; V. Roelcke, 'Unterwegs zur Pyschiatrie als Wissenschaft', in E. J. Engstrom and V. Roelcke, eds, *Pyschiatrie im 19. Jahrhundert* (Basel: Schwabe, 2003), 169–88; V. Roelcke, 'Psychiatrische Diagnosen im Wandel', in H. Freytag et al., eds, *Psychotraumatologische Begutachtung* (Frankfurt: Fischer, 2011), 25–48.
2 J. Andrews et al., *The History of Bethlem* (London/New York: Routledge, 1997); S. Cherry, *Mental Health Care in Modern England* (Woodbridge: Boydell, 2003); J. Crammer, *The History of Buckinghamshire County Pauper Lunatic Asylum, St John's* (London: Gaskell, 1990); J. Gardner, *Sweet Bells Jangled Out of Tune* (Brighton: James Gardner, 1999); D. Gittens, *Madness in Its Place* (London/New York: Routledge, 1988); P. Michael, *Care and Treatment of the Mentally Ill in North Wales* (Cardiff: University of Wales Press, 2003), 121.
3 V. Hess and B. Majerus, 'Writing the History of Psychiatry in the 20th Century', *History of Psychiatry* 22 (2011): 139–45; 139.
4 Michael, *Care and Treatment*, 121.
5 Ibid., 122. The comparability of these data sets is likely to be restricted on account of possibly different calculation practices. For example, the Ranchi data include the number of those classified as 'recovered or not yet diagnosed'. It is not clear from the Denbigh data if the same was the case there.
6 At Ranchi, confusional insanity was assigned to two per cent of male and four per cent of female inmates in 1926.
7 M. Grotjahn, 'Zur psychiatrischen Systematik und Statistik', *Allgemeine Zeitschrift für Psychiatrie* 99 (1933): 464–80. See also A. Dörries and J. Vollmann, 'Medizinische und ethische Probleme der Klassifikation psychischer Störungen dargestellt am Beispiel des "Würzburger Schlüssels" von 1933', *Fortschritte der Neurologie–Psychiatry* 65 (1997): 550–54; T. Beddies and A. Dörries, eds, *Die Patienten der Wittenauer Heilstätten in Berlin* (Husum: Matthiesen, 2001).
8 For an appraisal of the German classification, see Dörries and Vollmann, *Klassifikation*
9 Madras Report 1931.

10 G. E. Berrios et al., 'Schizophrenia', *International Journal of Psychology and Psychological Therapy* 3 (2003): 111–40.
11 The year of adoption varied. In Madras the form was not used until 1935.
12 In 1926, for example, only 13 categories were applied with a frequency greater than one per cent. By 1933 the situation was much the same as before and, what is more, similar to the pattern established in the new form from 1934 onward, still only 13 categories were used for men and 11 for women at a frequency of more than one per cent.
13 Doerries and Vollmann, *Klassifikation*.
14 See on this issue: E. J. Engstrom, 'Die Ökonomie klinischer Inskription', in C. Borck and A. Schäfer, eds, *Psychographien* (Zürich: Diaphanes, 2005), 219–40; M. Weber and E. J. Engstrom, 'Kraepelin's Diagnostic Cards', *History of Psychiatry* 8 (1997):375–85.
15 Berrios et al., 'Schizophrenia', 115.
16 Ibid., 116.
17 Ibid., 112.
18 Ibid.
19 Ibid., 113.
20 Ibid., 135.
21 Ibid., 129.
22 V. Roelcke et al., eds, *International Relations in Psychiatry* (Rochester: University of Rochester Press 2010); R. Noll, *American Madness* (New Haven: Harvard University Press, 2011).
23 Berrios et al., 'Schizophrenia', 127.
24 R. Siegel, *Galen on Psychology, Psychopathology and Functions and Diseases of the Nervous System* (Basel: Karger, 1973), 273.
25 G. E. Berrios, 'Of Mania', *History of Psychiatry* 15 (2004): 105–24; 108. See also, G. E. Berrios, 'Historical Aspects of Psychoses', *British Medical Bulletin* 43 (1987): 484–98.
26 Berrios et al., 'Schizophrenia', 116.
27 K. Koehler and H. Sass, 'Der Maniebegriff seit Kraepelin', *Der Nervenarzt* 52 (1981):19–25; 19: The German phrase in the original article is 'verwirrende Vielfalt von Symptomen'.
28 Ibid., 19–25.
29 Ibid., 19.
30 Ibid. '[...] dass viele oder sogar die meisten der zwischen 1900 und 1920 in Deutschland als Manie diagnostizierten Psychosen heute [in einer Schneider-orientierten Sicht] als Schizophrenien angesehen wuerden'.
31 J. E. Dhunjibhoy, 'Correspondence', *Journal of Mental Science* 77 (1931): 294–7; 295.
32 Ibid.
33 Report 1927, 11.
34 The subcategories for toxic psychosis were acute confusional insanity; alcoholic psychosis; cannabis indica psychosis; of endocrine origin; in relation to child bearing; in relation to other constitutional disease. The subcategories for organic psychosis were general; cerebral syphilis; arteriopathic and senile psychosis; encephalitis; other cerebral lesions.
35 The frequency of mania attributions apparently increased in the case of new admissions towards the end of the period, with between five and 25 patients being diagnosed with mania. The numbers involved are too low to allow us to identify any particular trend.
36 G. E. Berrios, 'Melancholia and Depression During the 19th Century', *British Journal of Psychiatry* 153 (1988): 298–304; 301.
37 Ibid., 302.
38 There was much debate about the need to disaggregate the various strands of melancholia lumped together under the label. The issue was whether the conditions that are now referred to as major and minor depression (or severe and common mental disorder) respectively, ought to be differentiated. This controversy was sparked off in the mid-1920s by general practitioners rather than institution-based psychiatrists. See on 'minor depression': G. Parker et al., 'Issues

for DSM-5: Whither Melancholia? The Case for its Classification as a Distinct Mood Disorder', *American Journal of Psychiatry* 167 (2010): 745–7; R. E. Kendell, 'The Classification of Depressions', *British Journal of Psychiatry* 129 (1976): 15–28; J. Cole et al., 'The Classification of Depression', *British Journal of Psychiatry* 192 (2008): 83–5; A. V. Horwitz, 'Creating an Age of Depression', *Society and Mental Health* 1 (2011): 41–54.

39 For an excellent historical account of melancholia that deals with ancient and modern meanings, see Berrios, 'Melancholia and Depression'. See also G. E. Berrios, R. Porter, 'Mood Disorders', in G. E. Berrios and R. Porter, eds, *A History of Clinical Psychiatry* (London: Athlone, 1995), 384–408; 409–20. For histories on pre-modern European meanings, see J. Schmidt, *Melancholy and the Care of the Soul* (Aldershot: Ashgate, 2007); H. D. Midelfort, *A History of Madness in 16th Century Germany* (Stanford: Stanford University Press, 1999); S. W. Jackson, *Melancholia and Depression* (New Haven: Yale University Press, 1992); T. H. Jobe, 'Medical Theories of Melancholia in the Seventeenth and Early Eighteenth Centuries', *Clio Medica* 11 (1976): 217–32; J. Starobinski, *A History of the Treatment of Melancholy from the Earliest times to 1900* (Basel: Geigy, 1962).

40 R. E. Siegel, *Galen on Psychology, Psychopathology and Function and Diseases of the Nervous System* (Basel: Karger, 1973), 274.

41 On mental disorders within the Ayurvedic tradition, see G. J. Meulenbeld, *A History of Indian Medical Literature*, 5 vols (Groningen: Egbert Forsten, 1999–2000).

42 Schmidt, *Melancholy and Care*, 1.

43 Starobinski, *Treatment of Melancholy*, 43.

44 R. Burton, *The Anatomy of Melancholy* (New York: AMS Press, 1973 [1621]), 456.

45 J. E. Esquirol, 'Melancolie', *Dictionnaire des Sciences Medicales* (Paris: Panckoucke, 1820), 148.

46 Esquirol suggested an alternative term: 'lypemania'. This came to be used in France and Spain, but not in any of the other northern European countries. See Berrios, 'Melancholia and Depression', 300–301.

47 Quoted in Berrios, 'Melancholia and Depression', 300.

48 S. W. Jackson, 'Melancholia and Partial Insanity', *Journal of the History of the Behavioral Sciences* 19 (1983): 173–84.

49 D. Healy, *The Antidepressant Era* (Cambridge, MA: Harvard University Press, 1997), 30.

50 Kendell, 'The Classification of Depressions', 16–17; Cole et al., 'The Classification of Depression', 83–5; Horwitz, 'Creating an Age of Depression'.

51 R. Hayward, 'Germany and the Making of "English" Psychiatry', in V. Roelcke et al., eds, *International Relations in Psychiatry* (Rochester: University of Rochester Press, 2010), 67–90; 67.

52 Quoted in Hayward, 'English' Psychiatry, 68.

53 Hayward mentions a similar phenomenon in regard to Jewish refugees working at the Maudsley who mixed British and German approaches. See Ibid., 80.

54 Subtypes: agitated, stuporous, hypochondriacal, associated with pregnancy, associated with parturition and lactation (puerperal), associated with old age, other forms.

55 An extra 30 patients can be accounted for in this way. Ten men and one woman from the agitated melancholia and one puerperal case as well as seven cases related to pregnancy and five men and six women suffering from melancholia associated with old age were integrated into the single melancholia group in 1934.

56 Kraepelin 1921, quoted in Berrios et al., 'Schizophrenia', 133.

57 Dhunjibhoy, 'Correspondence'.

58 G. Agich, 'Evaluative Judgment and Personality Disorder', in J. Z. Sadler et al., eds, *Philosophical Perspectives on Psychiatric Diagnostic Classification* (Baltimore: Johns Hopkins University Press, 1994), 233–45.

59 Based on J. E. Dhunjibhoy, 'A Brief *Resume* of the Types of Insanity Commonly Met with in India, with a Full Description of "Indian Hemp Insanity" Peculiar to the Country', *Journal of Mental Science* 76 (1930): 254–64; 255–7.

60 Berrios, 'Historical Aspects of Psychoses', 489.

61 Hayward, '"English" Psychiatry', 80.
62 The apparent sudden rise in the percentage rate for mania from 1933 to 1934, on occasion of the change of nomenclature, is an artefact of classification. The figures provided here for mania from 1925 to 1933 refer only to those cases subsumed under 'mania, other forms' and exclude the figures for mania associated with pregnancy; parturition and lactation; epilepsy; old age.
63 A. Lewis, 'Paranoia and Paranoid', *Psychological Medicine* 1 (1970): 2–12; K. Kendler, 'Delusional Disorder', in Berrios and Porter, *Clinical Psychiatry*, 360–71; I. Dowbiggin, 'Delusional Disorder', in Berrios and Porter, *Clinical Psychiatry*, 372–83.
64 Berrios, 'Historical Aspects of Psychoses'.
65 G. E. Berrios, personal communication, 23 August 2012.
66 Berrios, 'Historical Aspects of Psychoses'.
67 Kendler, 'Delusional Disorder', 363.
68 Kraepelin 1916, quoted in Ibid., 366.
69 Kraepelin 1907, quoted in Ibid., 364.
70 Ibid., 365.
71 Lewis, 'Paranoia and Paranoid', 5.
72 A. W. Overbeck-Wright, *Lunacy in India* (London: Bailliere, Tindall and Cox, 1921), 183.
73 H. Yellowlees, 'Obituary. Lewis Campbell Bruce', *British Journal of Psychiatry* 92 (1946): 857–9; 857.
74 Ibid., 585.
75 Ibid.
76 Overbeck-Wright, *Lunacy*, 183.
77 Based on Kraepelin's revised textbook of 1899.
78 Overbeck-Wright, *Lunacy*, 225.
79 Ibid.
80 Ibid.
81 G. E. Berrios, 'The Insanities of the Third Age: A Conceptual History of Paraphrenia', *Journal of Nutrition, Health and Aging* 7 (2003): 394–9.
82 Lewis, 'Paranoia and Paranoid', 4.
83 Ibid.
84 Ibid., 5.
85 Berrios, 'The Insanities of the Third Age', 397.
86 Dhunjibhoy, 'Indian Hemp Insanity', 257.
87 Ibid., 256.
88 Berrios, 'Paraphrenia', 396.
89 Berrios makes this suggestion in regard to dementia and delirium. See G. E. Berrios, 'Dementia During the Seventeenth and Eighteenth Centuries', *Psychological Medicine* 17 (1987): 829–37, 830; G. E. Berrios, 'Delirium and Confusion in the 19th Century', *British Journal of Psychiatry* 139 (1981): 439–49; D. Adamis et al., 'A Brief Review of the History of Delirium as a Mental Disorder', *History of Psychiatry* 18 (2007): 459–69. Berrios and Adamis et al. discuss delirium and confusion alongside each other.
90 Berrios, 'Dementia', 830, 836 and Adamis, 'Delirium', 459.
91 Lindesay et al., 1990, quoted in Adamis, 'Delirium', 460.
92 Lipourlis, 1983, quoted in Adamis et al., 461.
93 Ibid., 464.
94 Berrios, 'Delirium and Confusion', 438.
95 Ibid.
96 Adamis, 'Delirium', 466–7.
97 Berrios, 'Dementia', 836.
98 Dhunjibhoy, 'Indian Hemp Insanity', 257.

99 Similar restrictions applied to 'arteriopathic and senile psychosis' (previously 'senile arterial disease'). See D. Rothschild, 'The Clinical Differentiation of Senile and Arteriosclerotic Psychoses', *American Journal of Psychiatry* 98 (1941): 324–33.
100 Subdivisions: from organic cerebral diseases other than syphilitic, from arterial disease, senile, from epilepsy, from injury, and, the most frequently assigned, secondary or terminal dementia.
101 Berrios, 'Dementia', 830.
102 *The Nomenclature of Diseases Drawn up by a Joint Committee Appointed by the Royal College of Physicians of London*, 5th ed. (London: Thuscott, 1918).
103 Then a subcategory of 'dementia (primary or secondary)'.
104 Adamis, 'Delirium', 459.
105 *Nomenclature*, 17.
106 There was one new admission in 1929, and six (five male, one female) in 1925, when the hospital received its patients from the three old institutions.
107 Berrios, 'Delirium and Confusion', 440.
108 Ibid., 446.
109 Dhunjibhoy, 'Indian Hemp Insanity', 256.
110 C. Webster, 'Healthy or Hungry Thirties?', *History Workshop* 13 (1982): 110–29.
111 Dhunjibhoy, 'Indian Hemp Insanity', 256.
112 Ibid.
113 N. Scheper-Hughes, 'The Madness of Hunger', *Culture, Medicine and Psychiatry* 12 (1988): 429–58.
114 Twentieth Annual Report of the Board of Control for the Year 1933, quoted in 'Mental Disorders in 1933', *British Medical Journal* (1934): 640–41; 641.
115 The David Lewis Cheshire Care Home now provides education, therapy and support also for people with autism and complex learning disabilities.
116 See, for example, M. Thomson, *The Problem of Mental Deficiency* (Oxford: Oxford University Press, 1998); D. Wright and A. Digby, eds, *From Idiocy to Mental Deficiency* (London: Routledge, 1996); J. Melling and P. Dale, eds, *Mental Illness and Learning Disability* (London: Routledge, 2006); M. Jackson, *The Borderland of Imbecility* (Manchester: Manchester University Press, 2000).
117 Mental Deficiency Act, 1913, chapter 28, part 1, 5–6.
118 Dhunjibhoy, 'Indian Hemp Insanity', 256.
119 Figures from Tokanui Mental Hospital in New Zealand also show a prevalence of less severely affected patients, with imbecility the most common classification (45 per cent). See A. Hoult, 'Institutional Responses to Mental Deficiency in New Zealand'. PhD diss., University of Waikato, 2007, 39.
120 R. Scheerenberger, *A History of Mental Retardation* (Baltimore: Brookes, 1983), quoted in R. L. Schalock et al., 'The Renaming of Mental Retardation, Intellectual and Developmental Disabilites' 45 (2007): 116–24; 119.
121 Hoult, 'New Zealand', 52.
122 Dhunjibhoy, 'Indian Hemp Insanity', 256.
123 E. J. Engstrom, 'Kraepelin', *History of Psychiatry* 2 (1991): 111–32; E. J. Engstrom, 'Introduction to Classic Text', *History of Psychiatry* 18 (2007): 389–404; H. Pols, 'Emil Kraepelin on Ethnic and Cultural Factors in Mental Illness', *Psychiatric Times*, 22 June 2011. Online: http://www.psychiatrictimes.com/emil-kraepelin-cultural-and-ethnic-factors-mental-illness (accessed 14 August 2013).
124 On the development of psychoanalysis, see note 36 of Chapter 1 of this volume.
125 N. N., 'Notes and News', *Journal of Mental Science* 76 (1930): 917–21; 917.
126 Ibid., 918.
127 Eric Stroemgren, in M. Shepherd, ed., *Psychiatrists on Psychiatry* (Cambridge: Cambridge University Press, 1982), 152–69; 155. See also A. C. Catagnini, 'Wimmer's Concept of Psychogenic Psychosis Revisited', *History of Psychiatry* 21 (2010): 54–66.

128 N. N., 'Notes and News', 920.
129 Ibid.
130 Mass movements such as the Non-Cooperation Movement (1920–22) and the Civil Disobedience Movement (1929–31) were particularly important in this context.
131 S. Akhtar, 'Four Culture-Bound Psychiatric Syndromes in India', *International Journal of Social Psychiatry* 34 (1988): 70–74.
132 Kakar quoted in C. Hartnack, *Psychoanalysis in Colonial India* (New Delhi: Oxford University Press, 2001), 145.
133 A. Avasthi, 'Indianizing Psychiatry', *Indian Journal of Psychiatry* 53 (2011): 111–20.
134 See the article that has been credited with bringing the syndrome to the attention of Western psychiatrists: N. N. Wig, 'Problems of Mental Health in India', *Journal of Clinical Society, Medical College, Lucknow* 17 (1960): 48–53. In a subsequent, co-authored article, Wig described the syndrome in a somewhat sensationalist and truly Saidian Orientalist fashion as a 'sex neurosis of the orient'. See H. K. Malhotra and N. N. Wig, 'Dhat Syndrome: a Culture Bound Sex Neurosis of the Orient', *Archives of Sexual Behavior* 4 (1975): 519–28. More recently, the status of Dhat as a culture-bound condition has been questioned. See, for example, A. Sumathipala et al., 'Culture-bound Syndromes', *British Journal of Psychiatry* 184 (2004): 200–209.
135 Dhunjibhoy, 'Indian Hemp Insanity', 257.
136 Waddell reported: 'In 1907, out of 5474 insanes in Indian asylums, in 602 the insanity was ascribed to hemp drugs, in 135 to alcohol, and only 31 to opium.' See L. A. Waddell, *Lyon's Medical Jurisprudence for India*, 7th ed. (Calcutta: Thacker, 1921), 355. During the 1960s, the reported rate (on admission) was 3.2 per cent. Of 39,001 admitted between January 1959 and December 1969, 1,248 patients were considered to suffer from cannabis psychosis. See L. P. Varma, 'Cannabis Psychosis', *Indian Journal of Psychiatry* 14 (1972): 241–55; 242.
137 Dhunjibhoy presented his paper at the 7th Congress of the Far Eastern Association for Tropical Medicine in Calcutta, in December 1927, and at the Quarterly Meeting of the Royal Medico-Psychological Association on 4 February 1930. See N. N., 'Notes and News', 365–6.
138 A recent example is N. Ahuja, *A Short Textbook of Psychiatry* (New Delhi: Jaypee Brothers, 2006). He wrongly holds that cannabis psychosis was 'first described by Dhunjibhoy in 1930'.
139 *Report of the Drugs Enquiry Committee 1930–31* (Calcutta: Government Press, 1931).
140 I. C. Chopra and R. N. Chopra, 'The Use of Cannabis Drugs in India, 1957'. Online: http://www.unodc.org/unodc/en/data-and-analysis/bulletin/bulletin_1957-01-01_1_page003.html (accessed 13 August 2012). R. N. Chopra was a member of the WHO expert advisory panel on addiction-producing drugs as well as director of the Drug Research Laboratory in Jammu and Kashmir.
141 See on this aspect, for example: D. Wujastyk, 'The Evolution of Indian Government Policy on Ayurveda in the Twentieth Century', in D. Wujastyk and F. M. Smith, eds, *Modern and Global Ayurveda* (New York: SUNY, 2008), 43–76.
142 Dhunjibhoy, 'Indian Hemp Insanity', 263.
143 On eugenics see A. Bashford and P. Levine, eds, *The Oxford Handbook of the History of Eugenics* (Oxford: Oxford University Press, 2010). As the contributions to this handbook show, eugenics was a transnational phenomenon that informed scientific research as well as policy across the political spectrum. It was not exclusively linked to the Holocaust.
144 James Mills has explored aspects of the earlier context. See J. H. Mills, *Madness, Cannabis and Colonialism* (Houndmills: Macmillan, 2000).
145 S. Nigam, 'Disciplining and Policing the "Criminals by Birth"', *Indian Economic and Social History Review* 27 (1990): 131–64; M. Radhakrishna, *Dishonoured by History* (Hyderabad: Orient Longman, 2001).
146 Dhunjibhoy, 'Indian Hemp Insanity', 262–3.

147 Ibid., 263.
148 Personal communication, 26 August 2012.
149 V. R. Thacore and S. R. P. Shukla, 'Cannabis Psychosis and Paranoid Schizophrenia', *Archives of General Psychiatry* 33 (1976): 383–6. See also: M. Arendt et al., 'Cannabis-Induced Psychosis and Subsequent Schizophrenia-Spectrum Disorders', *British Medical Journal* 187 (2005): 510–15; D. M. Fergusson et al., 'Cannabis and Psychosis', *British Medical Journal* 332 (2006): 172–5; G. Watts, 'Science Commentary: Cannabis Confusions', *British Medical Journal* 332 (2006): 175.
150 D. Basu et al., 'Cannabis Psychosis and Acute Schizophrenia', *European Journal of Addiction Research* 5 (1999): 71–3; 71.
151 Personal communication, 19 September 2012.
152 Dhunjibhoy, 'Indian Hemp Insanity', 262.
153 Ibid.
154 Personal communication, 19 September 2012.
155 I. C. Chopra and R. N. Chopra, 'The Use of the Cannabis Drugs in India'.
156 Dhunjibhoy, 'Indian Hemp Insanity', 261.
157 P. Chatterjee, *A Princely Impostor?* (Princeton: Princeton University Press, 2002).
158 Dhunjibhoy, 'Indian Hemp Insanity', 261.
159 Chatterjee, *Impostor*, 200.
160 Ibid., 199.
161 N. Chevers, *A Manual of Medical Jurisprudence* (Calcutta: Bengal Military Orphan Press, 1856), 534.
162 Mills, *Cannabis*.
163 Chevers, *Manual*, 534.
164 *Report of the Indian Hemp Drugs Commission, 1893–1899*, vol. I (Simla: Government Central Printing Office, 1894), 264.
165 Waddell, *Medical Jurisprudence*, 369–70.
166 *Report of the Indian Hemp Drugs Commission*, 264.
167 Chevers, *Manual*, 134.
168 Dhunjibhoy, 'Indian Hemp Insanity', 261.
169 Ibid., 260.
170 W. Ernst, *Mad Tales from the Raj* (London/New York: Routledge, 1991; London: Anthem Press, 2010), 121–43; D. Arnold, ed., *Warm Climates and Western Medicine* (London: Rodopi, 1996).
171 G. F. W. Ewens, *Insanity in India* (Calcutta: Thacker, 1908), 102–3.
172 Overbeck-Wright, *Lunacy*, 299.
173 Ibid.
174 Ibid., 300.
175 Ibid., 3.
176 Ibid.
177 Ibid., 4.
178 Dhunjibhoy, 'Indian Hemp Insanity', 257.
179 Ibid.
180 Ibid.
181 E. J. Fitzgerald, 'Syphilis and the Mental Treatment Act', *British Journal of Venereal Diseases* 10 (1934): 117–37.
182 'Notes and News', *Journal of Mental Science* 76, (April 1930): 360–70; 365. Dublin lunatic asylum or 'Dottyville' and its one-time superintendent Conolly Norman were immortalised in fiction by James Joyce in his *Ulysses*: 'That fellow I was with […] last night, said Buck Mulligan, says you have g.p.i. He's up in Dottyville with Conolly Norman. General paralysis of the insane.' On Conolly Norman, see the section on confusional insanity.
183 'Notes and News', 365.

184 Ibid., 366.
185 Max-Planck-Institut für Psychiatrie: Letters by Silla Dhunjibhoy and J. E. Dhunjibhoy, September 1926, MPIP-HA: K24/1.
186 E. Shorter, *A Historical Dictionary of Psychiatry* (New York: Oxford University Press, 2005), 65.
187 Report 1927–29, 8.
188 Report 1927–29, 10.
189 Ibid., 28–30.
190 Report 1930, 40; Report 1931, 40; Report 1933, 42; Report 1934, 34. Statement on 'Aetiological Factors and Associated Conditions in the Patients Admitted'.
191 Report 1933, 36–7.
192 Resolution, 17.12.1930, para. 2, Report 1927–29.
193 Hartnack, *Psychoanalysis*, 36; O. Berkeley-Hill, 'A Wassermann Survey of the Inmates of the Ranchi European Lunatic Asylum', *The Indian Medical Gazette* 36 (1921): 89–94.
194 From 24 March 1935 to 31 December 1935.
195 Report 1933–35, 12.
196 Ibid.
197 E. M. Brown, 'Why Wagner-Jauregg Won the Nobel Prize for Discovering Malaria Therapy for General Paresis of the Insane', *History of Psychiatry* 11 (2000): 371–82; 379.
198 'Such contrasting results were reported by the early investigators that the 26 papers appearing before 1930 are not considered here. Since 1930, 11 publications have appeared, 10 of which state that malaria causes a false positive reaction for syphilis.' See F. Babin and A. D. Dulaney, 'Complement Fixation in Malaria and Syphilis', *American Journal of Epidemiology* 42 (1945): 167–73; 167.
199 Fitzgerald, *Syphilis*. Fitzgerald used the data discussed by E. T. Burke, *Scourges of To-day* (London: Faber/Gwyer, 1926).
200 W. Noyes, 'Review of *Acute Confusional Insanity* by Conally Norman', *American Journal of Psychology* 4 (1891): 326–8.
201 T. V. Sekher and N. Hatti, eds, *Unwanted Daughters* (Jaipur: Rawat, 2010); T. V. Sekher, 'Rural Demography of India', in L. J. Kulcsár and K. Curtis, eds, *International Handbook on Rural Demography* (Dordrecht: Springer, 2012), 169–89.
202 Dhunjibhoy, 'Indian Hemp Insanity', 256.
203 Ewens, *Insanity*, 111.
204 Meynert had 'added the psychosis occurring during physical exhaustion caused by loss of blood, lactation, or delivery', and Ewens referred to his category. Meynert 1890, referred to in M. Lanczik et al., 'Are Severe Psychiatric Disorders in Childbed of Endogenous or Organic Nature?', *Archives of Women's Mental Health* 9 (2006): 293; Dhunjibhoy, 'Indian Hemp Insanity', 299; 297.
205 Overbeck-Wright, *Lunacy*, 184.
206 Ibid., 206.
207 Ibid., 244.
208 Quoted in Varma, 'Cannabis Psychosis', 170.
209 Dhunjibhoy, 'Indian Hemp Insanity', 263; Chevers, *Manual*; Ewens, *Insanity*; Overbeck-Wright, *Lunacy*.
210 L. P. Varma, 'Cannabis Psychosis', *Indian Journal of Psychiatry* 14 (1972): 241–55; 243.
211 Ewens, *Insanity*, 31.
212 Overbeck-Wright, *Lunacy*, 265.
213 Varma, 'Cannabis Psychosis', 243.
214 Ewens, *Insanity*, 23.
215 Ibid., 128.
216 Overbeck-Wright, *Lunacy*, 131.
217 Dhunjibhoy, 'Indian Hemp Insanity', 256.
218 Ibid.

219 Overbeck-Wright, *Lunacy*, 131, 274.
220 W. Ernst, 'Alcohol in India', paper presented at the conference Under Control? Alcohol and Drug Regulation, Past and Present, London School of Hygiene and Tropical Medicine, London, 2013.
221 R. Porter, 'Epilepsy', in Berrios and Porter, *Clinical Psychiatry*, 164–92.
222 G. E. Berrios, 'Epilepsy', in Berrios and Porter, *Clinical Psychiatry*, 147–63.
223 E. Hare, 'The History of "Nervous Disorders" from 1600 to 1840, and a Comparison with Modern Views', *British Journal of Psychiatry* 159 (1991): 37–45.
224 *Saraa* in Arabic, meaning 'being knocked down'.
225 O. Somasundaram, 'Seizure Disorders', *Indian Journal of Psychiatry* 43 (2001): 12–15; B. V. Manyam, 'Epilepsy in Ancient India', *Epilepsia* 33 (1992): 473–5; S. W. Akhtar and H. Aziz, 'Perception of Epilepsy in Muslim History', *Neurology Asia* 9, Supplement 1 (2004): 59–60.
226 G. J. Meulenbeld, *A History of Indian Medical Literature*, 5 vols (Groningen: Egbert Forsten, 1999–2002); D. Wujastyk, *The Roots of Ayurveda* (New Delhi: Penguin, 1998); K. Zysk, *Religious Medicine* (New Brunswick: Transaction, 1993); F. Zimmermann, *The Jungle and the Aroma of Meats* (Berkeley: University of California Press, 1987).
227 For an exploration of the varied understandings of *apasmara* in different ayurvedic treatises, see H. Fabrega, *History of Mental Illness in India* (Delhi: Motilal Banarsidass, 2009).
228 Berrios, 'Epilepsy', 155–6.
229 Ewens, *Insanity*, 142.
230 Ibid., 150.
231 Ibid., 146.
232 Ibid.
233 Overbeck-Wright, *Lunacy*, 294.
234 Ibid., 295.
235 Ibid., 5.
236 Ewens, *Insanity*, 145.
237 Overbeck-Wright followed Bruce's approach. He pointed out that 'as to the nature of the toxine [*sic*], this is still a matter of conjecture'. See Overbeck-Wright, *Lunacy*, 288–9. His suggestions were uric acid poisoning (following Haig) and irritation by carbamate of ammonia (in line with Krainsky).
238 Ibid., 5.
239 Berrios, 'Epilepsy', 147.
240 M. Thomson, 'Though Ever the Subject of Psychological Medicine', in G. E. Berrios and H. Freeman, eds, *150 Years of British Psychiatry, ii, The Aftermath* (London: Athlone, 1996).
241 For India, see: S. P. Saha et al., 'A Prospective Incidence Study of Epilepsy in a Rural Community of West-Bengal', *Neurology Asia* 13 (2008): 41–8; R. Sridharan and B. N. Murthy, 'Prevalence and Pattern of Epilepsy in India', *Epilepsia* 40 (1999): 631–6.
242 P. N. Banerjee and W. A. Hauser, 'Incidence and Prevalence', in J. Engel and T. A. Pedley et al., eds, *Epilepsy* (Philadelphia: Wolters Kluwer, 2008), 45–56; 47.
243 Dhunjibhoy, 'Indian Hemp Insanity', 257.
244 J. D. McHugh and N. Delanty, 'Epidemiology and Classification of Epilepsy', *International Review of Neurobiology* 83 (2008): 11–26; 11.
245 K. S. 'Mani, Epidemiology of Epilepsy in Karnataka', *Neuroscience Today* 1 (1997): 167–74
246 Sridharan and Murthy, 'Prevalence and Pattern', 166. See also N. E. Bharucha, 'Epidemiology of Epilepsy in India', *Epilepsia* 44 (2003): 9–11.
247 S. Baviskar et al., 'Gender Disparities in Health Seeking Behaviour of Epilepsy Patients in Tertiary Care Facility of Rural Karnataka', *Current Neurobiology* 2 (2011): 113–16; 113. On the use of traditional healers see also: D. K. Pal et al., 'Help-seeking Patterns for Children with Epilepsy in Rural India', *Epilepsia* 43 (2002): 904–11.

248 International League Against Epilepsy, 'History: Epilepsy is still a Puzzle'. Online: http://www.ilae.org/ (accessed 5 October 2012).
249 J. Radden, 'From Melancholic States to Clinical Depression', in J. Radden, ed., *The Nature of Melancholy from Aristotle to Kristeva* (Oxford: Oxford University Press, 2000), 3–51; J. Schiesari, *The Gendering of Melancholia* (Ithaca: Cornell University Press, 1992).
250 L. Hock, 'Women and Melancholy in Nineteenth-Century German Psychiatry', *History of Psychiatry* 22 (2011): 448–64; 449.
251 B. V. Davar, 'Mental Illness Among Indian Women', *Economic and Political Weekly* 30 (1995): 2879–86; 2879.
252 Ibid., 2880.
253 Dhunjibhoy, 'Indian Hemp Insanity', 255.
254 Ewens, *Insanity*, 59.
255 Ibid., 60.
256 Ibid., 61.
257 G. Asha, 'Review of *Mental Health of Indian Women* by B. V. Davar', *Journal of International Women's Studies* 3 (2001): 281–7; 282.
258 Ewens, *Insanity*, 61.
259 Report 1927–28, 8.
260 Ewens, *Insanity*, 68.
261 Ibid., 67–8.
262 Ibid., 68.
263 On the difficulty of comparing data from different institutions, see W. Ernst, 'The Limits of Comparison', *History of Psychiatry* 23 (2012): 404–18.
264 Report 1928, 1.
265 **Figure 4.8.** Percentage of men (lower graph) and women (upper graph), resident at end of year, assigned the diagnosis dementia praecox/schizophrenia, including dementia praecox, 1925–1939

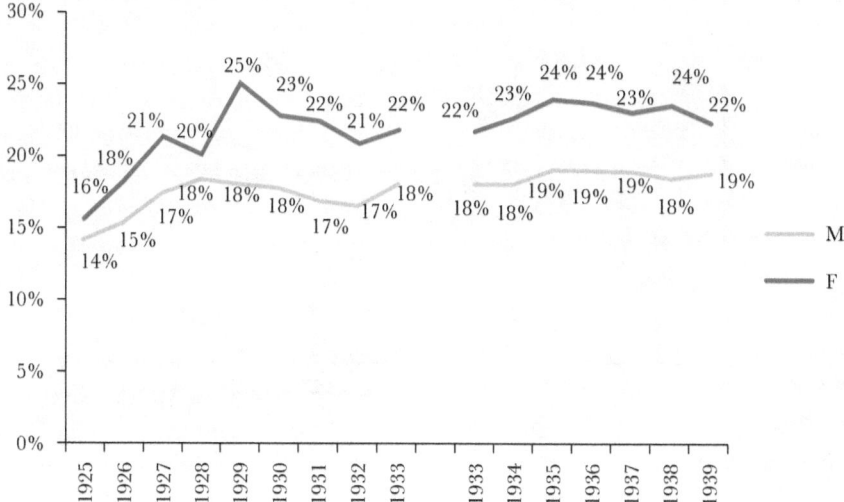

266 Ewens, *Insanity*, 157.
267 Ibid., 156.
268 Ibid., 161.
269 Ibid., 150.
270 Ibid.

271 **Figure 4.9.** Percentage of men (upper graph) and women (lower graph), resident at end of year, assigned the diagnosis delusional insanity (acute or chronic)/paranoia and paranoid states, 1925–1939

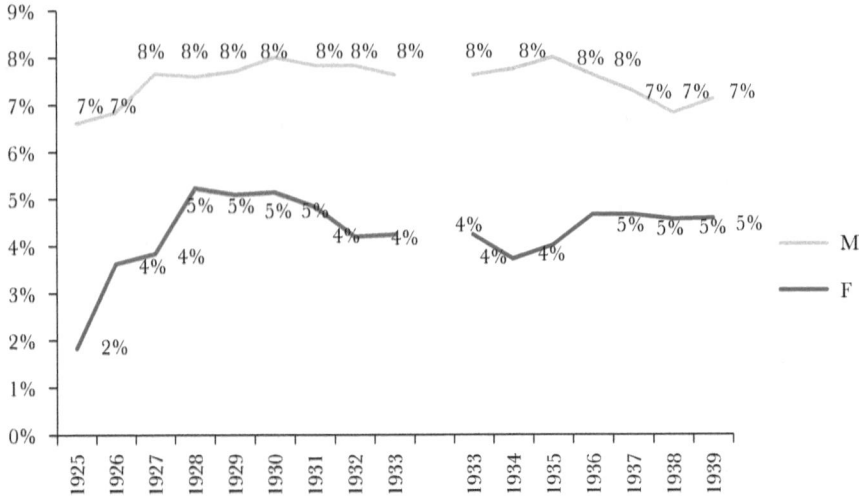

272 Overbeck-Wright, *Lunacy*, 225–6. The figures referred to all Indian lunatic asylums in 1913.
273 Ibid., 225.
274 **Figure 4.10.** Percentage of men (lower graph) and women (upper graph), resident at end of year, assigned the diagnosis circular insanity/manic depressive psychosis, 1925–1939

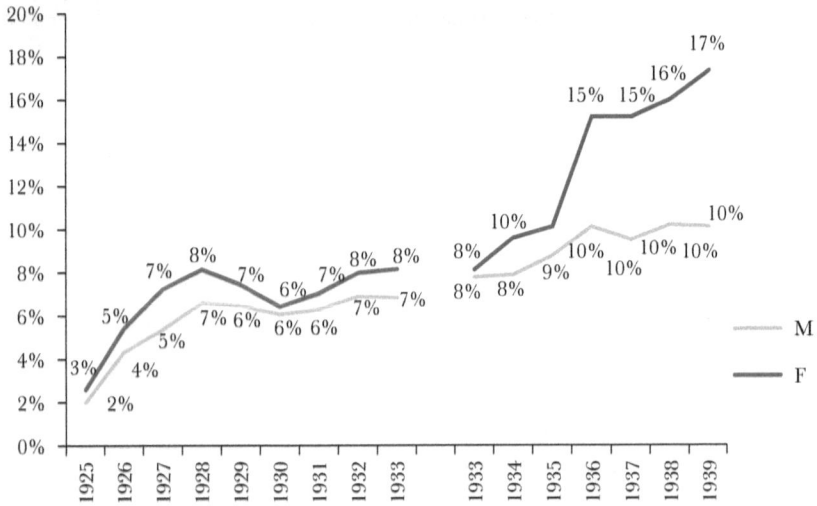

275 Ewens, *Insanity*, 214.
276 Ibid.
277 Ibid., 214–15.
278 Ibid., 247.
279 Overbeck-Wright objected to Kraepelin's classification but suggested that his description of katatonia, if contrasted to Kahlbaum's of 1874, was 'undoubtedly the more scientific of the two'. See Overbeck-Wright, *Lunacy*, 252–3.
280 Ranchi, 1933: 17 per cent for men, 13 per cent for women; 1939: 23 per cent for men, 28 per cent for women.

281 Report 1937, 9.
282 Ibid.
283 Ewens, *Insanity*, 19–20.
284 Ibid., 20.
285 Report 1937, 9.
286 Report 1930–32, 12.
287 C. A. Mercier (1852–1919), Consulting Physician for Mental Diseases, Charing Cross Hospital, and Past President of the Medico-Psychological Association. On Mercier, see the contemporary obituaries in *British Medical Journal* 2, 3063 (1919): 363–5.
288 Ewens, *Insanity*, 20.
289 On Bruce, see section on delusional insanity and paranoia, above.
290 Cited in Overbeck-Wright, *Lunacy*, 115.
291 Ibid.
292 Ewens, *Insanity*, 19.
293 D. Seitler, 'Queer Physiognomies', *Criticism* 46 (2004): 71–102; 79.
294 Overbeck-Wright, *Lunacy*, 116.
295 Ibid. (emphasis in the original).
296 Report 1930–32, 10.
297 Ibid. (emphasis in the original).
298 Ibid.
299 Ibid., 11.
300 Overbeck-Wright, *Lunacy*, 121.
301 Ibid.
302 Ibid., 118.
303 Ibid., 118–19.
304 Ibid., 119.
305 Report 1930–32, 11.
306 M. Thomson, 'Race, Culture and Mind in Britain', in W. Ernst and B. J. Harris, eds, *Race, Science and Medicine* (London: Routledge, 1999), 235–58.
307 Report 1930–32, 11.
308 Ibid., 12.
309 Ibid.
310 Ibid., iii.
311 Ibid., v.
312 Ibid.
313 Report 1937, 9.
314 Ibid., 10.
315 Ibid.
316 Ibid., 9.
317 Ewens, *Insanity*, 20.
318 Report 1930–23, 10.
319 Ibid.
320 Ewens, *Insanity*, 19.
321 Overbeck-Wright, *Lunacy*, 117.
322 Ibid., 124.
323 Report 1925, 21.
324 Report 1931, 8.
325 Overbeck-Wright, *Lunacy*, 114.
326 Ibid.
327 Ibid.
328 On Daktari medicine see P. B. Mukharji, *Nationalizing the Body* (London: Anthem Press, 2009).
329 Ewens, *Insanity*, 21.

330 Ibid., 22.
331 Overbeck-Wright, *Lunacy*, 118.
332 Even Overbeck-Wright had conceded that the nine per cent reported by him for 1913 were a 'very much lower proportion than has been previously expounded, and the greater figures previously quoted were probably due to individual provinces being taken as the basis of calculations instead of all India'. See Overbeck-Wright, *Lunacy*, 118.
333 Ibid.
334 Report 1940, 8.
335 Report 1931, 8. Report 1930–32, 10.
336 Overbeck-Wright, *Lunacy*, 117 (emphasis in the original in bold).
337 Ibid.
338 Ibid., 117–18.
339 Ibid., 118 (emphasis in the original in bold).
340 Ibid. (emphasis in the original in bold).
341 Report 1930–32, 12.
342 Ibid.

Chapter 5   Treatments

1 Report 1930–32, 14.
2 Report 1936, 24.
3 There were also journals relevant to Indian practitioners, such as the *Indian Medical Gazette* (from 1927), the *Antiseptic: A Monthly Medical Journal – Madras* (1927), and the *Calcutta Medical Journal* (1935). There is clear evidence that Dhunjibhoy actually read the literature and did not simply display it in the book cabinet. For example, in 1938 he provided a discussion of the failure of 'antirabic vaccine in the treatment of Epilepsy', referring to the relevant literature, as discussed, for example, in the *American Journal of Psychiatry*.
   Report 1937, 10 and 28 (in reference to the *British Medical Journal*, 1937, and Typhoid Bacilli)
4 Report 1934, 11.
5 Report 1936, 12.
6 Report 1933, 12.
7 Ibid., 12–13.
8 Report 1936, 25.
9 Ibid., 11–12.
10 Ibid., 12.
11 Ibid.
12 R. Hiltunem and Y. Holm, eds, *Basil: The Genus Ocimum* (Amsterdam: Taylor and Francis, 2005).
13 Report 1936, 8.
14 Report 1933–35, 11.
15 Ibid.
16 Ibid.
17 Report 1936, 11.
18 Dhunjibhoy had done so also in regard to basil, when he used an adulterated version of the Sindhi term. This can be explained by the fact that Dhunjibhoy came from Bombay province.
19 S. P. K. Gupta, 'Rustom Jal Vakil (1911–1974)', *Journal, Indian Academy of Clinical Medicine* 3 (2002): 100–104; 101. See also W. Sneader, *Drug Discovery* (Chichester: John Wiley, 2005).
20 M. M. G. Sen, 'The Scientific Basis of Ayurveda', in *Lectures of M. M. Gananatha Sen Saraswati* (Varanasi: Chowkhamba Sanskrity, 2002), 2.
21 G. Sen and K. Bose, 'Rauwolfia Serpentine, A New Indian Drug for Insanity and Blood Pressure', *Indian Medicine World* 2 (1931): 194; quoted in Gupta, 'Vakil', 102.

22 R. N. Chopra et al., 'The Pharmacological Action of an Alkaloid Obtained from Rauwolfia Serpentina Benth', *Indian Journal of Medical Research* 21 (1933): 261–71.
23 Gupta, 'Vakil', 101.
24 Gupta indicates that Chopra's team may have 'lacked the required analytical methods, devices and tools'. Chopra was a Cambridge-trained pharmacologist. Arguably, he may also have lacked the specialist expertise of experienced Ayurvedic practitioners, such as those harnessed by M. M. G. Sen. See G. Sen and K. Bose 'Rauwolfia Serpentine' and Gupta, 'Vakil', 102.
25 Report 1936, 11.
26 S. Isharwal and S. Gupta, 'Rustom Jal Vakil', *Texas Heart Institute Journal* 33 (2006): 161–71.
27 N. S. Kline, 'Use of Rauwolfia serpentina Benth in Neuropsychiatric Conditions', *Annuals New York Academy of Science* 59 (1954): 107–32; R. N. Noce et al., 'Reserpine (Serpasil) in the Management of the Mentally Ill and Mentally Retarded', *Journal of the American Medical Association* 156 (1954): 821–4.
28 G.W. Christison et al., 'When Symptoms Persist', *Schizophrenia Bulletin* 17 (1991):217–45; M. J. Aminoff, 'Pharmacologic Management of Parkinsonism and Other Movement Disorders', in: B. G. Katzung, ed., *Basic and Clinical Pharmacology*, 9th ed. (Singapore: McGraw-Hill, 2004), 447–6.
29 Report 1933–35, 2.
30 G. Windholz and L. H. Witherspoon, 'Sleep as Cure for Schizophrenia', *History of Psychiatry* 4 (1993): 83–93; F. López-Muñoz et al., 'The History of Barbiturates a Century after Their Clinical Introduction', *Neuropsychiatric Disease and Treatment* 1 (2005): 329–43.
31 Report 1933, 12.
32 Ibid.
33 Report 1928, 5. Its application to post encephalitis lethargica cases was also reported. The following year Dhunjibhoy noted that 'the results were not discouraging'. See Report 1929, 8.
34 Dhunjibhoy's use of generic and brand names is inconsistent. He also sometimes used both –al and –ol variations, such as Luminal and Luminol. It is difficult to say if these are printing errors or indicate different formulations or derivatives of the same drug.
35 López-Muñoz et al., 'History of Barbituates', 332.
36 Report 1930, 11.
37 Ibid. Dhunjibhoy's method differed from Klaesi's. He gave 'heroic doses of Sodium Luminal gr XII per day [...] by mouth or by deep intramuscular injections in the buttock'. This was continued for over a fortnight.
38 Ibid.
39 Report 1932, 14.
40 Report 1937, 14.
41 Ibid., 15.
42 Ibid.
43 Report 1938, 11. Dhunjibhoy suggested that this may be due to 'overdosage or idiosyncrasy of the drug'.
44 Ibid. As 'the best antidote' he suggested 'strychnine in doses as high as one-tenth grain hypodermically and prolonged artificial respiration'. He noted that 'The paraldehyde dose should be one dramme per stone of patient's total body weight and our experience has taught us to give always two drammes less than the total dose of the body weight.'
45 Report 1937, 15.
46 H. Weese and W. Scharpf, 'Evipan, ein neuartiges Einschlafmittel', *Deutsche Medizinische Wochenschrift* 58 (1932): 1205–7. Windholz and Witherspoon, 'Sleep as Cure'.
47 Report 1936, 11.
48 Ibid.
49 Report 1928, 5.
50 Report 1929, 8.
51 Report 1930–32, 16.

52 Report 1938, 10.
53 I. Finkleman et al., 'Rabies Vaccine in the Treatment of Epilepsy', *American Journal of Psychiatry* 94 (1938): 1363–8.
54 C. Perris, 'Leonhard and the Cycloid Psychoses', in G. E. Berrios and R. Porter, eds, *A History of Clinical Psychiatry* (London: Athlone, 1995), 421–32.
55 Report 1938, 10.
56 Report 1932–35, 13.
57 Ibid.
58 Ibid.
59 Report 1936, 12.
60 E. A Strecker et al., 'Hermatoporphyrin as a Therapeutic Agent in the Psychoses', *American Journal of Psychiatry* 90 (1934): 1157–73.
61 Ibid., 1157.
62 Report 1937, 14.
63 Ibid.
64 M. Borell, 'Brown-Sequard's Organotherapy and its Appearance in America at the End of the Nineteenth Century', *Bulletin of the History of Medicine* 50, 3 (1976): 309–20; 309–10.
65 Ibid., 313.
66 J. B. Sheppard, 'Organotherapy', *Journal of the National Medical Association* 15 (1923): 31–3; 33.
67 Leonard Williams, cited in Sheppard, 'Organotherapy', 31.
68 Kraepelin 1919, cited in R. Noll, 'Kraepelin's "Lost Biological Psychiatry"?', *History of Psychiatry* 18 (2007): 301–20; 311.
69 Report 1928, 5.
70 Reports 1933, 15; Report 1934, 13.
71 Report 1930–32, 16.
72 Report 1928, 5.
73 Report 1931, 12.
74 Ibid.
75 Report 1930–32, 16; Report 1933, 15.
76 Ibid.
77 Noll, 'Biological Psychiatry', 311.
78 Report 1928, 5.
79 Ibid.
80 Report 1937, 16.
81 Report 1936, 13.
82 Ibid.
83 Ibid.
84 Report 1931, 11.
85 Ibid.
86 Report 1933, 13.
87 Report 1930–32, 15.
88 Ibid., 16.
89 Ibid., 15.

Table 5.2. Results of experiments on 140 cases, with sulphur injections, 1930–1932

Number of patients	Type of mental diseases	Stationary or not improved	Improved	Recovered
62	Manic depressive psychosis	28	25	9
58	Dementia praecox	25	28	5
2	Paranoia & paranoid reactions	1	–	1

(Continued)

Number of patients	Type of mental diseases	Stationary or not improved	Improved	Recovered
3	Psycho-Neurosis	–	1	2
1	Dissiminated schlerosis [sic]	1	–	–
2	Encephalitis lethargica (Parkinsonian type)	2	–	–
4	Stupors	1	3	–
8	Epileptic insanity	8	–	–
Total		66	57	17

90 Report 1933, 13. For details on the European Mental Hospital and Berkeley-Hill see C. Hartnack, *Psychoanalysis in Colonial India* (Oxford: University Press, 2001) and A. R. Basu, 'The Birth of Psychology in India', in G. Mishra, ed., *Psychology and Psychoanalysis* (New Delhi: Centre for Studies in Civilizations, forthcoming).
91 Report 1934, 12.
92 Report 1937, 15.
93 Ibid.
94 Ibid.
95 Ibid.
96 For an excellent critical appraisal of the history of insulin coma therapy, see T. Walther, *Die 'Insulin-Koma-Behandlung'* (Berlin: Peter Lehmann Antipsychiatrieverlag, 2004). There is debate on whether Sakel's treatment ought to be described as 'shock' or 'coma' or 'convulsion' therapy; see for example: E. Shorter and D. Healy, *Shock Therapy*, (New Brunswick: Rutgers University Press, 2007), 13.
97 Report 1936, 25.
98 Nor did Dhunjibhoy practise leucotomy, which was developed by Egas Moniz in the mid-1930s. See Z. Kotowicz, 'Gottlieb Burckhardt and Egas Moniz', *Gesnerus* 62 (2005): 77–101.
99 Report 1939, 9.
100 Report 1937, 14.
101 Ibid.
102 Report 1936, 12. The spelling of names as given in the original source has been retained. Dhunjibhoy refers to Ladislaus von Meduna.
103 Report 1936, 13.
104 Ibid.
105 Ibid.
106 Report 1937, 13.

Table 5.3. Result of Cardiazol experiments in 42 cases of schizophrenia

No. of Cases	Types of Schizophrenia	Full remission	Improved	Stationary
15	Katatonic	7	4	4
17	Hebephrenic	5	9	3
8	Dementia Paranoides	1	2	5
2	Simple Dementia	–	–	2

107 Ibid., 14.
108 Ibid., 13.
109 Report 1938, 9.
110 Ibid.
111 Ibid.
112 Ibid., 10.
113 As Shorter and Healy have pointed out, there occurred in the US at this time a shift of focus from schizophrenia to depression and the view prevailed that 'insulin coma was to be reserved

for what everyone was calling "schizophrenia" and Metrazol should be used for affective disorders'. Shorter and Healy, *Shock Therapy*, 63.
114 M. Whitrow, 'Wagner-Jauregg and Fever Therapy', *Medical History* 34 (1990): 294–310. E. M. Brown, 'Why Wagner-Jauregg Won the Nobel Prize for Discovering Malaria Therapy for General Paresis of the Insane', *History of Psychiatry* 11 (2000): 371–82.
115 Report 1927–29, 8.
116 Ibid.
117 Report 1934, 14.
118 Ibid.
119 Ibid., 13.
120 Report 1934, 14.
121 Report 1933–35, 13.
122 Report 1936, 12.
123 Report 1937, 16.
124 Report 1939, 7–8.
125 Ibid., 9.
126 Ibid.
127 Ibid.
128 Ibid.
129 His colleague Berkeley-Hill, who led the neighbouring mental hospital for Europeans until 1933, was well-known for his psychoanalytic interests. However, Berkeley-Hill seems to have applied Cardiazol too and Hartnack points out that he 'was not enthusiastic about the use of psychoanalysis in a psychiatric institution'. Hartnack, *Psychoanalysis*, 36.
130 Shorter and Healy comment on the alarm caused by some treatments among the profession. See Shorter and Healy, *Shock Therapy*, 63.
131 Report 1940, 10.
132 Report 1939, 9.
133 Report 1927–29, 8.
134 Report 1934, 13.
135 Report 1930, 12.
136 Ibid.
137 Ibid., 13.
138 Report 1937, 16.
139 Dhunjibhoy omitted reference to the other key requisites of psychodynamic diagnostics and therapeutics: expertise and experience. Given that he had few opportunities to engage in psychoanalytic practice, it is likely that he was not able to build up a high level of professional competence in it.
140 Resolution, Government of Bihar and Orissa, 24.1.1931, Report 1927–29, 1–2.
141 Ibid., 1.
142 Report 1930, 13.
143 Ibid.
144 See, for example J. Bradley, 'Medicine on the Margins?', in W. Ernst, ed., *Plural Medicine, Tradition and Modernity* (London: Routledge, 2002), 19–39.
145 Report 1924–26, 5.
146 Ibid.
147 Report 1931, 10.
148 Report 1933, 16.
149 Ibid.,12.
150 Report 1938, 9.
151 Ibid. Immersion times fluctuated considerably, depending on the other treatments that were administered. In 1939, the 'average hours of immersion per patient were 97.5 hours'. Report 1939, 7.

152 Ibid.
153 Report 1939, 7.
154 Report 1940, 9.
155 Report 1938, 20.
156 Ibid., 20–21.
157 The founder of the Bratacharia Movement was G. S. (Gurusaday) Dutt (1882–1941), Secretary to the Government of Bengal in the Local Self-Government Department in 1938. In 1929, he founded the *Lok-nritya Samiti* (Folk Dance Society), and in 1931 the *Palli-sampad Rakshya Samiti* (Society for the Preservation of Rural Heritage) and the *Gram-mandali* (Village Association). The latter grew into the Bratachari Movement, founded in 1932. He also established the *Nikhil Bharat Lok Giti aur Lok Nritya Samiti* (All India Folk Song and Folk Dance Association) in 1932. He used popular rhymes and songs, attempting to preserve rural heritage and crafts. He started the *Saroj Nalini Nari Mangal Samiti* (Saroj Nalini Association for Women's Welfare), named after his wife, and *Bangalakshmi* magazine. He opened branches of the Bratachari Movement in Hyderabad, Mysore, Madras, Bengal and London. For details see Subodhchandra Sengupta and Anjali Basu, eds, *Samsad Bangali Charitabhidhan* (Calcutta: Shishu Shahitya Samsad, 2002), 135.
158 For a history of occupational therapy, see A. A. Wilcock, ed., *Occupation for Health*, vol. II (London: British Association and College of Occupational Therapists).
159 Report 1938, 20–21.
160 Report 1939, 20–21.
161 Report 1927, 5; Report 1925, 6–7.
162 Report 1931, 15 (emphasis in the original in bold).
163 Report 1932, 15.
164 Report 1931, 15 (emphasis in the original in bold).
165 Ibid. For Roman Catholics, Rev. Father G. Martin, S. J. , held regular services from 1931 onwards.
166 Report 1934, 17.
167 Report 1935, 17.
168 Report 1940, 13.
169 Report 1931, 10.
170 Report 1926, 5.
171 Ibid.
172 Ibid.
173 Ibid.
174 Ibid.
175 Ibid.
176 Report 1927, 4.
177 Ibid., 6.
178 Ibid.
179 Ibid., 40; total cost of medicines: Rs.3,782-3-6.
180 Ibid., 6.
181 Report 1928, 6.
182 Ibid.
183 Report 1933, 17.
184 Report 1929, 8.
185 Ibid., 11.
186 Ibid., 12. The annual cost per patient including Public Works Department charges (for water and electrical works) was calculated at Rs.606.
187 Report 1930, 9.
188 Report 1933, 17.
189 Ibid.

190 Ibid.
191 Ibid.
192 Report 1936, 9.
193 Report 1933, 18.
194 Ibid.
195 Report 1934, 14–15.
196 Ibid., 15.
197 Report 1936, 17.
198 Report 1933–35, 13.
199 Ibid., 14.
200 Ibid.
201 Ibid., 15.
202 Report 1936, 10.
203 Ibid., 9.
204 Report 1937, 12
205 Ibid.
206 Report 1939, 15.
207 Ibid.
208 Report 1926, 7.
209 Report 1924–26, 9.
210 Report 1925, 5.
211 The issue was clearly considered highly important, as is indicated by the presence of high-ranking officials such as the minister and secretary of the local self-government department, the inspector-general of civil hospitals of Bihar and Orissa, the secretaries of the finance and the education departments, the deputy director of agriculture and the chief engineer of roads and buildings. See Report 1924–26, 9.
212 W. Ernst, 'The Establishment of "Native Lunatic Asylums" in Early Nineteenth-Century British India', in J. Meulenbeld and D. Wujastyk, eds, *Studies on Indian Medical Traditions* (Groningen: Egbert Forsten, 1987; Delhi: Motilal, 2001), 169–204.
213 Report 1928, 8.
214 Report 1927, 5.
215 Report 1927–29, 8. For the following year, the reported average weight gain was 2 lb. for men and 0.85 lb. for women. See Report 1930, 9.
216 Report 1926, 7.
217 Report 1932, 19.
218 Report 1925, 6.
219 Ibid.
220 Ibid.
221 Report 1930, 9. See also Report 1929, 8.
222 Report 1938, 12.
223 Report 1937, 18.
224 Report 1925, 4.
225 Report 1926, 6.
226 Report 1929, 8.
227 Report 1926, 6.
228 Report 1929, 9.
229 Ibid.
230 Report 1925, 5. Libraries for patients and staff were common features from the early nineteenth century in mental hospitals in Western countries and in some institutions in British India.
231 Report 1926, 6.
232 Report 1927, 4.

233 Report 1929, 8.
234 Report 1928, 6.
235 Ibid.
236 Report 1933–35, 16.
237 Report 1926, 6.
238 Report 1933–35, 16.
239 Report 1926, 6.
240 Ibid.
241 Ibid.
242 Ibid.
243 Report 1927, 5.
244 Report 1929, 9.
245 Report 1927, 5.
246 Report 1931, 15; Report 1933, 18.
247 Report 1928, 7.
248 Report 1939, 14; Report 1940, 11.
249 Report 1937, 18.
250 Report 1928, 6.
251 Ibid.
252 Ibid., 7.
253 Ibid., 12.
254 Report 1930–32, 19.
255 Report 1928, 7.
256 Report 1936, 23. The Co-op had 335 members in 1936.
257 Report 1940, 11.
258 Report 1926, 6.
259 F. K. Prochaska, *The Voluntary Impulse* (London: Faber, 1988).

Conclusion

1 Report 1930–32, 14.
2 R. Dhunjibhoy, personal communication, 2009.
3 R. Dhunjibhoy, 2009.
4 Video of interview with R. Dhunjibhoy by Heinrich Böll Stiftung, The Green Political Foundation, 28 April 2011.
5 R. Dhunjibhoy, 2009.
6 Ibid.
7 Ibid.

BIBLIOGRAPHY

Archival Sources

British Library, London, Asia, Pacific and Africa Collections
  Annual and Triennial Reports of the Indian Mental Hospital, Ranchi, 1925–40.
  Annual Reports of the Mental Hospitals in the Madras Presidency, 1928–31.
Geheimes Staatsarchiv Preussischer Kulturbesitz, Berlin
  HA Rep 208 A Nr 96, 1, A. M. Vacha.
Max-Planck-Institut für Psychiatrie, Munich
  MPIP-HA: K24/1, Letters by Silla Dhunjibhoy and J. E. Dhunjibhoy, September 1926.

Published Primary Sources

Babin, Frances, and Anna Dean Dulaney. 'Complement Fixation in Malaria and Syphilis'. *American Journal of Epidemiology* 42 (1945): 167–73.
Berkeley-Hill, Owen. 'A Wassermann Survey of the Inmates of the Ranchi European Lunatic Asylum'. *Indian Medical Gazette* 36 (1921): 89–94.
_____. *All Too Human*. London: Peter Davies, 1939.
Boycott, A. E. and J. S. Haldane. 'An Outbreak of Ankylostomiasis in England'. *Journal of Hygiene* 3 (1903): 95–136.
_____. 'Ankylostomiasis'. *Journal of Hygiene* 1 (1904): 73–111.
Brock, A. J. 'Correspondence'. *British Medical Journal* 3535 (1928): 634–5.
Bulsara, Jal Feerose. *Parsi Charity Relief and Community Amelioration*. Bombay: Bulsara, 1935.
Burke, Edmund Tytler. *Scourges of To-day*. London: Faber/Gwyer, 1926.
Chevers, Norman. *A Manual of Medical Jurisprudence*. Calcutta: Bengal Military Orphan Press, 1856.
Chopra, R. N., J. C. Gupta and B. Mukerjee. 'The Pharmacological Action of an Alkaloid Obtained from Rauwolfia serpentina Benth'. *Indian Journal of Medical Research* 21 (1933): 261–71.
Darukhanawala, H. D. *Parsis and Sports*. Bombay: Darukhanawala, 1935.
Desai, Sapur Faredun. *A Community at the Crossroad*. Bombay: New Book, 1948.
Devine, H. 'Review'. *Journal of Mental Science* 70 (1924): 453–4.
Dhunjibhoy, J. E. 'Letters, Notes'. *British Medical Journal* 3555 (1929): 382.
_____. 'A Brief *Resume* of the Types of Insanity Commonly Met with in India, with a Full Description of "Indian Hemp Insanity" Peculiar to the Country'. *Journal of Mental Science* 76 (1930): 254–64.
_____. 'Correspondence'. *Journal of Mental Science* 77 (1931): 294–7.
Eager, Richard. 'Review of Report of the Board of Control for 1937'. *Journal of Mental Science* 85, 355 (1939): 293–4.
Ewens, G. F. W. *Insanity in India*. Calcutta: Thacker, 1908.
Finkelman, Isidore, Alex J. Arieff and Maurice A. Schiller. 'Rabies Vaccine in the Treatment of Epilepsy'. *American Journal of Psychiatry* 94 (1938): 1363–8.
Fitzgerald, E. J. 'Syphilis and "The Mental Treatment Act"'. *British Journal of Venereal Diseases* 10 (1934): 117–37.
Greenwood, Major. *Medical Statistics from Graunt to Farr*. Cambridge: Cambridge University Press, 1948.

Grotjahn, M. 'Zur psychiatrischen Systematik und Statistik'. *Allgemeine Zeitschrift für Psychiatrie* 99 (1933): 464–80.
Gruning, J. F. *Recruitment of Labour for Tea Gardens in Assam.* Chilong, 1909.
Karkaria, Rustomji Pestonji. *India: Forty Years of Progress and Reform.* London: Henry Frowde, 1896.
Kotwal, N. B. R. *A Discourse! The Naked Truth! etc.* Bombay: Kotwal, 1937.
Lacey, W. G. *Census of India, 1931 Bihar and Orissa.* Vol. VII. Patna: Government Printing, 1932.
Livesay, A. W. B. 'Decreasing Mortality and Eliminating Phthisis in Mental Hospitals'. *British Medical Journal* 3937 (1936): 1246–9.
Manual of the International List of Causes of Death, as adapted for use in England and Wales, Scotland, and Northern Ireland. London: His Majesty's Stationery Office, 1926.
Markham, S. F. *A Report to the Sir Ratan Tata Trustees on Problems Affecting the Parsee Community.* Bombay: Sir Ratan Tata Trust, 1932.
Meyer, W. S., J. S Cotton, H. H. Risley and Richard Burn. *Imperial Gazetteer of India.* Oxford: Clarendon, 1880–1931.
Nomenclature of Diseases Drawn up by a Joint Committee Appointed by the Royal College of Physicians of London. 5th ed. London: Thuscott, 1918.
Noyes, W. 'Review of *Acute Confusional Insanity* by Conally Norman'. *American Journal of Psychology* 4 (1891): 326–8.
Overbeck-Wright, Alexander William. *Lunacy in India.* London: Bailliere, Tindall and Cox, 1921.
Pilcher, Ellen. 'Relation of Mental Disease to Crime'. *Journal of the American Institute of Criminal Law and Criminology* 21 (1930): 212–46.
Porter, A. E. *Census of India, 1931 Bengal and Sikkim.* Vol. V. Calcutta: Central Publication Branch, 1933.
Report of the Drugs Enquiry Committee 1930–31. Calcutta: Government Press, 1931.
Report of the Indian Hemp Drugs Commission, 1893–94. Vol I. Simla: Government Central Printing Office, 1894.
Rothschild, D. 'The Clinical Differentiation of Senile and Arteriosclerotic Psychoses'. *American Journal of Psychiatry* 98 (1941): 324–33.
Sen, P. K. *Penology Old and New.* London: Longmans, Green, 1943.
Shaw, W. S. J. 'The Heredity of Dementia Praecox'. *British Medical Journal* 3534 (1928): 566–8.
———. 'Correspondence'. *British Medical Journal* 3537 (1928): 728.
———. 'Some Observations on the Aetiology of Dementia Praecox'. *Journal of Mental Science* 76 (1930): 505–11.
Sheppard, J. B. 'Organotherapy'. *Journal of the National Medical Association* 15 (1923): 31–3.
Stokes, P. 'Cancer Mortality in Mental Institutions (Correspondence)'. *British Medical Journal* 3389 (1924): 1136.
Strecker, Edward A., Harold P. Palmer and Francis J. Braceland. 'Hematoporphyrin as a Therapeutic Agent in the Psychoses'. *American Journal of Psychiatry* 90 (1934): 1157–73.
Waddell, L. A. *Lyon's Medical Jurisprudence for India.* 7th ed. Calcutta: Thacker, 1921.
Wadia, P. A. *Parsis Ere the Shadows Thicken.* Bombay: Wadia, 1949.
Weese, H. and W. Scharpf. 'Evipan, ein neuartiges Einschlafmittel'. *Deutsche Medizinische Wochenschrift* 58 (1932): 1205–7.
Yeatts, M. W. M. *Census of India 1941.* Simla: Government of India, 1943.
Yellowlees, H. 'Obituary. Lewis Campbell Bruce'. *British Journal of Psychiatry* 92 (1946): 857–9.
Yule, Henry. *Hobson-Jobson.* (1886). London: Murray, 1902.

Secondary Sources

Adamis, D., A. Treloar and F. C Martin. 'A Brief Review of the History of Delirium as a Mental Disorder'. *History of Psychiatry* 18 (2007): 459–69.
Agich, G. 'Evaluative Judgment and Personality Disorder', in J. Z. Sadler, Osborne P. Wiggins and Michael A. Schwartz, eds, *Philosophical Perspectives on Psychiatric Diagnostic Classification* (Baltimore: Johns Hopkins University, 1994), 233–45.
Ahmed, Rafiuddin. *The Bengal Muslims*. Delhi: Oxford University Press, 1988.
Ahuja, N. *A Short Textbook of Psychiatry*. New Delhi: Jaypee Brothers, 2006.
Akhtar, S. 'Four Culture-Bound Psychiatric Syndromes in India'. *International Journal of Social Psychiatry* 34 (1988): 70–74.
Akhtar, S. W. and H. Aziz. 'Perception of Epilepsy in Muslim History'. *Neurology Asia* 9, Supplement 1 (2004): 59–60.
Alaii, J. A., H. W. van den Borne, S. P. Kachur, K. Shelley, H. Mwenesi, J. M. Vulule, W. A. Hawley, B. L. Nahlen and P. A. Phillips-Howard. 'Community Reactions to the Introduction of Permethrin-Treated Bed Nets for Malaria Control During a Randomized Controlled Trial in Western Kenya'. *American Journal of Tropical Medicine and Hygiene* 68 (2003): 128–36.
Aminoff, M. J. 'Pharmacologic Management of Parkinsonism and Other Movement Disorders', in B. G. Katzung, ed. *Basic and Clinical Pharmacology*. 9th ed. Singapore: McGraw-Hill, 2004, 47–61.
Anderson, Olive. 'Did Suicide Increase with Industrialization in Victorian England?' *Past and Present* 86 (1980): 149–73.
_____. *Suicide in Victorian and Edwardian England*. Oxford: Oxford University Press, 1987.
Andrews, J. 'In her Vapours ... [or] indeed in her Madness?' *History of Psychiatry* 1 (1990): 125–43.
_____. *The History of Bethlem*. London/New York: Routledge, 1997.
Arendt, Mikkel, Raben Rosenberg, Leslie Foldager and Gurli Petro. 'Cannabis-Induced Psychosis and Subsequent Schizophrenia-Spectrum Disorders'. *British Medical Journal* 187 (2005): 510–15.
Arnold, D. 'Colonial Medicine in Transition'. *South Asia Research* 14 (1994): 10–35.
_____, ed. *Warm Climates and Western Medicine*. London: Rodopi, 1996.
Asha, G. 'Review of *Mental Health of Indian Women* by B. V. Davar'. *Journal of International Women's Studies* 3 (2001): 281–87.
Aspengren, H. C. 'Sociological Knowledge and Colonial Power in Bombay around the First World War'. *British Journal for the History of Science* (2010): 100–116.
Avasthi, A. 'Indianizing Psychiatry'. *Indian Journal of Psychiatry* 53 (2011): 111–20.
Ballhatchet, K. *Race, Sex and Class*. London: Weidenfeld, 1980.
Bandyopadhyay, S. 'Caste in the Perception of the Raj'. *Bengal Past and Present* 104 (1985): 56–80.
_____. 'Construction of Social Categories', in D. S. Singh, ed., *Ethnicity, Caste and People*. New Delhi: Manohar, 1992, 26–36.
_____. *Caste, Culture and Hegemony: Social Dominance in Colonial Bengal*. London: Sage, 2004.
Banerjee, P. N. and W. A. Hauser. 'Incidence and Prevalence', in J. Engel and T. A. Pedley, eds, *Epilepsy*. Philadelphia: Wolters Kluwer, 2008, 45–56.
Bara, J. *Colonialism, Christianity and the Tribes of Chhotanagpur in East India*. London/New York: Routledge, 2007.
_____.'Schooling the "Truant" Tribe'. *Studies in History* 26 (2010): 143–73.
Baran, P. A. *The Political Economy of Growth*. New York: Monthly Review Press, 1957.
Bashford, A. and P. Levine, eds. *The Oxford Handbook of the History of Eugenics*. Oxford: Oxford University Press, 2010.
Basu, A. R. 'The Coming of Psychoanalysis in Colonial India'. *Centre for Studies in Social Sciences Occasional Paper* 5 (1999): 36–54.
_____. 'The Birth of Psychology in India', in G. Mishra, ed., *Psychology and Psychoanalysis*. New Delhi: Centre for Studies in Civilizations, forthcoming.

Basu, D., A. Malhotra, A. Bhagat and V. K. Varma. 'Cannabis Psychosis and Acute Schizophrenia'. *European Journal of Addiction Research* 5 (1999): 71–3.

Bates, C. and M. Carter. 'Tribal and Indentured Migrants', in P. Robb, ed., *Dalit Movements and Meanings of Labour in India*. New Delhi: Oxford University Press, 1993.

Baume, C. A. and M. C. Marin. 'Intra-household Mosquito Net Use in Ethiopia, Ghana, Mali, Nigeria, Senegal, and Zambia'. *American Journal of Tropical Medicine and Hygiene* 77 (2007): 963–71.

Baviskar, S., V. Bhagat, R. Kirte and S. J. Sharanabasavaraj. 'Gender Disparities in Health Seeking Behaviour of Epilepsy Patients in Tertiary Care Facility of Rural Karnataka'. *Current Neurobiology* 2 (2011): 113–16.

Bayly, S. *Caste, Society and Politics in India from the Eighteenth Century to the Modern Age*. Cambridge: Cambridge University Press, 1999.

Beddies, T. and A. Dörries, eds. *Die Patienten der Wittenauer Heilstätten in Berlin*. Husum: Matthiesen, 2001.

Behal, R. P. 'Power Structure, Discipline, and Labour in Assam Tea Plantations under Colonial Rule'. *International Review of Social History* 51 (2006): 143–72.

Berrios, G. E. 'Delirium and Confusion in the 19th Century'. *British Journal of Psychiatry* 139 (1981): 439–49.

_____. 'Historical Aspects of Psychoses'. *British Medical Bulletin* 43 (1987): 484–98.

_____. 'Dementia During the Seventeenth and Eighteenth Centuries'. *Psychological Medicine* 17 (1987): 829–37.

_____. 'Melancholia and Depression During the 19th Century'. *British Journal of Psychiatry* 153 (1988): 298–304.

_____. 'Epilepsy', in G. E. Berrios and R. Porter, eds, *A History of Clinical Psychiatry*. London: Athlone, 1995, 147–63.

_____. 'Mood Disorders', in G. E. Berrios and R. Porter, eds, *A History of Clinical Psychiatry*. London: Athlone, 1995, 384–408.

_____. 'The Insanities of the Third Age'. *Journal of Nutrition, Health and Aging* 7 (2003): 394–9.

_____. 'Of Mania'. *History of Psychiatry* 15 (2004): 105–24.

Berrios, G. E., R. Luque and J. M Villagran. 'Schizophrenia'. *International Journal of Psychology and Psychological Therapy* 3 (2003): 111–40.

Béteille, André. *Caste, Class and Power*. Berkeley: University of California Press, 1965.

_____. *Castes: Old and New*. Bombay: Asia Publishing House, 1969.

Bhabha, Homi K. *The Location of Culture*. London/New York: Routledge, 1994.

Bhambra, G. K. *Rethinking Modernity*. Basingstoke: Palgrave Macmillan, 2009.

Bharucha, N. E. 'Epidemiology of Epilepsy in India'. *Epilepsia* 44 (2003): 9–11.

Borell, M. 'Brown-Sequard's Organotherapy and its Appearance in America at the End of the Nineteenth Century'. *Bulletin of the History of Medicine* 50, 3 (1976): 309–20.

Bose, Nirmal Kumar. *The Structure of Indian Society*. (1949). Hyderabad: Orient Longman, 1996.

Bradley, J. 'Medicine on the Margins?', in W. Ernst, ed., *Plural Medicine, Tradition and Modernity*. London: Routledge, 2002, 19–39.

Brown, E. M. 'Why Wagner-Jauregg Won the Nobel Prize for Discovering Malaria Therapy for General Paresis of the Insane'. *History of Psychiatry* 11 (2000): 371–82.

Brown, R. P., J. Sweeney and E. Loutsch. 'Involutional Melancholia Revisited'. *American Journal of Psychiatry* 141(1984): 24–8.

Busfield, Joan. *Men, Women and Madness*. Basingstoke: Macmillan, 1996.

Carrin-Bowez, M. 'Forest to Factories', in P. Robb, ed., *Dalit Movements and Meanings of Labour in India*. New Delhi: Oxford University Press, 1993.

Carroll, L. 'Caste, Social Change, and the Social Scientist'. *Journal of Asian Studies* 35 (1975): 63–84.

_____. 'Colonial Perceptions of Indian Society and the Emergence of Caste(s) Associations'. *Journal of Asian Studies* 37 (1978): 233–50.

Catagnini, A. C. 'Wimmer's Concept of Psychogenic Psychosis Revisited'. *History of Psychiatry* 21 (2010): 54–66.
Chakrabarti, P. 'Medicine and Nationhood in British India'. *OSIRIS* 24 (2009): 188–211.
Chatterjee, Partha. *A Princely Impostor?* Princeton: Princeton University Press, 2002.
Cherry, Steven. *Mental Health Care in Modern England.* Woodbridge: Boydell, 2003.
Choi, B. C. K. 'Future Challenges for Diagnostic Research'. *Journal of Epidemiology and Community Health* 56 (2002): 334–5.
Cohn, Bernard S. *Colonialism and Its Forms of Knowledge.* Princeton: Princeton University Press, 1996.
Cole, J., P. McGuffin and A. E Farmer. 'The Classification of Depression'. *British Journal of Psychiatry* 192 (2008): 83–5.
Condrau, Flurin and Michael Worboys, eds. *Tuberculosis Then and Now.* London: McGill, 2010.
Cooper, Fredrick. *Colonialism in Question.* Berkeley: University of California Press, 2005.
Corbridge, S. 'Outstating Singbonga', in P. Robb, ed., *Dalit Movements and Meanings of Labour in India*. New Delhi: Oxford University Press, 1993.
Crammer, John. *The History of Buckinghamshire County Pauper Lunatic Asylum, St John's.* London: Gaskell, 1990.
Christison, G. W., D. G. Kirch and R. J. Wyatt. 'When Symptoms Persist'. *Schizophrenia Bulletin* 17 (1991): 217–45.
Daniel, E. V. 'The Making of a Coolie', in H. Bernstein, E. V. Daniel and Tom Brass, eds, *Plantations, Proletarians and Peasants in Asia.* London: Frank Cass, 1992.
Davar, Bhargavi. V. 'Mental Illness Among Indian Women'. *Economic and Political Weekly* 30 (1995): 2879–86.
———. *Mental Health of Indian Women.* New Delhi: Sage, 1999.
Digby, A. and H. Sweet. 'Nurses as Culture Brokers in Twentieth-Century South Africa', in W. Ernst, ed., *Plural Medicine, Tradition and Modernity.* London/New York: Routledge, 2001), 113–29.
Dörries, A. and J. Vollmann. 'Medizinische und ethische Probleme der Klassifikation psychischer Störungen dargestellt am Beispiel des "Würzburger Schlüssels" von 1933'. *Fortschritte der Neurologie–Psychiatry* 65 (1997): 550–54.
Dowbiggin, I. 'Delusional Disorder', in G. E. Berrios and R. Porter, eds, *A History of Clinical Psychiatry*. London: Athlone, 1995, 372–83.
Dumont, Louis. *Homo Hierarchicus.* Paris: Gallimard, 1966.
Engstrom, E. J. 'Kraepelin.' *History of Psychiatry* 2 (1991): 111–32.
———. 'Nachwort zur Selbstschilderung', in W. Burgmair, E. J. Engstrom, M. M. Weber, eds, *Emil Kraepelin*, 73–97. München: Belleville, 2000.
———. 'Die Ökonomie klinischer Inskription', in C. Borck and A. Schäfer, eds, *Psychographien*. Zürich: Diaphanes, 2005, 219–40.
———. 'Introduction to Classic Text'. *History of Psychiatry* 18 (2007): 389–404.
Ernst, W. 'The Establishment of "Native Lunatic Asylums" in Early Nineteenth-Century British India', in J. Meulenbeld and D. Wujastyk, eds, *Studies on Indian Medical Traditions.* Groningen: Egbert Forsten, 1987; Delhi: Motilal, 2001, 169–204.
———. 'Mad, Bad and/or Subaltern?' Paper presented at the Situating the Subaltern in South Asian Medical History Workshop, University of Warwick, 2009.
———. *Mad Tales from the Raj.* London/New York: Routledge, 1991; London/ Delhi: Anthem, 2010.
———. 'The Limits of Comparison'. *History of Psychiatry* 23 (2012): 404–18.
———. 'Alcohol in India'. Paper presented at the conference Under Control? Alcohol and Drug Regulation, Past and Present, London School of Tropical Hygiene and Medicine, 2013.
Ernst, W. and B. J. Harris, eds. *Race, Science and Medicine.* London/New York: Routledge, 1998.
Eyler, John M. *Sir Arthur Newsholme and State Medicine.* Cambridge: Cambridge University Press, 1997.
Fábrega, Horacio. *History of Mental Illness in India.* Delhi: Motilal Banarsidass, 2009. Fanon, Frantz. *Black Skins White Masks.* New York: Grove, 1967.

Farewell, V., T. Johnson and P. Armitage. '"A Memorandum on the Present Position and Prospects of Medical Statistics and Epidemiology" by Major Greenwood'. *Statistics in Medicine* 25 (2006): 2161–77.

Farley, John. *To Cast Out Disease*. Oxford: Oxford University Press, 2004.

Fergusson, David M., Richie Poulton, Paul F. Smith and Joseph M. Boden. 'Cannabis and Psychosis'. *British Medical Journal* 332 (2006): 172–5.

Finnane, Mark. *Insanity and the Insane in Post-Famine Ireland*. London: Croom Helm, 1981.

Forbes, Geraldine. *Women in Modern India*. Cambridge: Cambridge University Press, 1996.

Freeman, Hugh. 'Infectious Lunacy'. Review of *Madhouse: A Tragic Tale of Megalomania and Modern Medicine*, by Andrew Scull. *Times Literary Supplement*, April 23, 2005.

Gardner, James. *Sweet Bells Jangled Out of Tune*. Brighton: James Gardner, 1999.

Gilroy, Paul, *Between Camps*. London: Allen Lane, 2000.

Gittens, Diana. *Madness in Its Place*. London/New York: Routledge, 1988.

Gove, W. R. and J. F. Tudor. 'Adult Sex Roles and Mental Illness'. *American Journal of Sociology* 78 (1972): 812–35.

Gove, W. R. and T. R. Herb. 'Stress and Mental Illness among the Young'. *Social Forces* 53 (1974): 256–65.

Groenhout, F. 'Loyal Feudatories or Depraved Despots?' in W. Ernst and B. Pati, eds, *India's Princely States*. London/New York: Routledge, 2007; New Delhi: Primus, 2010, 99–117.

Grotjahn, M. 'Zur psychiatrischen Systematik und Statistik'. *Allgemeine Zeitschrift für Psychiatrie* 99 (1933): 464–80.

Guay, Y. 'Emergence of Basic Research on the Periphery'. *Scientometric* 10 (1986): 77–94.

Guha, A. 'More about the Parsi Seths'. *Economic and Political Weekly* 19 (1984): 117–31.

Guha, S. 'The Importance of Social Intervention in England's Mortality Decline'. *Social History of Medicine* 7 (1994): 89–113.

Gupta, S. P. K. 'Rustom Jal Vakil (1911–1974)'. *Journal, Indian Academy of Clinical Medicine* 3 (2002): 100–104.

Hansen, V., E. Arnesen and B. K. Jacobsen. 'Total Mortality in People Admitted to a Psychiatric Hospital'. *British Journal of Psychiatry* 170 (1997): 186–90.

Harding, C. 'The Freud Franchise', in R. Clarke, ed., *Celebrity and Colonialism*. Newcastle: Cambridge Scholars, 2009.

Hardy, A. and M. E. Magnello. 'Statistical Methods in Epidemiology', in A. Morabia, ed., *A History of Epidemiologic Methods and Concepts*. Basel: Birkhaeuser, 2004.

Hare, E. 'The History of "Nervous Disorders" from 1600 to 1840, and a Comparison with Modern Views'. *British Journal of Psychiatry* 159 (1991): 37–45.

Harris, B. J. 'The Importance of Social Intervention in England's Mortality Decline'. *Social History of Medicine* 13 (2004): 379–407.

Harrison, Mark. *Public Health in British India*. Cambridge: Cambridge University Press, 1994.

Hartnack, Christiane. *Psychoanalysis in Colonial India*. Oxford: Oxford University Press, 2001.

Hayward, R. 'Germany and the Making of "English" Psychiatry', in V. Roelcke, P. J. Weindling and L. Westwood, eds, *International Relations in Psychiatry*. Rochester: University of Rochester Press, 2010, 67–90.

Healy, David. *The Antidepressant Era*. Cambridge, MA: Harvard University Press, 1997.

Hess, V. and B. Majerus. 'Writing the History of Psychiatry in the 20th Century'. *History of Psychiatry* 22 (2011): 139–45.

Hewer, W., W. Rössler, B. Fätkenheuer and W. Löffler. 'Mortality Among Patients in Psychiatric Hospitals in Germany'. *Acta Psychiatrica Scandinavica* 91 (1995): 174–9.

Hiltunem, Raimo and Yvonne Holm, eds. *Basil: The Genus Ocimum*. Amsterdam: Taylor and Francis, 2005.

Hochmuth, C. 'Patterns of Medical Culture in Colonial Bengal, 1835–1880'. *Bulletin of the History of Medicine* 80 (2006): 39–72.

BIBLIOGRAPHY

Hock, L. 'Women and Melancholy in Nineteenth-Century German Psychiatry'. *History of Psychiatry* 22 (2011): 448–64.
Home, Robert. *Of Planting and Planning*. London: Spoon/Chapman Hill, 1997.
Hook, E. W. and C. M. Marra. 'Acquired Syphilis in Adults'. *New England Journal of Medicine* 327 (1992): 959–61.
Horwitz, A. V. 'Creating an Age of Depression'. *Society and Mental Health* 1 (2011): 41–54.
Hoult, Adrienne. 'Institutional Responses to Mental Deficiency in New Zealand'. PhD dissertation, University of Waikato, 2007.
Hughes, H.'The Coolies Will Elbow Us Out of the Country'. *Labour History Review* 72 (2007): 155–68.
Hutchins, Francis G. *The Illusion of Permanence. British Imperialism in India*. Princeton: Princeton University Press, 1967.
Illich, Ivan. *Medical Nemesis*. New York: Random House, 1976.
Isharwal, S. and S. Gupta. 'Rustom Jal Vakil'. *Texas Heart Institute Journal* 33 (2006): 161–71.
Jackson, Mark. *The Borderland of Imbecility*. Manchester: Manchester University Press, 2000.
Jackson, S. W. 'Melancholia and Partial Insanity'. *Journal of the History of the Behavioral Sciences* 19 (1983): 173–84.
_____. *Melancholia and Depression*. New Haven: Yale University Press, 1992.
Jain, S. and P. Murthy. 'Madmen and Specialists'. *International Review of Psychiatry* 18 (2006): 345–54.
Jeffery, R. 'Recognizing India's Doctors: The Institutionalization of Medical Dependency, 1918–1939'. *Modern Asian Studies* 13 (1979): 301–26.
Jobe, T. H. 'Medical Theories of Melancholia in the Seventeenth and Early Eighteenth Centuries'. *Clio Medica* 11 (1976): 217–32.
Kak, Shakti and Biswamoy Pati, eds. *Exploring Gender Equations*. New Delhi: Nehru Memorial Museum, 2005.
Kakar, Sudhir. *Culture and Psyche*. New York: Psyche, 1997.
Kapila, S. 'Masculinity and Madness'. *Past and Present* 187 (2005): 121–56.
_____. 'Freud and His Indian Friends', in Sloane Mahone and Megan Vaughan, eds, *Psychiatry and Empire*. Basingstoke: Palgrave Macmillan, 2007, 124–52.
Kendell, R. E. 'The Classification of Depressions'. *British Journal of Psychiatry* 129 (1976): 15–28.
Kendler, K. 'Delusional Disorder', in G. E. Berrios and R. Porter, eds, *A History of Clinical Psychiatry*. London: Athlone, 1995, 360–71.
Khalid, A. '"Subordinate" Negotiations', in Biswamoy Pati and Mark Harrison, eds, *The Social History of Health and Medicine in Colonial India*. Delhi: Primus, 2011, 45–73.
Kline, N. S. 'Use of Rauwolfia serpentina Benth in Neuropsychiatric Conditions'. *Annuals New York Academy of Science* 59 (1954): 107–32.
Koehler, K. and H. Sass. 'Der Maniebegriff seit Kraepelin'. *Der Nervenarzt* 52 (1981):19–25.
Kotowicz, Z. 'Gottlieb Burckhardt and Egas Moniz'. *Gesnerus* 62 (2005): 77–101.
Kumar, Deepak, ed. *Science and Empire*. Delhi: Anamika Prakashan, 1991.
Kureishi, M. 'Christmas Letter to My Sister', in M. Shamsie, ed., *A Dragonfly in the Sun. An Anthology of Pakistani Writing in English*. Karachi: Oxford University Press, 1997, 67–8.
Kushner, Howard I. *Self-Destruction in the Promised Land*. New Brunswick: Rutgers University Press, 1989.
Lal, B. V. 'Veil of Dishonour'. *Journal of Pacific History* 20 (1985): 135–55.
Lanczik, M, A. Bergant and C. Klier. 'Are Severe Psychiatric Disorders in Childbed of Endogenous or Organic Nature?' *Archives of Women's Mental Health* 9 (2006): 293–9.
Lewis, A. 'Paranoia and Paranoid'. *Psychological Medicine* 1 (1970): 2–12.
López-Muñoz, Francisco, Ronaldo Ucha-Udabe and Cecilo Alamo. 'The History of Barbiturates a Century After Their Clinical Introduction'. *Neuropsychiatric Disease and Treatment* 1 (2005): 329–43.
Luhrmann, T. M. *The Good Parsi*. Cambridge, MA: Harvard University Press, 1996.

_____. 'The Traumatized Social Self', in A. C. G. M. Robben and M. M. Suarez-Orozco, eds, *Cultures under Siege*. Cambridge: Cambridge University Press, 2002, 158–93.

Lyons, M. 'The Power to Heal', in D. Engels and S. Marks, eds, *Contesting Colonial Hegemony*. London: German Historical Institute, 1994, 202–23.

MacDonald, M. and T. R. Murphy. *Sleepless Souls*. Oxford: Oxford University Press, 1990.

Mackenzie, Charlotte. *Psychiatry for the Rich*. London/New York: Routledge, 1992.

Malhotra, A. *Gender, Caste and Religious Identities*. Delhi: Oxford University Press, 2002.

Malhotra, H. K. and N. N. Wig. 'Dhat Syndrome: A Culture Bound Sex Neurosis of the Orient'. *Archives of Sexual Behavior* 4 (1975): 519–28.

Mani, K. S. 'Epidemiology of Epilepsy in Karnataka'. *Neuroscience Today* 1 (1997): 167–74.

Manyam, B. V. 'Epilepsy in Ancient India'. *Epilepsia* 33 (1992): 473–5.

Matthews, J. R. *Quantification and the Quest for Medical Certainty*. Princeton: Princeton University Press, 1995.

McHugh, J. D. and N. Delanty. 'Epidemiology and Classification of Epilepsy'. *International Review of Neurobiology* 83 (2008): 11–26.

Mehta, P. 'The Import and Export of Psychoanalysis'. *Journal of American Academy of Psychoanalysis* 25 (1997): 455–71.

Meller, Helen. *Patrick Geddes*. London/New York: Routledge.

Melling, J. and P. Dale, eds. *Mental Illness and Learning Disability*. London: Routledge, 2006.

Melling, J. and B. Forsythe, eds. *Insanity, Institutions and Society*. London/New York: Routledge, 1999), 223–42.

Memmi, Albert. *The Colonizer and the Colonized*. Boston: Beacon, 1965.

Metcalf, Thomas R., *An Imperial Vision*. Berkeley: University of California Press, 1989.

Meulenbeld, G. J. *A History of Indian Medical Literature*. 5 vols. Groningen: Egbert Forsten, 1999–2000.

Michael, Pamela. *Care and Treatment of the Mentally Ill in North Wales, 1800–2000*. Cardiff: University of Wales Press, 2003.

Midelfort, H. D. *A History of Madness in 16th Century Germany*. Stanford: Stanford University Press, 1999.

Mills, J. H. *Madness, Cannabis and Colonialism*. London: Macmillan, 2000.

Mohanty, A. and N. Hazary. *Indian Prison Systems*. New Delhi: Ashish, 1990.

Mukharji, Projit B., *Nationalizing the Body*. London: Anthem Press, 2009.

Naidu, V. *The Violence of Indenture in Fiji*. Suva: University of the South Pacific Press, 1980.

Nakayama, T. et al. 'Clinicians and Epidemiologists View Crude Death Rates Differently'. *British Medical Journal* 318 (1999): 395.

Nandi, D. N., S. P Mukherjee, S. Sinha, G. C. Boral, G. Banerjee, P. Dutta, P. S. Nandi and M. Palik. 'Demographic Characteristics and Mental Morbidity amongst Different Castes in West Bengal'. *International Journal of Social Psychiatry* 29 (1983): 21–8.

Nandy, Ashis. *The Intimate Enemy*. Delhi: Oxford University Press, 1983.

_____. *The Savage Freud*. New Jersey: Princeton University Press, 1995.

Nayak, J. K. 'Hubback's Memoirs'. *The Telegraph*. Calcutta, 29 November 2010.

Newell, J. 'Unseen Power'. *The Muslim World* 92 (2007): 640–56.

Nigam, S. 'Disciplining and Policing the "Criminals by Birth"', *Indian Economic and Social History Review* 27 (1990): 131–64.

Njuna, K. J., S. M. Magesa, T. J. Wilkes, A. E. Mnzava, J. Myamba, M. D. Kivuyo, N. Hill, J. D. Lines and C. F. Curtis. 'Trial of Pyrethroid Impregnated Bednets in an Area of Tanzania Holoendemic for Malaria'. *Acta Tropica* 49 (1991): 87–96.

Noce, R. N., David B. Williams and Walter Rapaport. 'Reserpine (serpasil) in the Management of the Mentally Ill and Mentally Retarded'. *Journal of the American Medical Association* 156 (1954): 821–4.

Noll, R. 'Kraepelin's "Lost Biological Psychiatry"?' *History of Psychiatry* 18 (2007): 301–20.

_____. *American Madness*. Cambridge, MA: Harvard University Press, 2011.

Pal, D. K., T. Das, S. Sengupta and G. Chaudhury. 'Help-Seeking Patterns for Children with Epilepsy in Rural India, *Epilepsia* 43 (2002): 904–11.
Pati, B. and C. P. Nanda. 'The Leprosy Patient', in B. Pati and M. Harrison, eds, *Social History of Health and Medicine in Colonial India*. London/New York: Routledge, 2009, 113–28.
Peduzzi, R. and U. C. Piffaretti. 'Ancylostoma Duodenale and the Saint Gothard Anaemia.' *British Medical Journal* 287 (1983): 1942–5.
Perris, C. 'Leonhard and the Cycloid Psychoses', in G. E. Berrios and R. Porter, eds, *A History of Clinical Psychiatry*. London: Athlone, 1995, 421–32.
Pols, H. 'Emile Kraepelin on Ethnic and Cultural Factors in Mental Illness'. *Psychiatric Times*, 22 June 2011.
Porter, Roy. *Mind-Forg'd Manacles*. London: Athlone, 1987.
_____. 'Foucault's Great Confinement', in A. Still and I. Velody, eds, *Rewriting the History of Madness*. London/New York: Routledge, 1992, 119–25.
_____. 'Epilepsy', in G. E. Berrios and R. Porter, eds, *A History of Clinical Psychiatry*, London: Athlone, 1995, 164–92.
_____. Mood Disorders, in G. E. Berrios and R. Porter, eds, *A History of Clinical Psychiatry*. London: Athlone, 1995, 409–420.
Prochaska, F. K. *The Voluntary Impulse*. London: Faber, 1988.
Radden, J., ed. *The Nature of Melancholy from Aristotle to Kristeva*. Oxford: Oxford University Press, 2000.
Radhakrishna, Meena. *Dishonoured by History*. Hyderabad: Orient Longman, 2001.
Raina, D. and S. I. Habib, eds. *Domesticating Modern Science*. New Delhi: Tulika, 2004.
Ramana, C. V. 'On the Early History and Development of Psychoanalysis in India'. *Journal of the American Psychoanalytical Association* 12 (1964): 110–34.
Rao, S. 'Caste and Mental Disorders in Bihar.' *American Journal of Psychiatry* 9 (1966): 1045–55.
Renwick, C. 'The Practice of Spencerian Science'. *Isis* 100 (2009): 36–57.
Risse, G. 'Cause of Death as a Historical Problem'. *Continuity and Change* 12 (1997): 175–88.
Roelcke, Volker. 'Unterwegs zur Psychiatrie als Wissenschaft', in E. J. Engstrom and V. Roelcke, eds, *Psychiatrie im 19. Jahrhundert*. Basel: Schwabe, 2003, 169–88.
_____. 'Psychiatrische Diagnosen im Wandel', in H. Freytag et al., eds, *Psychotraumatologische Begutachtung*. Frankfurt: Fischer, 2011, 25–48.
Roelcke, Volker, Paul Julian Weindling and Louise Westwood, eds. *International Relations in Psychiatry*. Rochester: University of Rochester Press 2010.
Roy, Asim. *Islam in South Asia*. New Delhi: South Asia Publishing, 1996.
Saha S. P., Sushanta Bhattacharya, Biman Kanti Roy, Arindam Basu, Trishit Roy, Bibekananda Maity and Shyamal K. Das. 'A Prospective Incidence Study of Epilepsy in a Rural Community of West-Bengal'. *Neurology Asia* 13 (2008): 41–48.
Sarkar, S. '"Kaliyuga", "Chakri" and "Bhakti"'. *Economic and Political Weekly* 27 (1992): 1543–66.
_____. *Writing Social History*. Delhi: Oxford University Press, 1997.
Schalock, R. L. et al. 'The Renaming of Mental Retardation'. *Intellectual and Developmental Disabilities* 45 (2007): 116–24.
Scheerenberger, R. *A History of Mental Retardation*. Baltimore: Brookes, 1983.
Schiesari, Juliana. *The Gendering of Melancholia*. Ithaca: Cornell University Press, 1992.
Schmidt, Jeremy. *Melancholy and the Care of the Soul*. Aldershot: Ashgate, 2007.
Scull, A. T. *Museums of Madness*. (1979). Harmondsworth: Penguin, 1982.
_____. 'Psychiatrists and Historical Facts.' *History of Psychiatry* 6 (1995): 387–94.
_____. *Madhouse*. New Haven: Yale University Press, 2005.
Scull, A. T. and J. Schulkin. 'Psychobiology, Psychiatry, and Psychoanalysis'. *Medical History* 53 (2009): 5–36.
Scheper-Hughes, N. 'The Madness of Hunger'. *Culture, Medicine and Psychiatry* 12 (1988): 429–58.
Seitler, D. 'Queer Physiognomies'. *Criticism* 46 (2004): 71–102.

Sekher, T. V. 'Rural Demography of India', in L. J. Kulcsár and K. Curtis, eds, *International Handbook on Rural Demography*. Dordrecht: Springer, 2012, 169–89.
Sekher, T. V. and Neelambar Hatti, eds. *Unwanted Daughters*. Jaipur/New Delhi: Rawat, 2009.
Sen, A. 'Many Faces of Gender Inequality'. *Frontline* 18, 22 (2001).
Sen, M. M. G. 'The Scientific Basis of Ayurveda', in *Lectures of M. M. Gananatha Sen Saraswati*. Varanasi: Chowkhamba Sanskrity, 2002.
Sen, S. *Women and Labour in Late Colonial India*. Cambridge: Cambridge University Press, 2006.
SenGupta, P. C. 'Soorjo Coomar Goodeve Chuckerbutty'. *Medical History* 14 (1970): 183–91.
Sengupta, S. and A. Basu, eds. *Samsad Bangali Charitabhidhan*. Calcutta: Shishu Shahitya Samsad, 2002.
Sharan, A. 'From Caste to Category'. *Indian Economic and Social History Review* 40 (2003): 279–310.
Sharma, J. '"Lazy" Natives, Coolie Labour, and the Assam Tea Industry'. *Modern Asian Studies* 43 (2009): 1287–1324.
Shepherd, A. and D. Wright. 'Madness, Suicide and the Victorian Asylum'. *Medical History* 46 (2002): 175–96.
Shorter, Edward. *A Historical Dictionary of Psychiatry*. New York: Oxford University Press, 2005.
Shorter, Edward and David Healy. *Shock Therapy*. New Brunswick: Rutgers University Press, 2007.
Siegel, Rudolph E. *Galen on Psychology, Psychopathology and Functions and Diseases of the Nervous System*. Basel: Karger, 1973.
Singer, M. and B. S. Cohn, eds. *Structure and Change in Indian Society*. Chicago: Aldine, 1968, 3–28.
Sinha, M. K. *In My Father's Footsteps*. Delhi, 1981.
———. 'Britishness, Clubbability, and the Colonial Public Sphere'. *Journal of British Studies* 40 (2001): 489–521.
Sinha, S. S. 'Adivasi Women in Transition', in Kak, S. and B. Pati, eds, *Exploring Gender Equations*. New Delhi: Nehru Memorial Museum, 2005, 175–202.
Sircar, K. K. 'Coolie Exodus from Assam's Chargola Valley'. *Economic and Political Weekly* 22 (1987): 184–93.
Sneader, Walter. *Drug Discovery*. Chichester: John Wiley, 2005.
Somasundaram, O. 'The Indian Lunacy Act 1912'. *Indian Journal of Psychiatry* 29 (1987): 3–14.
———. 'Seizure Disorders'. *Indian Journal of Psychiatry* 43 (2001): 12–15.
Sridharan, R. and B. N. Murthy. 'Prevalence and Pattern of Epilepsy in India'. *Epilepsia* 40 (1999): 631–6.
Srinivas, M. N. 'A Note on Sanskritization and Westernization'. *Far Eastern Quarterly* 15 (1956): 481–96.
———. *Caste in Modern India*. Bombay: Media Promoters, 1962.
Starobinski, Jean. *A History of the Treatment of Melancholy from the Earliest Times to 1900*. Basel: Geigy, 1962.
Stokes, E. *The English Utilitarians and India*. (1959). Delhi: Oxford University Press, 1982.
Stroemgren, Eric. 'Eric Stroemgren', in M. Shepherd, ed., *Psychiatrists on Psychiatry*. Cambridge: Cambridge University Press, 1982, 152–69.
Sumathipala, A., S. H. Siribaddana and D. Bhurga. 'Culture-Bound Syndromes'. *British Journal of Psychiatry* 184 (2004): 200–209.
Thacore, V. R. and S. R. P. Shukla. 'Cannabis Psychosis and Paranoid Schizophrenia'. *Archives of General Psychiatry* 33 (1976): 383–6.
Thomson, M. 'Though Ever the Subject of Psychological Medicine', in G. E. Berrios and H. Freeman, eds, *150 Years of British Psychiatry: Vol. II, The Aftermath*. London: Athlone, 1996.
———. *The Problem of Mental Deficiency*. Oxford: Oxford University Press, 1998.
———. 'Race, Culture and Mind in Britain', in W. Ernst and B. J. Harris, eds, *Race, Science and Medicine*. London: Routledge, 1999, 235–58.

Tidemalm, D., M. Waern, C. Stefansson, Stig Elofsson and Bo Runeson. 'Excess Mortality in Persons with Severe Mental Disorder in Sweden'. *Clinical Practice and Epidemiology in Mental Health* 4 (2008): 1–9.

Tinker, H. *A New System of Slavery*. London/New York: Oxford University Press, 1974.

Tokuhata, G. K. and V. A. Stehman. 'Mortality in State Mental Hospitals of Michigan'. *Public Health Reports* 73 (1958): 750–64.

Tunstall-Pedoe, H. 'Crude Rates, Without Standardisation for Age, Are Always Misleading'. *British Medical Journal* 317 (1998): 475–8.

Vaidyanathan, T. G. and J. J. Kripal, eds. *Vishnu on Freud's Desk*. Delhi: Oxford University Press, 2003.

Valenti, M. S. Necozione, G. Busellu, G. Borrelli, A. R Lepore, R. Madonna, E. Albotelli, A. Matei, P. Torchio, G. Corrao and F. Di Orlo. 'Mortality in Psychiatric Hospital Patients'. *International Journal of Epidemiology* 26 (1997): 1227–35.

Varma, L. P. 'Cannabis Psychosis'. *Indian Journal of Psychiatry* 14 (1972): 241–55.

Varma, N. 'Coolie Acts and the Acting Coolies'. *Social Scientist* 33 (2005): 49–72.

Walther, T. *Die 'Insulin-Koma-Behandlung'*. Berlin: Peter Lehmann Antipsychiatrieverlag, 2004.

Watts, G. 'Science Commentary: Cannabis Confusions'. *British Medical Journal* 332 (2006): 175.

Weaver, J. and D. Wright. 'Suicide, Mental Illness, and Psychiatry in Queensland'. *Health History* 11 (2009): 102–27.

Weber, M. and E. J. Engstrom. 'Kraepelin's Diagnostic Cards'. *History of Psychiatry* 8 (1997): 375–85.

Webster, C. 'Healthy or Hungry Thirties?' *History Workshop* 13 (1982): 110–29.

White, K. L. 'Contemporary Epidemiology'. *International Journal of Epidemiology* 3 (1974): 295–303.

Whitrow, M. 'Wagner-Jauregg and Fever Therapy'. *Medical History* 34 (1990): 294–310.

Wilcock, Anne Allart, ed. *Occupation for Health*. Vol II. London: British Association and College of Occupational Therapists.

Windholz, G. and L. H. Witherspoon. 'Sleep as Cure for Schizophrenia'. *History of Psychiatry* 4 (1993): 83–93.

Wolfe, D. A. and E. J. Mash, eds. *Behavioral and Emotional Disorder in Adolescents*. New York: Guildford, 2006.

Wright, D. and A. Digby, eds. *From Idiocy to Mental Deficiency*. London: Routledge, 1996.

Wright, D. and J. Weaver, eds. *Histories of Suicide*. Toronto: University of Toronto Press, 2009.

Wujastyk, D. *The Roots of Ayurveda*. New Delhi: Penguin, 1998.

_____. 'The Evolution of Indian Government Policy on Ayurveda in the Twentieth Century', in D. Wujastyk and F. M. Smith, eds, *Modern and Global Ayurveda*. New York: SUNY Press, 2008, 43–76.

Yang, Anand A. *Bazaar India*. Berkeley: University of California Press, 1999.

York, S. 'Alienists, Attendants and the Containment of Suicide in Public Lunatic Asylums'. *Social History of Medicine* 25 (2012): 324–42.

Zimmermann, Francis. *The Jungle and the Aroma of Meats*. Berkeley: University of California Press, 1987.

Zysk, Kenneth G. *Religious Medicine*. New Brunswick: Transaction, 1993.

INDEX

Note: Page numbers in bold refer to figures and tables.

A

absconding *see* escapes
access to institution xviii, 64
accidents 91–4, 197
administration 2, 10, 35, 38, 97
   colonial 52, 65, 164
admission
   by gender **44**, **63**
   patterns of 33
   physical condition on 74
   policies xviii
aetiology xviii, 159–72, 206
   see also causes
age
   and gendered trend in admissions 43–4
   of patients 41–5
   and senile dementia 45
Agich, G. 117
Agra
   institutional death rates in **68**
   Medical School 121
   Mental Hospital 121, 137, 145–6
agriculturalists 49–50
ahirs 54
Ahmedabad 153
   circular insanity at **158**
   MDP at 156, **157–8**
   melancholia at **152**, **156**, **158**
   trends in gendered diagnoses at 155–6
Ainsworth, H. 4, 84
ajmaline 176
alcohol abuse 131, 160–61
alcohol insanity, and gender 143–5
All too Human (Berkeley-Hill) 140
alternating insanity 109, 115
   see also circular insanity
ambivalence 17–20
America, dementia in 13, 42, 113
American Foundation for Mental Hygiene 172

amnesia, temporary 134
amok 137
amphetamines 180
anaemia 76, 86, 90, 100, 181
Anatomy of Melancholie (Burton) 115
Anderson, O. 95
Andrews, J. 105
Anglo-Indians (British in India) 2
Animists 55–6
ankylostomiasis (hookworm) 76, 78, 86–90
anoxia 187
anti-depressants 180
antirabic vaccine 179
anxiety 170
apasmara (loss of recollection/consciousness) 145–6
Aristotle 115
arsenic 185
Arya Samaj 56
asthenia 76
asylums, disciplinary function of 27–8
Atharva Veda 136
atropine 179
attendants 22–3
Austria 69, 107, 120
Avasthi, A. 129–30, 132–3
Ayurveda 130, 145–6, 170, 174–6

B

Baba, H. T. 28
Bachelor of Medicine and Surgery (MBBS) 3, 5, 25, 113
bacterial toxaemia 121, 155
Ballhatchet, K. 1
Bankipore Club, Patna 7
barbiturates xix, 178–80
Basilicum citratum 174
Basu, D. 132–3
bauls 54

Baviskar, S. 148
Bengal xviii, 16, 29, 134, 155, 205
　age distribution of population **45**
　caste barriers in 53–4
　Christian women in 64
　criminalisation of mentally ill in 40
　female–male ratio in **61**, 62
　Government of 3
　institutional death rates in 68
　lunatics detained in **35**
　religious affiliation of patients in 55, **58**–9
　socio-cultural traditions of 8
Bengal Club, Calcutta 7
benzederine 180
Berhampore 4, 29, 112, 131
　coolies in 50
　criminal patients in **36**
　GPI at 138
　malaria at 84
　Mental Hospital 3, 40
　mortality rates in 69–71
　occupational categories in 47–8
　religious affiliation of patients in 59
Berkeley-Hill, O. 5, 9–11, 71, 134, 140, 183
　Indian wife of 10
Berrios, G. E. 110–11, 122, 124–5
Bertillon, J. 77
Bhabha, H. 18
bhadralok status 52
bhang 131
　see also cannabis
Bhawal case 134
Bhowanipur Mental Observation Ward 25
Bihar xviii, 4, 29, 50, 155, 176, 205
　age distribution of population **45**
　caste barriers in 53–4
　Christian women in 64
　female–male ratio **61**, 62
　Government of 10
　lunatics detained in **35**
　prison reform committee 42
　religious affiliation of patients in 55, **58**, 59
　socio-cultural traditions of 8
Bilharz, T. 89
Bills of Mortality (Graunt) 77
Biraud, Dr Y. M. 194
Birla, R. B. D. 202
Bisva Tulasi 174
　see also *Ocimum*
Black Skin, White Masks (Fanon) 3
Bleuler, E. 105, 111, 113, 120

Bombay (Mumbai) 6, 155
　governor of 6
　Medical College 3
　Medical Union 7, 13
　Parsi in 11
Bose, Dr C. L. 198
Bose, G. 128
Bose, K. C. 176
Bossier de Sauvages de Lacroix, F. 77
Brahmo Samaj 56
Bratachari Movement 25, 191–2, 343n157
　see also Dutt, G. S.
Brazil 126
Britain
　decline of mortality in 78–9
　institutional histories of 105
　mental hospitals in xvii
　unlawful confinement in 28
　see also England; Northern Ireland; Scotland; Wales
British India
　agriculturalists in 49
　criminal lunatics in 35
　history of psychiatry in 3
　institutional statistics in 155–9
　institutional trends in 42, 64
　lunatic asylums in 27
　medical marketplace in 6
　mortality statistics in 67, 69
　Parsi decline in 15
　provision for children in 43
　responsibility for health and welfare in 79
　standard report forms in 108
　unlawful confinement in 28
British Medical Association (BMA) 3, 7, 13
British Medical Journal (BMJ) 6, 11, 13–14, 71, 74–5, 77, 116
Broadmoor Hospital, UK 35–7, 67, 205
Brock, A. 12–14
Brown-Sequard, C. 180
Bruce, L. C. 121, 137, 161–3, 170
Budapest 184
Bulsara, J. F. 16
Burton, R. 115
Busfield, J. 44

C

Calcinol 181
Calcium gluconate 181

INDEX

Calcutta (Kolkata) 2, 64
  All-Bengal Bratachari Training Camp 191
  Medical College, professor of *materia medica* at 1
  School of Tropical Medicine (CSTM) 130, 175, 177
  University of 4, 25
  Westernisation of 8
Calicut
  circular insanity at **158**
  Hospital 144–5
  MDP at 156, **157–8**
  melancholia at **152**, **156**, **158**
  trends in gendered diagnoses at 155–6
cannabis xviii, 171
  indica 109, 117, 131, 170, 185
  insanity xviii, 107–9, 117, 124, 128–37, 141, 170
  Cardiazol treatment of 185
  and gender 143–5, 154
  symptoms of 131, 133
Cardiazol 9, 187
  experiments with 185, 241n105
  shock therapy 183–5
caste 45–55, 195, 218n111
  typologies of 129
causes xviii
  classification of 160
  of death 67, 70, 74–6, 80
  nomenclature 77
  of decline in morality 78–9
  of disorders 109
  exciting 160, 162, 166–7, 169, 171
  of female under-representation 62
  hereditary 164–5
  of infections 161
  of mental breakdown 159–60, 165, 169–71
  moral 167–8
  non-organic 123
  pathological 41
  physical 169
  predisposing 160, 166–7, 169, 171
  preventable 162
  racial differences in 169–70
  of schizophrenia 14
  social 164
  of toxaemia 161
  of trends 61
  unascertained 167–9
  in women 171
Central Institute of Psychiatry (CIP) 9

cerebro-spinal fluid (CSF) 138, 140, 185
certification, irregularities in 40–41
Chadwick, E. 79
Chakrabarti, P. 6
charmakar 53
Chatterjee, P. 134
Chatterji, Rev. A. C. 188, 193
Chaudhuri, D. R. 202
Chennai *see* Madras
Cherry, S. 105
Chesler, P. 149
Chevers, N. 133–6
chickenpox 70, 81
child marriages 171–2
children, intellectually disabled 43
chloral hydrate 98
chlorosis *see* ankylostomiasis
cholera 70, 74, 81, 87, 113, 197
Chopra, I. C. 133–4
Chopra, R. N. 130, 133–4, 177
chota chand 176
  see also *Rauvolfia*
Chota Nagpur 50, 52
  Christian women in 63–4
  religion in 55
Christians 54–6, 58–9, 63, 155, 188
  native 58
  services for 193
Chuckerbutty, S. G., career of 1, 209n3
cinema 201
circular (alternating) insanity 109, 113–20, **119**, 141
  gendered trends in 153–5, **158**, 236n274
classifications
  impact on treatment 109
  of insanity **118**
  ruptures and continuities in 108–41
  standardisation and variation of 106–8
clerks 52
closure, professional 11–14
Clouston, T. 170
Code of Criminal Procedure (1898) 35
Colaba Observatory 15
collaboration, psychological cost of 17
collaborators (compradors) 17–20
College of Physicians and Surgeons (CPS) 3
Colloidal calcium 181
colonial medicine, history of xvii
colonisation, psychopathology of 3
Colonizer and Colonized (Memmi) 7
commissions, appointments to 1

Committing Magistrates 39–41
competitors 17–20
compounders, salary of 22
compradors 209n8
   bourgeoisie 3
   thesis of 17
confinement
   gender issues 29–34
   long-term 30–33
   unlawful 28–9
   of women 30
confusional insanity 107–9, 122–6, 141–2
   and female reproduction-related
      disorders 142–3
   see also starvation
Congress of the Far Eastern Association of
   Tropical Medicine 113
control, of the socially undesirable xviii, 27–8
conversion hysteria 188–9
Cook, Col. L. 35–6, 164–5
coolies (labourers) 49–50
Cotton, H. A. 102
Crammer, J. 105
crannies (kerani) 52, 218nn105–106
Crime and Destiny (Lange) 139
crimes
   incidence and range of **38**
   petty 39–41
criminal lunatics 35–41, 151
   classes of 38
   gender of 37
Criminal Tribes Acts 28
Cullen, W. 77
cultivators 49–50
cures 99–104
   percentage of **101**
Cuttack 64
   Medical School 25

D

Dacca (Dhaka) 4, 29, 112
   criminal patients in **36**
   GPI at 138
   malaria at 84
   Mental Hospital 50, 59
   mortality statistics in 69–70
   occupational categories in 47–8
   religious affiliation of patients in 59
   University of 4, 25
Daktari 170
dance therapy xix, 191–2

   see also Bratachari Movement; Dutt, G. S.
Darbhanga Medical School 25
Darukhanawala, H. D. 15
Das, Dr P. C. 32–3, 100, 171, 187, 190, 202
   discipline regime of 24
   introduction of athletics by 200
   as locum for Dhunjibhoy 39, 85, 103,
      139, 166
   reporting of injuries by 91, 93
Davar, B. V. 150
David Lewis Colony, UK 118, 127–8, 148
day labourers 50
De, B. J. 194
death
   analysis of rates 67–8
   by gender 69–74
   causes of xviii, 74–6, 221n30
   nomenclature 77
debility 76, 86, 100
Degeneracy: Its Causes, Signs, and Results
   (Talbot) 161
degeneracy 161, 164
Delhi 2
   central government in 6
Delhi belly 87
delirium 116, 122–6
   acute 109
delirium tremens 131
delusional insanity 109, 116, 120–22, 141
   gendered trends in 153–4, 236n271
delusions 114–15, 120, 122, 132
dementia xviii, 32, 105–6, 122–6
   from epilepsy 146–8
   subcategories of 124
dementia paralytica see general paralysis of the
   insane (GPI)
dementia praecox (DP) 11, 13, 45, 108–13,
   117–22, 124, 141
   diagnosis of 181
   gendered trends in 153–5, 235n265
   heredity of 165
   organotherapy for 180
   sulphur treatment of 182
demographics, of patients 64–5
Denbigh Mental Hospital, UK 75, 88, 100,
   102, 105
   disorders attributed on admission
      106, 107–8
Denmark 182
Deo, R. R. N. B. 202
dependents 48–9

depression 115–16, 149–50
  and suicide 97
deprivation, food-related 142
dermatographia 181
Dermotubin 182
Devi 129
Devon Mental Hospital, UK 197
Dhaka *see* Dacca
Dhandhania, R. B. D. D. 202
Dharwar
  circular insanity, at **158**
  MDP at 156, **157–8**
  melancholia at **152**, **156**, **158**
  trends in gendered diagnoses at 155–6
Dhat-syndrome 130
dhatura (*Datura*) seeds 131
dhobi 53
Dhunjibhoy, J. E. xvii, 6, 32, 173, 206–7
  administrative standards of 23–4
  admission policies of 33–4
  analysis of offences by **38**
  appointment at Ranchi 3–4
  attention to patients' religion by 192–3
  career development 4
  classification used by **118**
  criticism of 4
  European travels of 4, 20, 114, 139, 174–6, 196–7
  hemp drugs expertise of 128–37
  as Indian outsider 8
  journals studied by 173
  marginalisation of 9, 17
  measures against malaria by 83–4
  military commission of 3
  nationalism of 19
  notes on mental defectives 41–2
  and the Parsi dementia debate 13–15, 17
  praising of staff by 95–7
  reflections on suicidal patients 95, 97
  retirement of 20, 207
  salary of 5
  self-experimentation by 134
  thoughts on aetiology 159–72
  training 3–4
  transnational influences on 120
  use of indigenous herbs by 174–8
  use of Kraepelin's scheme by 117–18, 120–22
  use of modern drugs by 178–80
  use of wonder cures by 180–82
  views on attendants 22–3
  views on GPI 138–41
  wife of 20
Dhunjibhoy, R. (daughter) 8, 11, 16, 18–20, 192, 207, 210n20
Dhunjibhoy, S. (wife) 139
diagnoses, longitudinal gendered trends in 155–9
diagnostic categories, and gender 141–59
Diagnostic and Statistical Manual of Mental Disorders (DSM-V) 120
diagnostic styles, variation in 108
Dial 178
diarrhoea 70, 76, 78, 88–9
diet 197–9
disability, intellectual 41–5
discharge
  lack of desire for 99
  rates of 32–3
discipline 24
discrimination 4, 71
  gendered 31
  professional 8–11
diseases xviii
  airborne 78–80, 84–7, 206
  classification of xviii, 77–9
  of digestive system 86
  ecology of 78
  intestinal 88
  other classified 79–80
  parasitic 78, 80–81, 87–90, 206
  prevalence of 81–94
  respiratory 69, 74–5, 78, 84–5, 223n66
  waterborne 69–70, 78–81, 87–90, 206
disempowerment, of the socially undesirable xviii
disorders
  gender-specific trends in xviii
  types of 105–72
Dolcoath Mine, UK 90
dome 53
dome-chamar 53
Dowbiggin, I. 120
dramatic performances 200–201
drugs, modern 178–80
Drugs Act (1940) 130
Drugs Enquiry Committee 130
Dutt, G. S. 191–2, 243n157
  see also Bratachari Movement
Dutton, Lt. Col. H. R. 4
dysentery 70, 78, 87–90, 151

E

eczema 182
Edinburgh, University of 4, 12, 25
education 52–3
  Western 12
Egypt 136
elation 114
Ellis, H. 161
encephalitis lethargica 76
endogamy 15, 17
England 120
  criminal lunatics in 35
  cure rates in 102
  dementia in 13, 42, 113
  dysentery in 88
  female–male ratio in 37
  gender trend in 43
  health on admission in 74
  institution death rates in 68
  intellectual disability in 127
  legislation in 35, 42–3
  medical coding in 109
  mortality nomenclature in 77
  New Poor Law in 128
  overcrowded hospitals in 30
  patient types in 27
  specialist facilities in 35–6, 67
  suicide in 95–6
  use of sedation in 98
entertainment 199–203
environment 160, 165
epilepsy 92, 113, 124, 127
  drugs for 179
  and gender 145–9
  sulphur treatment of 182
Epilepsy (Muskens) 179
epileptic insanity 147
escapes xviii, 94–9
Esquirol, J. E. 115, 120
eugenics 12–13, 42–3, 165–6
Europe xviii, 46, 100, 111, 113, 153, 205–6
  aetiology in 163, 169–70, 172
  classifications in 107, 115, 117–18
  epilepsy in 146–7
  gendered social control in 28, 149–50
  GPI in 91, 138, 185
  hydrotherapy in 189
  mortality in 78
  patients in 27
  sulphur treatment in 183
  training in 22

European Club, Patna *see* Bankipore Club
European Mental Hospital, Ranchi 67–8, 182–3
  administration of 10
  death rates at **68**, 71
  senior staff at 21
  syphilis at 140
Evipan 179
  Sodium 177
Ewens, G. F. W.
  classification used by 142, 154, 160
  views on aetiology 160–61, 163, 167–70, 172
  views on epilepsy 146–8
  views on GPI 137
  views on hemp drugs 135, 144
  views on melancholia 150–51, 153–5
exhaustion 143
  insanity 142–3
exploitation 193

F

fakirs see *faquirs*
famine 70, 99, 142
Fanon, F. 3, 16–17
faquirs (fakirs) 54–5, 144, 174–5
Farr, W. 77
feasts 192–3
females *see* women
Finnane, M. 99
fits
  Cardiazol-induced 184
  epileptic 146, 148
  of rage 112, 151
Fitzgerald, E. J. 138, 141
force feeding 97–8, 151, 199
Foucault, M. 27, 206
France 13, 113, 120
French North Africa 3, 17
Freud, S. 128–9, 140, 162–3, 188

G

Gandhi, M. K. 19, 192
ganja *see* cannabis indica
Gardner, J. 105
Geddes, P. 12–13
gender
  admissions by **44**, **63**
  and age 43–4
  and alcohol 143–5
  and cannabis 143–5
  of criminal lunatics 37

INDEX 265

and cure rates 103
death and illness by 69–74
of dependents 49
and epilepsy 145–9
of influenza patients **81**
longitudinal trends in diagnosis 155–9
maladies related to 141–59
and mania 149–55
and melancholia 149–55
and preferential rearing 60–61
and readmissions 103
and religious affiliation 59–60, **60**, 219nn133–34
and reported sickness **72**, 73
and respiratory diseases 85
and schizophrenia 149–55
Genera Morborum (Linnaeus) 77
general paralysis of the insane (GPI) 76, 91, 107–8, 114, 186
   a culture-bound syndrome 137–41
   treatment with malaria 185
   treatment with sulphur 182
Germany 116, 119–20
   causes of death in 75
   classification in 107, 109
   dementia in 13, 42, 113
   mania in 113
Gillespie, R. D. 129
girls, intellectually defective 43–4
Gittins, D. 105
glandular therapy 181
goala (gwala) caste 46, 54
Government of India Act (1935) 52
Grahas 146
grand mal 148
Graunt, J. 77
Greenwood, Major 67, 78
Groenhout, F. 28
Grotjahn, M. 107, 109
Guha, A. 15–16, 18
Gujarat 16
Gupta, S. 177
Gütersloh hospital, Germany 197

H

hakims 174
Haliverol 181
Hall, Dr G. E. 187
hallucinations 120, 132–3
hallucinatory insanity 142
Hardless, H. 1

Harper Nelson, J. J. 71
Hassan Imam's root 176
   see also *Rauvolfia*
Health and Conduct (Brock) 12
Healy, D. 116
heart failure 70
hebephrenia 121, 154–5, 184
Heidegger, M. 105
hemp drugs 131, 160, 170
hemp insanity *see* cannabis insanity
Henderson, D. K. 129
Hensman, Dr H. S. 5–6, 9
heredity 160–62, 164–7
Hess, V. 105
Hewer, W. 75
hijras 54
Hindus 15, 53–60, 62–3, 155
   culture of 129
   feasts of 192
   opium and hemp use by 136
   and organotherapy 181
Hippocrates 123
Hochmuth, C. 22
Hock, L. 149
hoematopophyrin 180
holy basil 175
   see also *Ocimum*
hookworm *see* ankylostomiasis
Hoult, A. 128
Hubback, Miss C. 10
Hubback, Sir J. A. 10
Hungary 69
hunger, madness of 126, 171
Hyderabad
   circular insanity, at **158**
   MDP at 156, **157–8**
   melancholia at **152**, **156**, **158**
   trends in gendered diagnoses at 155–6
hydrotherapy xix, 187, 189–91, 196
hygiene xviii
   see also mental hygiene; racial hygiene
hyoscine hydrobromide 178
hyperactivity 114
Hypnol 178, 190
hypnosis 188
hypnotics 195
hypochondria 115

I

Ibn al-Baitar al-Malaqi (Iban Beitar) 136
identity, questions of 3

idiocy *see* intellectual disability
Idiots Act (1886) 127
Ilbert Bill (1883) 7
Illich, I. 28
illness
 by gender 69–74
 causes of xviii, 159–72
imbecility *see* intellectual disability
imperial order, reconstituted 7
impetigo 182
inbreeding 12–13, 17, 172
Incretone 181
India
 anticolonialism in 129
 female–male ratio **61**
 types of insanity in **118**
 see also British India
Indian competition 8
Indian Gentleman's Guide to Etiquette, The (Hardless) 1
Indian hemp *see* cannabis indica; hemp drugs
Indian Hemp Drugs Commission 135
Indian Lunacy Act (1912) 35
Indian Lunatic Asylums Act (1858) 35
Indian Medical Gazette 137, 140, 182, 185
Indian Medical Service (IMS) xvii, 3, 6, 207
 competition in 21
 European lobby in 10
 monopoly 6–7
 pay scales of 5
Indian National Congress 2, 19
Indian pharmacopoeia 130
Indian Psychiatric Society 130
Indian Psychoanalytic Society 128
Indian Railways Act (1890) 39
Indian snakeroot 174–6
 see also *Rauvolfia*
Indianisation xvii, 2, 207
 and histories of medicine 20–21
 move towards 3–4
 and subordinate staff 5
Indians, anti-British sentiments of 11
indigenous herbs 174–8
inequities, structural 5–6
influenza 69–70, 74, 80–84, 206
 by gender **81**
injuries 80, 86, 91–4, 197
insania universalis see mania
insanity *see* alcohol; alternating; cannabis; circular; confusional; delusional; epileptic; exhaustion; hallucinatory; hemp; partial; princely; and puerperal insanity
institutions, comparison of 155–9
insulin 9, 187
 coma 183–5
intellectual disability 41–5, 109, 126–8
interest groups 10
intermediaries, role of 3
International Classification of Diseases (ICD) 77, 130, 132, 222n43
International Congress of Medicine 147
International Fever Therapy Conference 183
International League against Epilepsy (ILAE) 147–8, 179
International List of Causes of Death 76–7, 79–80, 89
International Neurological Congress 147
International Statistical Congress 77
intoxication groups 161
Ionia State Hospital, USA 37
Ireland 99, 138, 142
Isharwal, S. 177
Islam 46, 57
Italy 13, 69, 113

J

jails, lunatics detained in **35**
Jains 15
Japan 182
jati categories 46
Jeffery, R. 6
Jharkhand *see* Chota Nagpur
Journal of Mental Science (*JMS*) 4, 14, 117–18
Journal of the National Medical Association 180
Jung, C. 129, 162–3, 188

K

Kabuli, escape by 96
Kakar, S. 129
kala-azar 76
Kapila, S. 28
Karachi 9, 19–20, 171
Karkaria, R. P. 15
katatonia 121–2, 154–5, 184
kayasthas 54
Kendell, R. E.. 116
Kendler, K. 120
kerani 52
kerosene oil 73, 88

khalasi 71
Khan, H. A. 176
King George's Medical College
    Lucknow 121
Kiyoshi, T. 182
Klaesi, J. 178
Knight, Lt. F. E. 4
Knoll, Messrs A. G. 183
Koehler, K. 113
Kolkata *see* Calcutta
Kotwal, N. B. R. 15
Kraepelin, E. 105, 113, 128–9, 139, 155
    classification of 116–22
    influence of 111
    use of organotherapy by 180–81
    views on postpartum psychoses 143
Krafft-Ebing, R. von 120, 142
Kunhimanny, K. 10
Kureishi, M. 11, 18, 212n82

L

laboratory testing 89
labourers 52
    see also coolies
Lacey, W. G. 48
lactation 113, 142–3
    psychosis 143
Lahore, institutional death rates in **68**
Lancet, The 182, 185
Lange, J. 139
League of Nations 35–6, 172, 194
Leonhard, K. 105, 179
leprosy 76, 78
Lewis, A. 120–21
Licentiate in Medicine and Surgery
    (LMS) 5
Lindesay, J. 123
Linnaeus, C. von 77
Livesay, A. W. B. 74
Lloyd, G. 6
Loewenstein, E. 182
London, University of 4, 25
Lord, J. R. 129
Luhrmann, T. M. 17
Luminal 178
Lunacy in India (Overbeck-Wright) 121, 161
lunatics, criminal 35–41, 151
Luque, R. 110
Lyon's Medical Jurisprudence for India
    (Waddell) 133
lypemania *see* melancholia

M

Macaulay, T. B. 2–3
Mackelvie, Lt. Col. M. 4
Mackenzie, C. 96
McKeown, T. 78–9
Macpherson, J. 129, 160–61, 163
Madras (Chennai) 5–6, 144, 155
    circular insanity at **158**
    institutional death rates at **68**
    MDP at 156, **157–8**
    melancholia at **152**, **156**, **158**
    Mental Hospital 5, 9
    disorders attributed on admission 108
    trends in gendered diagnoses at 155–6
Maduna, Dr L. v. 184
Majerus, B. 105
majum 131
malaria 69, 80–84, 86, 88–90, 186, 206
    fever therapy 182
    patients with **83**, 223n63
    shock therapy 9, 185–6
    and syphilis 138, 141
males *see* men
Malinowsky, B. 129
mania xviii, 105–6, 108, 110, 115–19, 141
    associated with epilepsy 146–7
    cannabis-induced 133
    female 149–55
    gendered trends in 153
    identification of 112–14
    puerperal 143
    treatment with malaria 185
manic depression 13
manic depressive insanity (MDI) 109,
    113–20, **119**, **157**
manic depressive psychosis (MDP) 117–19,
    141, 149
    Cardiazol treatment of 185
    gendered trends in 153–6, **157–8**, 159,
        236n274
    heredity of 165
    sulphur treatment of 182
Manual of Medical Jurisprudence
    (Chevers) 133
Mapother, E. 23, 25, 116
Al-Maqrizi (Makrizi) 136
Margaret Morris Movement 191
Markham, S. F. 15
matrons, salary of 22
Maudsley Hospital, UK 116, 119
mazdoor 53

measles 81
medical market 8
Medical Nemesis (Illich) 28
medical politics 6–8
medicine, histories of 20–21
Medinol 178
melancholia xviii, 105–8, 111–12, 114–20, 141
    diagnosis of **152**, **156**, **158**
    drugs for 180
    gendered trends in 153, 155–6, 159
    male 149–55
    puerperal 143
    symptoms of 150–51
Memmi, A. 7, 17
men
    maladies of 141–59
    melancholia in 149–55
    occupational categories of **51**, 52–3
    ratio to females **61**
    religious affiliations of 59–60
mental deficiency *see* intellectual disability
Mental Deficiency Act (1913) 127–8
Mental Deficiency Act (1927) 42–3
Mental Deficiency (Amentia) (Tredgold) 127
Mental Derangements in India
    (Overbeck-Wright) 121
mental disorder, category form (1934) **114**
mental hygiene 14, 42, 162, 164–7
mental illness
    classification of 105–72
    prevalence data for 149
mental institutions, as means of control 27–8
mental stress *see* stress
Mental Treatment Act (1930) 109
mentally ill
    criminalisation of 39–41
    early treatment of 103
Mercier, C. A. 160–61
mercury iodide 179
Metatone 181
Metcalf, T. R. 2
Meyer, A. 105, 111
Meynert's amentia 142
Michael, P. 75, 105
Michigan, mental hospitals in 75
middles, role of 3
Mills, J. 27
mind, unconscious 9
mirgi (small death) 145–6
missionary fervour, psychological
    pressures of 64

mochi 53
Modern Methods in Psychiatry (Pacheco) 140
Mohammedans, *see* Muhammadans
monomania 120
Montague-Chelmsford Reforms 6
Moore, H. 139
Moos, Dr N. A. F. 15
moral deficiency 167
moral imbecility 127
morbidity 77–80, 206
    aggregate disease categories **79**
Morel, B. 111
mortality 68–9, 78–80, 206, 220n8
    aggregate disease categories **75**
    nomenclature of 77
    rates of 31, 34, 67
mosquitoes, breeding of 83
Mott, F. 116
Muhammadans 56–7
    feasts of 192
    opium and hemp use by 136
Mukharji, Sir R. N. 202
Mumbai *see* Bombay
murderers 37
Murray, Colonel J. P. 10
music 201
    and movement 191–2
Muskens, L. J. J. 179
Muslims 19, 53–63, 155
    opium and hemp use by 136
    and organotherapy 181
Muthu, Dr D. G. 87
Mysore 90

N

Nagpur
    institutional death rates in **68**
    Mental Hospital 28
Nandy, A. 18
nayee 53
Nembutal 178, 190
Netherlands 107
neurosyphilis 140–41, 185–6
New Jersey State Hospital, USA 102
New Zealand 128
Nikitin, Dr 179
nitrogen inhalation sub-shock 187–8
Noguchi, J. W. 139
Noll, R. 181
nomads 57
nomenclature, change in 110, 168, 206

Nomenclature of Diseases 124–5, 127
Norman, C. 142
North America xviii, 4, 91, 180, 205–6
   aetiology in 163
   gendered social control in 28
   GPI in 91
   patients in 27
   see also United States
Northern Ireland, mortality nomenclature in 77
Nosologia Methodica (Bossier) 77
nurses 22–3
   salaries of 22

O

occupational background 45–55
occupational therapy (OT) 193–7
Ocimum
   sanctum 175
   basilicum 174
offences, petty 40
Ojha, A. L. 202
old age 113
Opium Wars 131
organotherapy xix, 180–81
Orissa xviii, 4, 10, 29, 155, 205
   age distribution of population **45**
   Christian women in 64
   female–male ratio **61**, 62
   lunatics detained in **35**
   religious affiliation of patients in 55, **58**, 59
   socio-cultural traditions of 8
Ostelin, D. 181
Overbeck-Wright, A. W.
   classification of 121–2, 153–5
   superintendent at Agra 121
   views on aetiology 160–63, 168–72
   views on alcohol abuse 145
   views on confusional insanity 142–3
   views on epilepsy 146–8
   views on GPI 137–8
   views on hemp drugs 135, 144
overcrowding 29, 73, 113
   and airborne diseases 84
   and cure rate 101
   and influenza 82
   and readmissions 103

P

Pacheco, J. N. J. 22, 32, 50, 147, 200
   hygiene precautions of 88
   as locum for Dhunjibhoy 21, 49, 70–72, 85, 90, 103, 166
   reports on accidents by 94
   reports of GPI by 91, 140–41
   tests on Indian snakeroot by 176–8
   treatment of staff by 95–6
   use of occupational therapy by 196
   use of radium therapy by 179
   use of Swift-Ellis method by 185–6
pagal-ki-dawa 176
Pakistan 9, 19, 155
paracetamol 178
paraldehyde 178
paranoia 109, 120–22, 149, 154
   Cardiazol treatment of 185
   gendered trends in 153, 236n271
paraphrenia 122
paretic dementia *see* general paralysis of the insane (GPI)
Parsi community 155
   ambivalence of 17–20
   decline of 15–17
   pathologisation of 11–14
   racial purity of 16
Parsis and Sport (Darukhanawala) 15
partial insanity 120
parturition 113
   causing insanity 169
patients 27–65
   ages of 41–5
   bedding for 199
   caste of 45–55
   chronic 30–33
   CI/MDI in **119**
   clothing for 198–9
   criminal xviii, 35–41, 96
   demographics of 64–5
   discharge of 32–3
   exploitation of 193
   freedom of movement of 94–9
   intake of 67
   with malaria **83**
   occupational background of 45–55
   physical illness of 102–3
   private and public 33–4
   rehabilitation of 199–203
   religious background of 57–8, 192–3
   reported sickness of **72**, **82**
   rewarding of 196
   socialisation of 199–203
   socio-demographics of xvii–xviii, 29

transfer of 4
upper class 54
violent attacks by 92–3
Patna 4, 29, 112
   coolies in 50
   criminal patients in **36**
   GPI at 138
   Medical College 4, 23
   mortality statistics in 69
   occupational categories in 48
   religious affiliation of patients in 59
   University, training courses in 25, 113
pay scales 5
Peel, Lord W. 6
Penology Old and New (Sen) 42
peons 168
Perth District Mental Hospital, UK 121
petit mal 148
phenyle 73, 88
Photodyne 180
phthisis *see* tuberculosis
plague 74, 78
Plasmodium falciparum 90
pneumonia 69–70, 74–5, 78, 84–7, 91
political prisoners 38–9
politics, medical 6–8
Poona (Pune) 11–12
possession 169
Prasad, Dr R. 19
pregnancy 113
prejudice *see* racial prejudice
Prince of Wales Medical College 25
Princely Impostor, A (Chatterjee) 134
princely insanity 28
Prison Act (1894) 38
Prisoners Act (1900) 35
priya 175
Prochaska, F. K. 203
protozoans 90
provincialisation 6–7, 10, 21
psychiatry
   in a colonial setting xvii
   history of xvii, 3
psychoanalysis 9, 188–9
psychoneuroses
   Cardiazol treatment of 185
   psychoanalysis treatment of 188
psychoses 112, 227n34
   cannabis-induced 133
   post-epileptic 146
puerperal insanity 113, 142–3, 171
purdah (seclusion) 62

R

Race, Sex and Class (Ballhatchet) 1
racial hygiene 14, 17, 139, 163
racial prejudice 1, 6–8, 21
racial typologies 129
racism 71, 207
   financial 5
Radden, J. 149
radium therapy 179
Raj
   careers in 2
   folklore 87
Ranchi Indian Mental Hospital xvii, 205–6
   admissions by gender **44**, **63**
   airborne diseases at 85–6
   children's ward at 43
   cinema at 201
   circular insanity at **158**
   classification schemes at 106, 110
   confusional insanity at 143
   criminal patients in **36**
   cure rates at 101–2, **101**
   discipline at 24
   disorders attributed on admission **106**, **107–8**
   dramatic performances at 200–201
   first superintendent of 3
   fund raising by 202
   identity of patients at 29
   intellectual disability in 127
   international recognition of 183
   library facilities at 200
   Mapother visit to 23–4
   MDP at 156, **157–8**
   melancholia at **152**, **156**, **158**
   morbidity patterns at 80, 206
   mortality rates at 31, 68–9, **68**, 70, 206
   music at 201
   new report form in 109–10, **114**
   occupational categories in 47–8
   overcrowding at 29, 73, 82, 84, 113
   patient numbers at 29
   profile of 9
   religious affiliation of patients 57–9, **58**
   reported sickness in **72**, 73
   salary inequities in 5, 22
   self-sufficiency of 194, 197–8
   senior staff at 22
   sport at 200
   staff benefits at 24–5
   staff–patient ratios at 24

staffing deficiencies at 24
suicide at 95–6
trends in gendered diagnoses at 155, 159, 206
Ranchi Institute of Neuro-Psychiatry and Allied Sciences (RINPAS) 9
Ranchi Mansik Aryogyashala 53
Ranchi TB Sanatorium 87
Rangoon, institutional death rates in **68**
Rao, S. 53
Rauvolfia 177
  serpentina 174–5, **176**, 177
Rauwolfia 176–7
readmissions 103
relapse 99
religion 46, 55–65
  gender ratios **60**
religious sages, confinement of 28
religious suggestion 188
religious therapy 192–3
remissions 100
repression, mechanisms of 9
reserpine 177
Risley, H. H. 129
Risse, G. 78
Rockefeller Foundation hookworm programme 90
Rohypnol 178
Rorschach diagnostics 181, 188
roundworm 89
Royal Army Medical Corps (RAMC) 6
Royal College of Physicians, Diploma or Licentiate of (LRCD) 5
Royal College of Surgeons, Diploma or Licentiate of (MRCS) 5
Royal Commission on the Care and Control of the Feeble-Minded (1904–1908) 127
Royal Hungarian State Mental Hospital 184
Royal Medico-Psychological Association 118, 128–9, 138

S

Sabji (Sabajhi; Subji) 174
  see also *Rauvolfia*
Sadhus 174–5
Sahay, Mr K. B. 42
Sakel, M. J. 183
salaries, inequities in 5–6, 22
Salversan 185–6
Sanitary Conditions of the Labouring Population, The (Chadwick) 79

sanitation 87–8
Santpoort Hospital, Holland 197
sanyasins 54–5
Sarkar, B. D. C. 201
Sarkar, S. 52
Sarnalpur 64
Sass, H. 113
Scandinavia 107
scarlet fever 81
Scheerenberger, R. 128
Scheper-Hughes, N. 126
Schiesari, J. 149
schizophrenia xviii, 45, 108–13, 120, 124, 141
  and cannabis use 132–3
  Cardiazol treatment of 184
  drug treatment of 177
  female 149–55
  gendered trends in 153, 235n265
  heredity of 12–13, 165
  insulin treatment of 183–4
  sub-shock nitrogen inhalation treatment 187
  tuberculin treatment of 182
Schneider, K. 113
schools 52–3
Schroeder, K. 182–3
Scotland, mortality nomenclature in 77
Scroggie, W. R. J. 6
Scull, A. 27
secondary dementia 110
sedation xix, 97–8, 196
  by paraldehyde 9
  justification of 186–8
Seitler, D. 161
Seligman, C. G. 129
Sen, Dr P. K. 42
Sen, M. M. G. 176
senile dementia 106–7
  and age 45
senility 76
service people 52
sexuality 9, 140
  perverse 127
Shaw, Lt. Col. W. S. J. 11–17
Shenley Mental Hospital, UK 74
Shepherd, A. 95–6
shock therapies xix, 182–6, 196
  justification of 186–8
Shorter, E. 139
Showalter, E. 28
Siddha 130, 174–5
Siddiqui, R. H. 176

Siddiqui, S. 176
Siegel, R. E. 112
Sikhs, opium and hemp use by 136
Sikkim 64
Sind 155
Sinha, A. K. 7
Sinha, M. K. 7
Sir Cowasji Jehangir Mental Hospital 155
   see also Hyderabad
Sir Ratan Tata Trust 15
skin disease, sulphur treatment of 182
sleep therapy 178
smallpox 70, 74, 81, 113
snake venene 179
social control, gendered 28
social standing 195
socio-economic status
   and caste/occupation 47
   and criminal activity 38
sodium luminol 178
Somnifene 178, 190
Soneryl 178, 190
sources xix
Spain 81
sports 199–203
St Andrew's Mental Hospital, UK 44–5, 74, 102
St Gotthard Tunnel, Switzerland 90
standardisation
   and institutional trends 67–104
   move towards 76–8
starvation 142–3, 171
   see also confusional insanity
status epilepticus 148
sterilisation 42–3
Stokes, Dr P. 74
Stott, Lt. Col. H. 86–7
stramonium 131
stress 160, 165–7, 170–72
Stromgren, E. 129
students 52–3
Studies in Clinical Psychiatry (Bruce) 121
stupor 109, 116–19
sub-assistant surgeons 2, 92
subalterns 21–5
   role of 3
suicide xviii, 94–9
   and depression 97, 151
Sulfosin therapy 182–3
sulphonol 178
sulphur, injection of 182, 240n89

surgeons
   patient numbers of 24
   salaries of 22
   sub-assistant 2, 92
sweet basil 174, 178
Swift-Ellis method 185
Switzerland 107
syndromes 124
   culture-bound 137–41
   culture-specific 128–37
Synopsis Nosologiae Methodicae (Cullen) 77
syphilis 91, 108, 137–41, 160–61
   and malaria 138, 141, 182, 186

T

tabes dorsalis, treatment with sulphur 182
Talbot, E. 161
Tata, J. 19
temperaments, racial 129
Tezpur, institutional death rates in **68**
Thatcher, Mrs M. 79
therapies xix, 9
   Cardiazol shock 183–5
   dance 191–2
   insulin coma 183–5
   malaria fever 182
   malaria shock 185–6
   occupational (OT) 193–7
   religious 192–3
   shock 182–6, 196
   Sulfosin 182–3
   work 98, 193–7
   see also treatments
thyroid treatment 121
Toronto, University of 187
toxic theory 161
transmission, modes of 78
treatments xviii–xix, 173–203
   dermatographia 181
   early 103
   glandular therapy 181
   impact of classifications on 109
   indigenous herbs 174–8
   modern drugs 178–80
   organotherapy 180–81
   outcomes of xviii
   for physical symptoms 102–3
   psychiatric 9
   tuberculin therapy 182
   wonder cures 180–82
   see also therapies

INDEX 273

Tredgold, A. 127
trends, and standardisation 67–104
Triazol 187
tribal leaders, confinement of 28
tribals *see* Animists
trionol 178
Tryparsamide 185–6
tuberculin therapy 182
tuberculosis (TB) 91, 100, 141, 151
  aetiology of 161
  airborne 84–7
  heredity of 160
  laboratory testing for 89
  mortality from 69–70, 74–5, 78, 139
  organotherapy for 180
tulasi 175
typhoid fever 90

U

Unani 130, 170, 174–5
Unani and Ayurvedic Tibbia College, Delhi 176
United States 37, 43, 120
  classification in 107, 120, 128, 182
  vaccine treatment in 179
  see also North America
University College London, UK 74
unmada (insanity) 146
Use of the Cannabis Drugs in India (Chopra) 133

V

vaccine therapy 121
Vacha, A. M. 20
Vacha, S. 20
vaidyas 174
Vakil, R. J. 177
Varma, L. P. 144
veronol 178
Vienna 183
Villagran, J. M. 110
violence, by patients 92

W

Waddell, L. A. 133–5
Wagner-Jauregg, J. 182, 185
Wales
  classification in 107–8
  criminal lunatics in 35
  cure rates in 102
  disorders attributed on admission in 106–7
  dysentery in 88
  female–male ratio in 37
  gender trend in 43
  GPI in 91
  institution death rates in 68
  intellectual disability in 127
  legislation in 35, 42–3
  medical coding in 109
  mortality nomenclature in 77
  New Poor Law in 128
  overcrowded hospitals in 30
  suicide in 95
  use of sedation in 98
Walsh, O. 39
Waltair
  circular insanity at **158**
  Hospital 144–5
  MDP at 156, **157–8**
  melancholia at **152**, **156**, **158**
  trends in gendered diagnoses at 155–6, 159
warrant officers 1
Wassermann reaction 91, 138–41, 185–6
Weygandt, W. 122
White, K. L. 78
Wimmer, A. 129
women
  Christian 63
  intellectually defective 43–4
  maladies of 141–59
  mania and schizophrenia in 149–55
  occupational categories of 51
  ratio to males **61**
  readmission of 103
  religious affiliations of 59–60
  repression of 30
  reproduction-related disorders of 142–3
Women and Madness (Chesler) 149
work therapy 98, 193–7
World Health Organization (WHO) 130
worms, parasitic 76
worry 170
Wright, K. L. 95–6
Würzburger Schlüssel, Germany 117

Y

yadav 54
Yeatts, M. W. M. 56–7, 61–2
Yeravda 152–3
  circular insanity at **158**

institutional death rates at **68**
MDP at 156, **157–8**
melancholia at **152**, **156**, **158**
trends in gendered diagnoses at 155, 159

Z

Zoroastrian community *see* Parsi community
Zoroastrianism 15

www.ingramcontent.com/pod-product-compliance
Lightning Source LLC
Chambersburg PA
CBHW021820300426
44114CB00009BA/257